CLASSIC CASES
IN MEDICAL ETHICS

CLASSIC CASES IN MEDICAL ETHICS

Accounts of the Cases
That Have Shaped
Medical Ethics, with
Philosophical, Legal, and
Historical Backgrounds

Gregory E. Pence, Ph.D.

School of Medicine
and Department of Philosophy

University of Alabama at Birmingham

McGRAW-HILL PUBLISHING COMPANY
New York St. Louis San Francisco Auckland
Bogotá Caracas Hamburg Lisbon London Madrid
Mexico Milan Montreal New Delhi Oklahoma City Paris
San Juan São Paulo Singapore Sydney Tokyo Toronto

CLASSIC CASES IN MEDICAL ETHICS

Copyright © 1990 by McGraw-Hill, Inc. All rights reserved. Printed in the
United States of America. Except as permitted under the United States
Copyright Act of 1976, no part of this publication may be reproduced or distributed
in any form or by any means, or stored in a data base or retrieval system, without
the prior written permission of the publisher.

2 3 4 5 6 7 8 9 0   DOC   DOC   9 4 3 2 1 0

ISBN 0-07-038092-9

This book was set in Palatino by the College Composition Unit
in cooperation with General Graphic Services, Inc.
The editors were Phillip A. Butcher, Cynthia Ward, and Bernadette Boylan;
the production supervisor was Leroy A. Young.
The cover was designed by Eric Baker.
R. R. Donnelley & Sons Company was printer and binder.

Library of Congress Cataloging-in-Publication Data

Pence, Gregory E.
    Classic cases in medical ethics: accounts of the cases that have shaped medical
ethics, with philosophical, legal, and historical backgrounds / Gregory E. Pence.
        p.   cm.
    Includes bibliographical references.
    ISBN 0-07-038092-9
    1. Medical ethics—Case studies.   I. Title.
    [DNLM: 1. Ethics, Medical.   W 50 P397c]
    R724.P36   1990
    174' .2—dc20
    DNLM/DLC
    for Library of Congress   89-14504

About
the Author

Gregory E. Pence holds joint appointments in the School of Medicine and Department of Philosophy at The University of Alabama at Birmingham. He serves on university committees on human experimentation, AIDS, and animal research, as well as on the executive board of Birmingham AIDS Outreach. He is also the author of *Ethical Options in Medicine* (1980). His articles have appeared in the *Journal of the American Medical Association, American Philosophical Quarterly,* The *New York Times, Newsweek,* and the *Wall Street Journal.*

Contents
in Brief

CONTENTS

CHAPTER 3

Mercy Killing in Holland   45

PART 2

CLASSIC CASES ABOUT THE BEGINNING OF LIFE   65

CHAPTER 4

Baby Louise Brown's In Vitro Fertilization   67

CHAPTER 5

The Baby M Case   89

CHAPTER 6

Abortion and the Trial of Kenneth Edelin   114

CHAPTER 7

The Baby Jane Doe Case   136

PART 3

CLASSIC CASES ABOUT RESEARCH   165

CHAPTER 8

The Philadelphia Head-Injury Studies on Primates   167

CHAPTER 9

The Tuskegee Syphilis Study   184

CHAPTER 10

Christiaan Barnard's First Heart Transplant   206

CHAPTER 11

Barney Clark's Artificial Heart   225

CHAPTER **12** _____

Baby Fae   251

PART 4 _____

CLASSIC CASES ABOUT INDIVIDUAL RIGHTS VS. THE PUBLIC GOOD   263

CHAPTER **13** _____

Mayor Koch, Joyce Brown, and Involuntary Psychiatric Commitment   265

CHAPTER 14

Preventing Undesirable Teenage Pregnancies   286

CHAPTER 15 _____

Nancy Wexler and Genetic Markers   303

CHAPTER 16 _____

Mandatory Testing for AIDS   320

Preface

Recent interest in medical ethics began when Christiaan Barnard transplanted the first human heart into Louis Washkansky in 1967. In 1973, the U.S. Supreme Court declared as unconstitutional state laws prohibiting abortions. Two years later, in 1975, there occurred perhaps the most famous case of all in American medical ethics, Karen Quinlan's coma and alleged "death." These three key cases raised new ethical issues about organ transplantation, abortion, and standards of death. They also launched medical ethics as a new area of popular interest and scholarship.

Medical ethics as it is known and taught today is little over two decades old. Each generation must impart its wisdom to the next, and to do so, it seems best to focus on the landmark cases which have shaped our laws, ethics, and public consciousness. The rationale of this book is that such cases can introduce readers to medical ethics and to show them the impressive amount which has been accomplished.

To allow readers to understand not only the legal history of abortion but also its difficult controversies, Kenneth Edelin's case from 1973–1975 is a wonderful teaching tool. About the same time (in 1972), the world first learned of the infamous Tuskegee Study of untreated syphilis in black men living in Alabama. Knowledge of this study is absolutely essential in understanding how modern regulation of medical experimentation through IRBs (institutional review boards) came about, as well as in examining racism in medicine. This chapter also discusses the topic (oft-neglected in medical ethics) of the crimes of Nazi physicians such as Josef Mengele. Is there anyone who believes that every student, premed or otherwise, should not know something about those cases?

Not all the landmark cases occurred in the 1970s; the 1980s also saw their share: Elizabeth Bouvia, the decriminalization of mercy-killing in Holland, the break-ins by the Animal Liberation Front at the University of Pennsylvania and elsewhere, and most controversially, the "Baby Doe" cases—including the Baby Jane Doe case at Stony Brook in 1983. This last case shows why most chapters describe recent history: Who could understand the Baby Jane Doe case without understanding the background of the "Baby Doe" regulations?

The recent past also brought us Barney Clark and the implantation of the Jarvik-7, Baby Fae and the heart transplanted from the baboon Goobers, and the infamous Baby M case involving "surrogate mother" Mary Beth Whitehead. Descriptions and commentaries on this last case, as well as the two other cases involving sex and procreation (Kenneth Edelin and Louise Brown), show the powerful passions entering discussion when the topics involve sex, mother-hood, babies, or the family. In so far as is humanly possible the author has attempted to maintain a neutral tone in writing about such cases.

Finally, we move from the present to the future burdened with several kinds of cases which are unlikely to go away: the million annual teenage pregnancies in America, the rise of genetic markers for asymptomatic victims of hereditary conditions such as Huntington's disease, the problem of involuntary but benef-icent treatment of the mentally-ill homeless, and the problems of AIDS. Each of these general topics is discussed through a case: the unwed teenage Bertha in West Virginia, Huntington's researcher Nancy Wexler's decisions about testing herself for Huntington's, Joyce Brown's battle with Mayor Ed Koch, and the prob-lem of whether to require mandatory testing for HIV in general populations .

Although this last chapter does not focus on a case about a specific person, it is clear today that AIDS itself is a major—if not *the* major—topic of medical eth-ics. If there is such a thing as malpractice against professors who teach medical ethics, it would be for a course which did not discuss AIDS. The issues raised by AIDS—about homosexuality, about fear, and about proportioning reasoning to evidence—are central to any modern education in medical ethics.

Most of the following chapters contain four parts: an historical introduc-tion, presentation of the case itself (in much greater detail than other "case-study" books), discussion of the ethical issues raised by the case, and an up-date. Although generally brief, the updates frequently reveal interesting or surprising details, such as how Louise Brown is faring today and some mod-ern problems about *in vitro* fertilization. The updates also trace the subsequent course of the debate, e.g., how the issues of abortion most recently have fo-cused on maternal neglect of semi-viable fetuses.

Acknowledgments

This book developed over ten years and its author has many debts. For over a decade, I have met one evening every three weeks with three physicians—Max Michael, C. Kirk Avent, and Bill Goetter—to discuss a piece of medical ethics, philosophy, or literature. They read and discussed much of this book and invaluably enriched both me and it. I owe them a lot.

In the Philosophy Department, I am intellectually most in debt to Jim Rachels, whose own work in medical ethics has been widely recognized. Even where I disagree with him, I have been enriched by studying his views. He has read most of this book and his general support has been much appreciated. G. Lynn Stephens has also been a major influence on my views, especially for his knowledge of history and his general erudition. Harold Kincaid also improved several chapters, as did Scott Arnold. Marjorie Price, Lila Luce, George Graham, Theodore Benditt, and James A. Pittman, Jr. provided key references. Harel Reach Chancellor proofread the entire manu-script and typed many chapters.

Several physicians at the University of Alabama at Birmingham read chapters. They include Paul Palmisano (pediatrics), Wayne Finley (medical genetics), Harriet Dustan (medicine), Benjamin Freidman (emeritus, internal medicine), and Sarah Polt (pathology). Surgeon Roy Gandy in Birmingham read the three chapters on cardiac surgery. Norman Fost of the University of Wisconsin Medical School greatly improved the chapter on Baby Jane Doe, as did psychiatrist Luis R. Marcos of New York City who greatly improved the chapter on Joyce Brown. (Both of these physicians participated in some of the events described in the relevant chapters.) I would also like to thank the staff at the National Reference Center for Bioethics Literature at the Kennedy Institute of Ethics and also at the Hastings Center. Seymour Glick of the Ben Gurion Medical School made valuable suggestions on Nazi experimentation. To all these physicians, I am indebted.

Many scholars improved various chapters, including Peter Singer (Centre for Bioethics, Monash, Australia) who introduced me to the problems of animal research while supervising my doctoral thesis, Shi Da Pu (Vice President, Xian Medical University, Xian China), Todd Savitt and Loretta Kopelman (Medical Humanities, East Carolina Medical School), Clifton Perry, (Philosophy, Auburn University), Jonathan H. Dick (University of London), Richard Mohr (Philosophy, University of Illinois), John Fletcher (Medical Humanities, University of Virginia), Baruch Brody (Center for Ethics, Baylor), Bonnie Steinbock (Philosophy, SUNY-Albany), Margaret Battin (Philosophy, University of Utah), Rose Gastner (Society for the Right to Die), William Ruddick (Philosophy, New York University) and David Ozar (Philosophy, Loyola University of Chicago).

Alfred Garwood kept me from losing sight of what the intelligent lay person wants to know. Karen Bell, California State University; Nora Bell, University of South Carolina; Howard Ducharme, University of Akron; Daniel Farrell, The Ohio State University; Chris Hackler, University of Arkansas for Medical Sciences; Joshua Halberstam, New York University; and David McNaron, NOVA University Fort Lauderdale, Florida all improved the book considerably by their careful reviews.

At McGraw-Hill, I am indebted to Stephanie Happer, Phillip Butcher, Lesley Denton, Cynthia Ward and Bernadette Boylan for their assistance. Their sensitivity, tact, and encouragement are much appreciated.

My wife, Patricia Rippetoe, provided many insights from her work as a clinical psychologist. Her support over many years for this book has been wonderful. Fellow members of the executive board of Birmingham AIDS Outreach have also increased my sensitivity about AIDS.

Finally, several hundred medical, and a few hundred undergraduate, students have read early versions of this book over the last three years. It is impossible here to recognize the many individuals for their comments on the book, but Troy Dillard, Derek Jones, Dennis Davin, and Mary Whall stand out.

Gregory E. Pence

CLASSIC CASES
IN MEDICAL ETHICS

PART 1

CLASSIC CASES ABOUT THE END OF LIFE

CHAPTER 1

Karen Quinlan

Karen Quinlan represents one of America's most famous cases of medical ethics. The case first came to media attention in 1975, when Karen's parents were fighting for legal guardianship of her with the intent of removing a respirator so that she could die. She has since become a larger-than-life symbol of tragic dying and her name is now a household word. Nevertheless, many people never understood the real issues of her case, issues which were not solved by the resulting court decision and which still haunt medicine today.

THE KAREN QUINLAN CASE

Misunderstandings of the Quinlan case occurred because details about the case were hidden in various ways. First, during the beginning months of the case in late 1975, *The New York Times* only ran the story in its "New Jersey" section, and even this coverage did not begin until 5 months after Karen lost consciousness.[1] Second, Mr. and Mrs. Quinlan only allowed one reporter to see their adopted daughter, Karen. Like any other parents, they wanted to present their daughter in the best possible light. Third, neither the media nor the nation was neurologically sophisticated enough to understand Karen's state, reports of which ran the gamut from "brain death" to "sleeping beauty." Some of these early misleading impressions became fixed in public perceptions. By the time the New Jersey Supreme Court ruled in 1976 and the Quinlan-Battelle book appeared in 1977, the media's attention had long since shifted to other topics.[2]

As the Quinlans tell their story, on April 11, 1975, Karen Quinlan was a perky, 21-year-old when she comforted her mother Julia as she left her family house around dinnertime. Karen was intensely independent and this was the familiar scene of an adult child moving out against her family's wishes. Karen had adventuresomely rented a room, a few miles away, with two male friends.

Karen's parents paint her as a saint, albeit an independent one, saying she once made children cease making fun of a local Down boy. She helped a pregnant friend whose parents wanted Karen's friend to abort. The family priest said Karen was generous.

Others saw Karen as a wild, free spirit. According to this view, Karen took illegal drugs and lived in the fast lane. She had once lost control of her car going around a curve, went over a cliff, slid down a ravine, walked away unhurt, hitched a ride home, and told her parents it was no big deal. A friend claims Karen had previously taken heroin, cocaine, and methadone. Karen's parents deny it.

A few nights after moving out, Karen celebrated a friend's birthday at a local bar. After a few gin and tonics, she suddenly appeared faint and was taken home. Her friends put her to bed, where she immediately slept. When they checked her fifteen minutes later, she wasn't breathing. Her friends never said why they felt the need to check her.

One roommate started mouth-to-mouth resuscitation while the other called an ambulance. Karen didn't respond, but a policeman later got her breathing. Although her color returned, she didn't regain consciousness. She was admitted after midnight as an emergency patient to the intensive care unit (ICU) of Newton Memorial Hospital in suburban New Jersey. A bottle of Valium was found in her purse with some pills missing.

To understand this case, a few points about pharmacology and drugs need brief discussion. Alcohol and barbiturates are *synergistic* in that each intensifies the other. A barbiturate (''downer'') is not an antianxiety drug such as diazepam (Valium, Ativan, Xanax). A barbiturate depresses the central nervous system in a way similar to alcohol, but taking the barbiturate with any alcohol can be much more potent than merely drinking many drinks. Alcohol *potentiates* both barbiturates and antianxiety drugs, depressing the nervous system much more than either taken alone.

Why Karen lost consciousness is often not discussed. What was in her bloodstream upon admission is disputed. The transcript of the later hearing has contradictory evidence. The attending physician, Morse, testified that, ''She had some barbiturates, which was normal, 0.6 milligrams percent; toxic is 2 milligrams, and the fatal dose is about 5 milligrams percent.''[3] Julius Korein, the consulting neurologist for the Quinlans, testified that Karen's medical chart said the drug screen on April 15, ''was positive for quinine, negative for morphine, barbiturates, and other substances. A subsequent test for Valium and Librium was positive.''[4] (Librium was not mentioned by anyone else.) Sussex County Prosecutor George Daggett said Karen had taken tranquilizers with alcohol shortly before her death.[5] The Quinlans deny that the drug screen showed barbiturates. They said, ''early urine and blood samples, taken on the day Karen was brought to the hospital, revealed only a 'normal therapeutic' level of aspirin and the tranquilizer Valium in her system.''[6]

Friends said Karen consumed three drinks. Most drinkers underestimate their drinking when talking to police (the drinks may have been doubles). Her friends initially panicked and lied, saying that Karen had been staying over while her parents were on vacation and that they had unexpectedly found her having difficulty breathing. Did they change other aspects of the real story?

Karen had also been dieting (maybe fasting) for several days before admission and weighed only 115 pounds. The diet would have intensified any drug's effects. If Karen indeed took barbiturates and Valium followed by alcohol, the cumulative effects probably suppressed her breathing and caused anoxia (loss of oxygen to the brain) and, then, irreversible brain damage.

Nine days after Karen's initial admission, her medical status was unchanged and she was transferred to St. Clare's hospital, a larger Catholic hospital in Denville, New Jersey. St. Clare's had the neurologists not present at Newton Memorial.

A small black respirator kept Karen breathing during her first few days at St. Clare's. The respirator was also necessary to prevent aspiration of vomit into her lungs; such aspiration is very dangerous and may cause pneumonia. Sometimes she exhaled when the machine was forcing air into her lungs and then she would choke, sounding an alarm. At such times, her arms flew out as she sat upright, her eyes opened wildly, and she appeared in intense pain. Eventually she breathed spontaneously but she didn't breathe deeply enough, so she was to be transferred to a special respirator, the MA-1, which would require a tracheotomy. The MA-1 would periodically expand her lungs fully to give her a "sigh volume," improving her lung function.

Mrs. Quinlan hated the idea of the tracheotomy. According to the Quinlans, Karen had twice said that if anything terrible happened, she didn't want to be kept alive as a vegetable on machines. She had premonitions that she wouldn't live long, perhaps because she took chances. At this point, four days after Karen's admission, Mrs. Quinlan claimed no one had mentioned brain damage. Reluctantly, she agreed to the tracheotomy and new respirator.

Contrary to popular belief, Karen was not brain dead under New Jersey law. She had "slow-wave" electroencephalograms (EEG's) but her EEG was not isoelectric (or "flat"). Although Karen was in a coma, her eyes opened and she would suddenly cry or laugh. Her eyes however were *disconjugate*, i.e., they moved in different, random directions at the same time. Karen was also thought to be *decorticate:* her brain couldn't receive any input from her eyes, although her eyes still worked. She was technically in *persistent vegetative state* (abbreviated as "PVS"), a generic term covering a type of deep unconsciousness which is almost always irreversible. Indeed, one modern standard equates PVS with brain death.

Karen's sister, Mary Lou, knew Karen was unconscious but wasn't expecting what she found when she went to see Karen:

> Whenever I thought of a person in a coma, I thought they would just
> lie there very quietly, almost as though they were sleeping. Karen's
> head was moving around, as if she was trying to pull away from that
> tube in her throat, and she made little noises, like moans. I don't know
> if she was in pain, but it seemed as though she was. And I thought—if
> Karen could ever see herself like this, it would be the worst thing in the
> world for her.[7]

Over the next five months, Karen's posture began to show the kind of neurological damage seen in stroke victims. Her left wrist cocked at right angles to her hand so that it looked as if her fingernails were digging into her wrist; her left foot twisted inward; her left elbow drew into her body. These positions were held rigidly. Physical therapists employed counteractive traction but the muscle contraction was too strong, and Karen's body became rigid.

Karen's weight dropped, and because her muscles were so rigid that IV feeding couldn't be used, a naso-gastric (N-G) feeding tube was used. By September, Karen's mother had become very upset at the feeding tube:

> They were feeding her a high caloric diet—which seemed completely unreasonable, especially since her body didn't always accept the food. Often she would vomit....And she was more agitated than she'd ever been. I wouldn't have thought it possible that Karen's head could writhe so much. It was as though her body was in a vise, and her head was caught in a whirlpool.[8]

When Karen's case went to court (as described on page 10), Morristown lawyer Daniel Coburn was appointed by a local judge as Karen's legal guardian. His brief to Judge Muir described Karen in September of 1975:

> Her eyes are open and move in a circular manner as she breathes; her eyes blink approximately three or four times per minute; her forehead evidences very noticeable perspiration; her mouth is open while the respirator expands to ingest oxygen, and while her mouth is open, her tongue appears to be moving in a rather random manner; her mouth closes as the oxygen is ingested into her body through the tracheotomy and she appears to be slightly convulsing or gasping as the oxygen enters her windpipe; her hands are visible in an emaciated form, facing in a praying position away from her body. Her present weight would seem to be in the vicinity of 70–80 pounds....[9]

In this state, there was little chance that she would regain consciousness. On the other hand, St. Clare's was giving Karen that "one in a million" chance of recovery which some people want hospitals to take.

The question arose as to what should be done with Karen. Her body was moved from the ICU and put in a corner of the emergency room (ER), where staff could respond if she vomited. The father was upset and wanted her back in a private room or the ICU. Although her heart was strong and she no longer needed a cardiac monitor of the ICU, she needed more monitoring than was possible in a private room. A corner of the ER was the logical, if somewhat cold, solution.

The social worker on the case attempted to transfer Karen to a state psychiatric hospital. All such institutions lacked respirators and inhalation therapists. As an issue in public policy or distributive justice, where trade-offs are constantly made in allocating resources, absence of respirators in nursing homes expresses the judgment that chances of recovery in such patients are too low to be worth the investment in equipment which would keep them alive. Some administrators explicitly said this and questioned the wisdom of continuing care for Karen.

It took Joseph Quinlan, Karen's father, many months to accept his wife's and adult children's view that Karen would never regain consciousness. When he finally did, he felt guilty for his previous insistence on full treatment. Mr. Quinlan consulted Father Thomas Trapaso, his local priest, who told him that taking Karen off the respirator wasn't playing God but merely agreeing with God's will. Father Tom said continuing the respirator would be using "extraordinary means," which wasn't required, according to what Pope Pius XII had said in a 1957 address to anesthesiologists. The Quinlans felt relieved and ceased a crisis-watch lifestyle.

After many months, Joseph and Julia Quinlan and their two adult teenage children came to a unanimous decision. In their view, these were the facts: Karen was beyond hope; she was dead; her mind was gone; she would have never wanted her body to continue like this. Their family priest supported their decision. So the Quinlans decided to remove the respirator and let Karen die. They had no idea that their three-month struggle to achieve this familial unanimity would be the easy part.

LEGAL ISSUES

When the Quinlans asked for Karen's respirator to be disconnected, Robert Morse, Karen's attending physician at St. Clare's, had them sign a form absolving him of all liability. Morse was Catholic and the Quinlans naively assumed that because their priest was behind them, Morse would agree with their decision. According to the Quinlans, Morse soon had second thoughts, said he had a moral problem with disconnecting the respirator, and became irritable, uncommunicative, and distant. The Quinlans felt upset and abandoned.

Robert Morse, along with his colleague on the Quinlan case, Arshad Javed, was just beginning his medical career. Morse had completed his residency in neurology only ten months before. Javed had graduated from a Pakistani medical school and two years before Karen's admission had completed an American fellowship in pulmonary medicine. Neither had a lifetime of experience in dealing with unconscious, brain-injured patients and their families.

The legal environment before the Quinlan case needs to be explained, especially the effect of the Edelin case in Massachusetts. Abortion had been legalized by the U.S. Supreme Court's *Roe vs. Wade* decision in 1973, which said a fetus could not be aborted after "viability." In other words, after viability, a fetus was legally a person.

Like Morse and Javed a few years before, Edelin was a third-year resident. Edelin practiced at Boston City Hospital, where he was chief obstetrics resident in 1973. (Chapter 6 focuses on this case.) Edelin then had performed a very late, second-term abortion by hysterotomy at the request of a pregnant teenage girl and her mother. After a long, sensationalized trial, preparation of which took two years, and which culminated just a few weeks before Karen

Quinlan became unconscious, a jury convicted him of criminal negligence. Edelin was convicted because the jury believed he had not done everything possible to save a viable fetus and because the jury believed that the law said that a viable fetus was a person. He was not convicted of killing, in which case the charge would have been murder or manslaughter.

Edelin was sentenced to a year of probation and risked losing his medical license if his conviction was upheld on appeal. During late 1975 when Morse and Javed were assigned to the Quinlan case, an appeal was in process, but things looked bad for Edelin.

Edelin's conviction was influential in the Quinlan case. First, it would have been difficult for the lawyers of Morse and Javed not to have drawn parallels between the decision facing the two young physicians and the decision facing Edelin, i.e., the Quinlans were asking the two physicians to promote the death of someone who was legally still a person. Edelin had just been convicted of criminal negligence for exactly the same thing, i.e., for not aggressively trying to keep alive a being defined by law as a person with the right to life. Karen was not legally brain dead, and as such, was still a person under New Jersey law and entitled to protection. Moreover, as far as anyone knew at the time, Edelin's conviction was going to be upheld. As far as the physicians' lawyers probably saw it, Edelin may have stepped over the legal boundary separating a very late-term abortion from criminal negligence, and Morse and Javed were in a very similar predicament, being asked to disconnect a respirator to kill a non-brain-dead patient. Here was another fine line and it was clear that what the Quinlans were asking was, at the very least, not definitely legal. Because Karen was not brain dead under New Jersey law, she had to be treated like any other patient—unless some court said otherwise.

Confusing things even more was the widespread belief of the Catholic Church and the American Medical Association during this time that no moral difference existed between withdrawing life support from a patient such as Karen to "let" her die and actively killing her (see below and also the discussion at the end of Chapter 3 on Dutch mercy killing). Both "allowing to die" and "mercy killing" were condemned as "euthanasia." No legal decisions had yet begun to make distinctions or to clarify rights of patients in such cases.

Moreover, Morse worried about malpractice if the Quinlans changed their minds. One of the major standards of malpractice is departing from normal, community practice of physicians. Actively helping to kill a non-brain-dead patient violated then current standards of medical practice.

Dr. Morse discussed the case with his hospital's lawyer, Theodore Einhorn, whose job was to protect St. Clare's Hospital. Einhorn advised the Quinlans that Mr. Quinlan needed to be appointed Karen's legal guardian (since she was over 21) and even then, that St. Clare's wouldn't guarantee cooperation with disconnection. Einhorn almost certainly advised Morse that Karen wasn't brain dead under New Jersey law and was, hence, still a person. Mr. Quinlan then got a lawyer, Paul Armstrong. The Quinlans claim that when Dr. Morse found out, he pressured them to drop the lawyer.

The Quinlans found themselves in a Catch-22 situation, in that first, no one would do what they wanted without a court order—for which they needed a lawyer, but second, no one wanted the Quinlans to get a lawyer or have the courts involved. The physicians and hospital wanted the case handled privately without legal action but were unwilling to do what the Quinlans wanted.

Mr. Quinlan found Paul Armstrong at a Legal Aid office (the official client was his indigent daughter, Karen). The Quinlans portray Armstrong as a young, idealistic lawyer, but some critics say he botched the case. Instead of simply asking the court to appoint Mr. Quinlan legal guardian, Armstrong announced Mr. Quinlan's intention to have the respirator disconnected. As legal guardian, Mr. Quinlan could have moved Karen to another hospital where the family's wishes would have been carried out. Instead, Armstrong pushed the issue of letting Karen die, forcing the lower court judge Muir to appoint a guardian *ad litem* (advocate for an incompetent plaintiff) other than the Quinlans. Judge Muir was forced to do this because, had he appointed Mr. Quinlan as guardian for Karen (considering Mr. Quinlan's announced intention of wanting to "kill" his daughter) he would have been accused of prejudging the case.

As one legal commentator said,

> In the hands of a conscientious but regrettably inexperienced 30-year-old lawyer, Paul Armstrong, the Quinlan family got very dubious legal advice. For the question of *guardianship* could have been pursued prior to and separate from the question of *treatment refusal*.[10]

Armstrong also initially argued that Karen was brain dead and that, therefore, the Quinlans should be allowed to turn off her respirator. But after the judge made it clear that Karen did *not* meet the criteria of brain death in New Jersey, Armstrong quickly amended his brief.

Before going on, an overview of the stages the case went through may be helpful. Crimes such as homicide and manslaughter, as well as issues of guardianship, are defined by laws of states (such as the state of New Jersey). As such, definitions of homicide and its exceptions differ from state to state. In making such laws, states may not violate federal law as defined by the U.S. Constitution and its interpretations. Such interpretations are ultimately made by the U.S. Supreme Court, but—occasionally—by state supreme courts when the U.S. Supreme Court has rendered no decision. The first stage in hearing a case is in a local court, presided over by a "judge." In this case, it was Judge Muir in probate court. Next are various levels of appeal, or appellate courts, run by "justices." Finally, there is the state supreme court, presided over by a "chief justice" and his "associate justices." In the Quinlan case after Judge Muir's decision, the New Jersey Supreme Court agreed to hear the case immediately, without intermediate appeals, because it knew the case would set a precedent.

In the lower-court case, neurologists would soon testify that Karen's condition was "irreversible" and that the chances of her returning to consciousness were "minuscule." However, there is no stated right to die under the federal Constitution, and even if there were, it would likely be for voluntary, adult, competent patients, rather than for incompetents represented by the proxies of a family who *alleged* that the patient would have wanted to die.

There were three ways for Armstrong to argue without invoking the so far nonexistent right of patients to die: religious freedom, cruel and unusual punishment, and right to privacy. The first would allege that Karen's wish to die was part of her religious views. The second assumed that the physicians and hospitals, in their effort to keep Karen alive, were like jailers who punished prisoners. Finally, there was the "right to privacy." A constitutional right to privacy was first explicitly spelled out by the U.S. Supreme Court in 1965, in *Griswold vs. Connecticut,* which gave couples the right to get contraception from physicians. This phrase "right to privacy" is a misnomer; a better description would be the right to make personal decisions about one's life without interference from the State. The 1973 *Roe. vs. Wade* abortion decision was based on, and further expanded, this right.

Armstrong took a scattergun approach and put forth all three arguments. The physicians' lawyers countered by arguing that physicians should make such decisions and not have the courts involved, and second, that even if disconnection was ordered, immunity from prosecution and suit should be granted to physicians.

The lower-court case generated immense publicity, and several elected officials became involved: the Morris County District Attorney, New Jersey Attorney General Hyland, the hospital's lawyer, and Ralph Porzio, the lawyer for the two attending physicians. Some people wondered if the courts were the correct place to decide such issues. It was the consensus of the AMA and most physicians that they were not. The Quinlans must have agreed when they heard the opening remarks of Coburn, who had been appointed by Judge Muir as interim guardian for Karen. Coburn opened by saying:

> I have one simple role in this case...and that is, to do every single thing that I can do as a skilled professional to keep Karen Quinlan alive.

> We talk about facts. Karen Quinlan is not brain dead. She's nowhere near being "brain dead," if that's the accepted standard.

> There's another facet...there are thousands of Karen Quinlans out there. I've received phone calls from all over the world about people...where there was no hope, and they recovered. Certainly, they recovered. They have been brain damaged, and they are educable, although they may have some retardation. But they are still alive. These people don't want Karen Quinlan dead. I don't want Karen Quinlan dead.

> ...As to the theory that she's not really leaving this earth —that she's just getting to the next world a little bit sooner—in all frankness to the court, and I'm not trying to be flippant, my attitude is that if the Quinlans want an express; I'm going to take the local.

As far as the legal basis for this, I've heard "death with dignity,"
"self-determination," "religious freedom"—and I consider that to be a
complete shell game that's being played here. This is euthanasia.
Nobody seems to want to use the word. I'm going to use the word,
whether it's euthanasia or a variation of it.

One human being, by conduct, or lack of conduct, is going to cause the
death of another human being.[11]

The New Jersey Attorney General opposed letting Karen die because to
do so "would open the door to euthanasia" and allow parents such as the
Quinlans to obtain "death at will" for incompetents in their care. Soon came
Ralph Porzio, attorney for Morse, who had a reputation for oratory. Porzio
implored the Judge not to "impose an execution—a death sentence": "Now,
once you admit that a person is alive, legally and medically, and once you
make a determination that a life must come to an end, then where do you
draw the line?"[12] Repeating Coburn, Porzio claimed that "hundreds and thousands" of Karen Quinlans would be similarly killed if the Quinlans were successful. Moreover, they would be killed according to someone else's definition
of poor quality of life. "And fresh in our minds are the Nazi atrocities," he
said. "Fresh in our minds are the human experimentations. Fresh in our minds
are [sic] the Nuremberg Code."

Porzio asserted that sanctity of life was "the cornerstone of our Western
culture...and of our Western religions." Turning off Karen's respirator was
"like turning on the gas chamber." Agreeing to the Quinlan's request would
be "ordering an execution in a civil suit." Moreover, "I don't care where the
idea [of mercy-killing] comes from, whether it comes from Rome or from Mecca
or from Salt Lake City, the end result is still the same." He wanted to get rid
of distinctions and "those semantics," such as "whether 1000 angels can dance
on the head of a needle." He compared Dr. Morse's refusal to disconnect the
respirator to the civil disobedience of Socrates and Sir Thomas Moore, and
reminded the Court that, "We are not gods."

In closing, Porzio said:

So let us then, as in this hour of trial as we begin, so conduct ourselves
that when the eyes grow dim and when our own lives shall fade, and
when men and women in some distant day shall gather to warm their
hands over the fires of memory, they may look back—they may look
back and say of us: They searched for truth, they nurtured justice, they
knew compassion; but above all, above all, they walked with honor and
wore the garments of understanding.

Physician Robert Morse testified that no medical precedent allowed him
to discontinue Karen's respirator. Patients in New Jersey who met the Harvard
criteria of brain death could be taken off respirators but Karen did not meet
that criteria. He testified that if he could find some cases where other physicians had taken patients off respirators who did not meet the Harvard criteria,
he would do so.

Two neurologists testified in the case. For the Quinlans, Julius Korein testified that he had seen about 50 patients in PVS, all better off than Karen. During his testimony, Mrs. Quinlan left the courtroom when Korein described Karen's mental age as like that of "an anencephalic monster," who was humanoid and often accepted by the parents until they put the baby's head in front of a light (having no brain, light from behind the head comes out of the baby's pupils).[13] For the state, Plum confirmed Korein's diagnosis and said Karen "was lying in bed, emaciated, curled up in what is known as flexion contracture. Every joint was bent in a flexion position and making one tight sort of fetal position. It's too grotesque, really, to describe in human terms like fetal."[14]

During the wait for the lower-court verdict, the Quinlans were offered $10,000 by a national tabloid "as a starting point" in negotiations for a picture of Karen in her bed. The Quinlans refused. Karen had been very cute and her parents felt she would not have wanted to be remembered in her final grotesque form. The hospital hired private security men and a media relations expert to protect itself and Karen. For this reason, the public never saw the real extent of Karen's condition. Some artists even portrayed her as resting peacefully.

The decision by Judge Muir came on November 10, 1975, almost seven months after Karen's admission.[15] He ruled that Coburn should continue as her legal guardian because first, Karen's wishes were unknown because of lack of written evidence and second, because no constitutional right to die existed, much less one by which a parent could decide for an incompetent adult child. He also ruled that Karen was alive and not brain dead, and, perhaps most surprising in view of later court decisions, that physicians, not courts of law, should make such decisions in the future. He also ruled that appeals to religious freedom and "cruel and unusual punishment" did not apply to this case, because Karen's views could not be traced to her religious views and because she was not a prisoner who was being punished.

During the testimony of the appeal to the New Jersey Supreme Court several months later, the role of physicians in deciding matters of life and death underwent close scrutiny. The justices continually expressed surprise at the importance placed by physicians on the distinction between disconnecting a respirator and not starting it. According to the official position of the American Medical Association at the time, it was permissible not to put a patient on a respirator but prohibited to take a patient off a respirator once connected. The government district attorneys argued that duties "attached" to a physician once a patient was accepted, and from then on, a physician could only keep treating and protect life. Disconnection, they said, would be "euthanasia." The justices thought this acting and omitting distinction "rather flimsy."

Neurologist Korein countered the district attorney's argument by saying that physicians privately used "judicious neglect" to let terminal patients die and that this was an "unwritten standard" in medicine. The justices pressed the physicians' attorney about why they couldn't transfer Karen to other physicians and end their relationship with her. The physicians' lawyers finally said that the physicians and the hospital thought the Quinlans' decision was immoral, and that only physicians, not the family, should make such decisions.

The New Jersey Supreme Court, one of the leaders in the country in tackling such cases, ruled unanimously in January of 1976 (after two months) in favor of the Quinlans.[16] It decided that Mr. Quinlan, not Mr. Coburn, would be Karen's legal guardian; that at Mr. Quinlan's request, the respirator could be turned off and other support withdrawn; that legal immunity would be granted to physicians and hospital from charges of neglect or homicide; that Karen's constitutional right to privacy could be asserted by her father to allow her to die. The court also suggested, but did not require, that any further doubts could be resolved by a hospital ethics committee.

Because the U.S. Supreme Court had never decided a case about brain death or euthanasia, it was up to a state supreme court such as New Jersey's to issue a ruling in the vacuum. Now in 1976, the New Jersey Supreme Court had said that the right to privacy was broad enough to allow families to let their irreversibly unconscious relatives die.

The Case Continues

Five months later, Karen was still alive. By now her hip bones could be seen after decubitus ulcers ate through her flesh. When the Quinlans asked Dr. Morse to follow law and disconnect Karen's respirator, they claim he asked them to be patient because "this is something I will have to live with for the rest of my life."[17] When they asked the administrator, a Catholic nun, whether Karen would ever be allowed to die, they claim she said, "You have to understand our position, Mrs. Quinlan. In this hospital we don't kill people."[18] Whereupon Mrs. Quinlan replied, "Why didn't you tell me ten months ago? I would have taken Karen out of this hospital immediately."

Catholic hospitals saw *Quinlan* as another step down the slippery slope which had started two years previously, in 1973, in America with the legalization of abortion. During the Quinlan trial, a Vatican theologian, Gino Concetti, criticized the Quinlans, saying, "A right to death does not exist. Love for life, even a life reduced to a ruin, drives one to protect life with every possible care."[19] A pulmonary physician at Catholic University in Rome chimed in, saying that removal of the respirator "would be an extremely dangerous move by her doctors, and represents an indirect form of euthanasia."

Meanwhile, Morse and Javed attempted to wean Karen from the respirator. The hospital stood firm that Karen would not die within its walls and was determined to transfer her to a nursing home. No nursing home would accept her on a respirator because of the intensive nursing care required.

The passive Quinlans and their inexperienced lawyer did nothing and seemed not to have understood the implications of the weaning—implications which would become painfully apparent over the next ten years. The New

Jersey Supreme Court had ruled in January, but St. Clare's and the physicians stalled for three months because they didn't agree with the decision. The Quinlan's lawyer could have sought an immediate writ of *habeus corpus* ("to have the body") to transfer the body to a facility with more sympathetic personnel. Such a writ would have taken effect immediately, as it protects patients against the constitutional crime of false imprisonment.

Lawyer Armstrong wrote letters politely reminding the hospital of the court's decision to let Karen die. A month later, Javed had Karen off the respirator for 4 hours, and by working intently, had her off for 12 hours by May 18. On May 22, Karen was declared off the respirator for good. When the news came out, many in the public interpreted it as meaning she might regain consciousness.

The Quinlans claim that, immediately after this success, St. Clare's asked them to transfer Karen somewhere else. Having brought the body to the point where it could be maintained indefinitely, St. Clare's told the Quinlans that it would no longer keep her. The Quinlans interpreted the transfer order as callous.

For a few weeks, no physician would accept her. Finally, internist Joseph Fennelly agreed, after Medicaid officials forced a public nursing home to accept Karen. Fennelly said the medical profession had helped create the problem and that "it's up to us in the medical profession to resolve it." He said New Jersey's physicians were "too afraid of their medical skins" to act humanely.[20]

Condemnations of the Quinlans from the Vatican began to slow, both externally and internally. The Bishop of New Jersey, himself dying of cancer, assailed Vatican bureaucrats and asked how could Rome attack such a Catholic family who had tried to do the right thing in consultation with their priest. The Vatican compromised and took no official position.

On June 9, 1976, nearly 14 months after onset of unconsciousness, Karen was transferred to a nursing home. There she would be maintained for over a decade. During these years, the Quinlans made regular weekly and sometimes daily visits.

ETHICAL ISSUES IN THE QUINLAN CASE

Resolving Conflicts of Morals

Issues in medical ethics in such cases often arise over conflicting standards of morality. The Quinlan case illustrated one such conflict, as does each chapter of this book. Here, we only begin to discuss these conflicts, which we shall see again when we discuss issues such as abortion, Baby Doe cases, and AIDS.

In recent decades, a familiar pattern of such moral conflict in medical ethics has been where physicians have opposed the wishes of patients or where hospital administrators have opposed the decisions of families. The nun/administrators at St. Clare's and the Vatican appear to have believed that morality rested on unchanging standards given by God and to have refused to act on any other standard. The Quinlans and Father Trapasso also believed that morality rested on unchanging standards given by God—they just differed with St. Clare's about what those standards were.

Resolution of such conflict can occur philosophically through analysis of the nature of morality. Questions must be asked—such as Socrates' in the dialogue *Euthyphro*—as to whether morality depends on the existence of God or can exist independently. If one believes that morality rests on God, one must then specify how particular moral rules are known to be His Will. If one turns to a religious book such as the Bible, one needs to justify one's interpretation of it (many people take certain moral teachings to be biblical without realizing that the teaching is often relatively new in the history of Christianity and that it is an interpretation based on ambiguous, conflicting sources).

It is important to realize that one can be spiritual without being a follower of a particular religion or denomination. Many people today believe in God's existence but don't believe that Christianity, or any one religion, has the whole truth and nothing but the truth. Even people who reject God's existence or who are agnostics commonly accept values grounded in the great religious traditions, values such as compassion, equality, and service to others.

One common solution to the problem of moral conflict is to accept a certain amount of irreducible diversity or pluralism in everyday morality. Perhaps not everyone will ever accept the same standard of brain death. Perhaps there will never be a time when almost everyone agrees with such-and-such a policy about abortion. Perhaps people will always disagree about what is "natural" about sexuality and homosexuality.

One way to think about acceptance of such pluralism was proposed by John Stuart Mill in *On Liberty* in the 19th century. Mill drew a distinction between private and public morality. He believed that society must publicly stand "for" and "against" certain values in order to flourish as a society.[21] Such stands, however, were compatible with some private latitude of belief and action in personal affairs.

But where is the line to be drawn between public and private morality? Mill's rough rule of thumb was his so-called *harm principle:* that private morality encompassed those actions by an adult (or adults together) which were purely personal and which did not put other people at risk of harm. Thus even if some people thought that a certain form of sex between two adults was immoral, so long as no one else was affected, it was not—for Mill—a question of public morality.

In the next chapter about Elizabeth Bouvia, we will see more of the application of Mill's principle and its problems. Before ending this discussion, however, it is worth remarking that some people hold extreme views about morality, views which recognize no other moral view as being possibly correct. (Such views may also stem from certain types of personality.) When faced with this situation, no resolution of conflict is possible inside the moral realm. This is one reason why some cases in medical ethics go to court.

Communication and Control of the Case

When the Quinlans were initially asked to transfer Karen from Newton Memorial to St. Clare's Hospital, they didn't understand that the transfer confronted them with a gamble. When any patient goes from a local hospital with familiar physicians to a larger hospital staffed by specialists, the patient risks losing control. When a family allows the transfer of an incompetent patient from familiar physicians to unknown ones, it often finds that strangers have taken over medical care. With such strangers, one gets the luck of the draw. Moreover, various specialties have their own routines, which can establish momentum in certain directions—sometimes in divergence with what families would have wanted if options had been carefully discussed at the beginning.

Such cases arise frequently in medicine, and like the Quinlans, many families are ignorant of possible problems until too late. Robert and Peggy Stinson described such loss of control in *The Long Dying of Baby Andrew* when their severely imparred baby was transferred from a community hospital to a sophisticated neonatal ICU.[22] Once Baby Andrew entered the NICU, the Stinsons were never allowed to make decisions about his care.

The Quinlans faced another critical point when asked to sign consent papers for a tracheotomy on Karen and for putting her on the MA-1 respirator. If we believe the Quinlans, they were not informed about the consequences of this decision. More specifically, they were not informed of the hospital's policy of not removing patients from long-term respirators once they were placed on them.

It is possible that the hospital and physicians did inform the Quinlans. Sometimes relatives are in such shock and denial that they cannot "hear" painful information. For this reason, professionals who specialize in medical communications emphasize that such information must be repeated over and over again in the simplest language. Sometimes such information is spoken but physicians attribute more sophistication to relatives than they have, with resulting misunderstandings. These possibilities show the wisdom of writing down as much as possible, both to prevent misunderstandings and to document informed consent.

Standards of Brain Death

One ethical issue in this case was whether Karen was really dead; the initial question of whether withdrawing the respirator was a matter of letting Karen die or of merely terminating activity on a dead patient hinges on this point. To understand this issue, it will be helpful to distinguish four basic standards of death: whole-body, whole-brain, irreversible unconsciousness, and higher brain. Some of the ethical issues raised by these standards are: (1) What concept of death should be the legal standard in a state? (2) Should there be one national standard, or should we continue to let each state make its own definition? (3) What operations or tests should identify that concept of death? (4) Is there room in public policy for individual differences over personal definitions of death? and (5) What effect, if any, should other needs have on definitions of death, e.g., the need for transplantable organs?

People have always feared that they might be declared dead and buried while still alive. Gruesome 18th-century tales speak of exhumed bodies said to have clawed at the inside of coffin lids. In the 19th century, Kirchbaum connected a periscope to buried coffins whereby awakened corpses might signal above, and some legislatures required delays before burial.[23] Such fears contribute to the reluctance of people today to sign organ-donor cards.

For thousands of years, definitions of death focused on cessation of breathing and heartbeat. When breathing stopped, cardiac anoxia (lack of oxygen to an area) and ischemia (lack of blood flow to an area) resulted, causing the heart to stop. Ventilators and ICUs changed things, allowing artificial respiration of brain-damaged patients. This is the ancient "whole body" standard of death.

In 1967, Christiaan Barnard wanted to transplant a heart from the brain-damaged Denise Darvall to the dying patient Louis Washkansky.[24] The issue arose immediately of whether it would be right to go ahead, even though Denise's heart was still beating. Being cautious, Barnard waited until the heart stopped beating, even though it meant using a slightly damaged heart for transplantation to Louis Washkansky. Thus, Barnard used a whole body standard of death.

One year later in 1968, the *Harvard criteria* operationally defined brain death as a total unawareness of external stimuli, with no movements or spontaneous breathing, no reflexes, and a nearly flat (isoelectric) brain wave (electroencephalogram or EEG) repeated twice over a 24-hour period.[25] The Harvard criteria were exceedingly cautious and no one has ever regained consciousness after being declared dead by them. The Harvard criteria moved the definition of death from whole-body to whole-brain. They required loss of virtually all brain activity, including brain stem (and hence, breathing).

A difference exists between a concept and the operations used to define it. One can say death is the destruction of all of the brain, but neurologists want something more precise. The Harvard criteria was the first operational definition of whole-brain death.

Although it was good to have some way of declaring death short of cessation of heartbeat, transplant surgeons had hoped for a broader definition of death which would allow more declarations of brain death and, hence, more organs for transplantation. The important fact is that very few patients who are comatose for extended times meet the Harvard criteria.

If the whole-brain standard is one extreme of the many possible definitions of brain death, the other extreme is the *higher brain* definition. This standard holds that death occurs with the absence of thinking, rationality, and self-consciousness. So far, this standard has been considered too vague and too hard to define operationally. Nevertheless, many relatives and residents find it acceptable when a patient has become impaired and they remark, "He's really not there anymore." Such a patient is often called derogatory names by residents because of the frustration of caring for a patient who is legally a full person but who in other ways may not be.

In between the Harvard and higher-brain standards is the *irreversibility standard*, which holds that a person is dead when he or she will never return to self-consciousness—even though that person may be breathing and have moving eyes. This standard is often equated with PVS and was rejected in 1968 as too broad.

Eighteen years later in 1986, the American Medical Association (AMA) said that it was ethical for physicians to withdraw care from patients who met this standard. This decision didn't imply that such patients were actually dead, i.e., it did not explicitly equate PVS or irreversibility with brain death. Rather, it was motivated by the extremely low probability of a deeply comatose patient's return to normalcy. It is important to stress that while criteria for removal of care from comatose patients may be the same as criteria for brain death, they may differ. Put another way, the AMA's 1986 decision can be construed as either about brain death or as about withdrawing care from dying but not legally dead patients. This last issue is part of the killing and letting die controversy (see Chapter 3).

Since 1986, only a few states have adopted the irreversibility criterion, which, had it been in effect in 1975 in New Jersey, would have allowed Karen to have been declared brain dead.

After 1985, a few cases in which patients recovered from PVS states were verified. In these cases, relatives instructed physicians to disconnect respirators and feeding tubes from supposedly irreversibly unconscious patients. One was Jacqueline Coles, the wife of a minister, who was unconscious for six weeks.[26] Abiding by her stated wishes, her family petitioned for disconnection of her respirator. The judge rejected the petition and three days later, Jacqueline revived with some loss of intelligence. Mrs. Coles, who had clearly said previously that she didn't want to be maintained artificially in a coma, said her family had acted correctly in assuming she was dead. Another case involved a young man in his twentie's who seems to have suffered no loss of intelligence upon reawakening. This case was followed by others, e.g., in April 1989 in New York, 86-year-old Carrie Coons regained consciousness just before a court-ordered act took place to remove her feeding tube. Carrie had supposedly been in a state of irreversible unconsciousness for six months, but suddelnly she was having a conversation.

These counter examples raise the question of whether PVS over months is sufficient for brain death. Needs for organs for transplants partially fueled the push to the broader criteria of death seen in the AMA's 1986 recommendation, and such pressure will continue as long as needs for such organs outstrip supply. Such pressures, combined with the above counter examples, make some critics resist equating PVS with brain death.

Some states adopted the Harvard criteria and others went with irreversible loss of consciousness. Over 30 states adopted a version of the whole-brain standard specified in the *Uniform Brain Death Act,* which equated irreversible cessation of *all* functioning of the brain with brain death.[27] This Act did not, like the Harvard criteria, spell out exact operations for defining this cessation.

In summary, the number of cases of brain death increases in going from the Harvard standard to the Uniform Definition of Brain Death (UDBD)—both whole-brain standards. In turn, cases increase in moving up to the irreversibility standard, and from there to the higher-brain standard. Second, homicide and its exceptions are defined by state, not federal, law. Different states define brain death in different ways. It is possible to be brain dead at one hospital in one state and, when transferred to another hospital in another state to come "alive." The UDBD was sought to prevent just such paradoxes.

Ironically, although the UDBD has been accepted by over thirty states, if it had been accepted by New Jersey in 1975, Karen Quinlan could *not* have been declared brain dead. She had a functioning brain stem and could breathe on her own. She could be declared dead only on the more rarely adopted irreversibility criterion, not the commonly adopted, whole-brain standard of the UDBD act. The country is changing its standard of death, but very, very slowly.

Mercy

Another ethical issue in the Quinlan case concerned compassion. Many people would argue from mercy, as Karen's mother appeared to do in the early months. The issue of mercy arises in this way. It cannot be known for certain that Karen never felt pain. Karen constantly dislodged the tubes from her throat, indicating to some people that she felt pain on some level. In conscious patients, such endotracheal tubes are very irritating and painful. Although her limbs were tied to the bed, her head moved violently as if trying to dislodge the tube from her throat. Her mother and sister, who saw her frequently, and her court-appointed lawyer, all said she looked as if she were in pain, and Mrs. Quinlan told a reporter on April 27 that Karen, "seems as if she's in pain by her facial expressions." Later, she said, "They say she doesn't feel pain, but I wondered if they really knew."[28]

The philosophical question concerns whether Karen manifested "intentional behavior" in fighting off her tubes, or was this just reflex? Studies have shown surprising instinctual responses in animals, such as where severed lower torsos move and act as if directed by a conscious brain. The philosophical problem is that—whether in higher animals or in other adults, and as Descartes taught us—consciousness in others is always an *inference* from outward behavior. Lack of consciousness is similarly an inference. Some unconscious patients undergoing operations have later reported conversations during their surgery. Usually, consciousness or its absence is correctly inferred, but with Karen and other patients in PVS, the problem of correct inference becomes acute. To some people it is terrifying to imagine that inside that writhing body and those terrorized eyes, a flicker of self-consciousness might have once appeared.

In the similar Paul Brophy case decided in 1986, the American Academy of Neurology voiced an opinion:

> No conscious experience of pain and suffering is possible without the integrated functioning of the brain stem and cerebral cortex. Pain and suffering are attributes of consciousness, and PVS patients like Brophy do not experience them. Noxious stimuli may activate peripherally located nerves, but only a brain with the capacity for consciousness can transfer that neural activity into an experience.[29]

Nevertheless, this statement by the neurologists is still an inference, not a factual observation. Some families still believe that their PVS relative might experience something.

Ordinary vs. Extraordinary Care

Traditional Catholic moral theology contains certain absolute prohibitions. For example, a distinction was drawn between means and ends, and certain means were banned, no matter how worthy the end. For example, a fetus could not be aborted to save a mother's life. Active killing has been a prohibited means of acting in euthanasia cases, but not in others.

Another prohibited means was removing ordinary care, and such a prohibition figured in the Quinlan case. According to official doctrine, it was permissible to remove extraordinary, but not ordinary, care. Several philosophers and physicians have argued that the very least we owe any patient is food and water. The Quinlans seemed to have felt this way.

Implicit in the idea that "the very least we owe someone is food and water" is the assumption that something very simple and basic is being removed when we cease feeding a comatose patient. But that assumption needs careful scrutiny. Feeding tubes appear deceptively simple and mask very sophisticated medical knowledge needed to keep them inserted without infection and to provide nutritious liquid diets. Such tubes are relatively new in medicine, having appeared in the last two decades, and before them, patients who could not swallow or chew food simply died. Moreover, Karen's daily care required 24-hour nursing, giving expectorants and anticonvulsant drugs, changing tubes carrying urine and bodily wastes, flexing muscles to prevent contractions, washing her body, preventing dental cavities and correcting them (sepsis from acute mouth infections can kill). So providing "basic care" for PVS patient is a complex, expensive process.

"Active Euthanasia"?

Another prohibited means was "active" killing or (as some Catholic theologians of the time used the term) "euthanasia." Taking a patient off a respirator was considered to actively contribute to, or hasten, the death of the patient. If this view were accepted, once a patient was put on an iron-lung machine, respirator, or feeding tube, he or she could not be taken off (for that would be "active," or "euthanasia").

Exactly what counts as active killing and what does not is a major topic of medical ethics. Holland has recently decriminalized mercy killing by physicians, and since Quinlan, several (but not all) state supreme courts have allowed physicians to remove respirators, food, and even water from unconscious patients to hasten death. Since Chapter 3 is devoted to such cases of mercy killing and withdrawing care, discussion of these issues is postponed until then.

The Slippery Slope

The New Jersey Supreme Court's decision in *Quinlan* ran together different kinds of cases, and such confusion fuels worries that once society allows one kind of death to occur, it will plunge hither-thither down a "slippery slope" to mass, involuntary killings. The slippery slope is just a metaphor, but it is one of the most powerful ones in medical ethics.

To see the worry, consider that the natural place to make the first kind of legal decision about death would have been for adult, competent, patients such as Elizabeth Bouvia (see next chapter). In such a case, a court would know exactly what a patient wanted and then could determine if the law permitted such a patient to end his or her own life and by what means. Next and ideally, subsequent decisions might have addressed problems of voluntary death and degrees of incompetence (since many patients who want to die suffer from strokes and incapacitating diseases, and are thus only partially competent). Finally, after building up a foundation with these decisions, only later would the court have looked at cases involving incompetent patients— such as defective children, the retarded, and comatose victims like Karen Quinlan—and decided how much power to give families to make such decisions. In *Quinlan*, the New Jersey Supreme Court jumped right in and declared that families could make decisions to let incompetent patients die. The Court justified its ruling by appealing to the (implied) constitutional right of (competent adults) to privacy. This decision hastily lumped different kinds of cases together. In addition, the court said the respirator could be removed from a PVS patient. Had that standard been hastily applied to Mrs. Coles, or a few other "resurrected" PVS patients, they would never have regained consciousness.

Again, the slippery slope metaphor and its objections will be discussed more in Chapter 3 on mercy killing in Holland. For now, the point is that the worry behind the metaphor has some evidence at least, in that the *Quinlan* court seemed unable to distinguish carefully different kinds of cases.

Choosing Standards of Brain Death

The Quinlan case also raised the question of how certain must judgments be of "irreversible" unconsciousness and who should make them? Judging the odds is a *technical* question; judging the acceptable odds is an *evaluative* one. Philosopher Robert Veatch argues that each person should be allowed to choose his or her own standard of death and specify it in an advance directive.[30] Veatch argues that having only one standard, no matter what it is, imposes one religious or philosophical view on everyone. Surgeons who want more organs for transplantation say Veatch's idea would decrease donations. Nevertheless, the idea is intriguing: choosing the standard of death under which one might be declared dead. Although it would require much greater sophistication about neurology, perhaps Americans will one day be ready for this choice.

As emphasized before, Karen's persistent coma would have allowed her parents to declare her dead in some states, e.g., in Alabama, but not in the 31 states which follow the Uniform Brain Death Statute. Many states made standards too rigid and didn't allow families any choice about brain death. This may stem from a lingering belief, often matched with a similar belief about the other end of life, that there is some uniform, metaphysical event which marks death. This may be a mistake, because definitions of death may be decisions, rather than discoveries.

UPDATE

On June 13, 1986, more than 10 years after being transferred to the nursing home, Karen was declared dead. Karen's body died from pneumonia from months of increasing respiratory congestion, during which time the Quinlan family had asked that no antibiotics or blood pressure medication be given. Nevertheless, with today's antibiotics, no young body need die this way. (Deaths from AIDS are sometimes disguised as due to "pneumonia.") In the end, they decided to let Karen die. Joe and Julia Quinlan alternated a bedside vigil during the final five days, and Julia Quinlan was at her bedside at the death.

The death had been a very, very long time coming and when it did, it came to symbolize an inversion of values in medicine where mindless, antifamily technological medical science had replaced reflective, humane, family-centered medical art. In becoming such a symbol, Karen Quinlan's death goaded many people to rethink how medicine had come to such a point. Unintentionally, Karen Quinlan and her parents started an intense, international debate about ending life. It was the beginning of many court battles where physicians and patients clashed over differing views of proper care at the margins of personhood. Before 1975, right-to-die bills had been introduced in only 5 states; by 1987, 39 states had passed Living Will laws.

Paul Armstrong went on to become a famous lawyer and tried several further precedent-setting cases about euthanasia before the New Jersey Supreme Court. About a year after Karen died, and after practicing medicine for a decade, Robert J. Morse was killed in an airplane crash.

Because of the Quinlan decision and several subsequent decisions, advance directives such as *Living Wills* and durable powers of attorney have become important. Unfortunately, most Living Wills are too vague to be useful, vary in conditions from state to state (they may lose application when people move), and are signed by few people. They do, however, have moral force and usefully direct physicians in knowing the wishes of incompetent patients who were once competent.

Videotaped Living Wills are more effective, but have some of the same problems. The best strategy for a terminal but competent patient is to assign to a trusted person a *durable power of attorney,* a legal device assigning all decision-making power to another.

The Living Will legislation, however, marked a confused response to the Quinlan case because advance directives are made by competent, adult patients. Indeed, as the country moves into the last decade of the 20th century, significant confusion remains about key terms surrounding the issues of the Quinlan case. Both ordinary physicians and laypersons confuse words such as "coma" in their medical and common meanings. Phrases such as "irreversibly comatose" or "chronically comatose" are imprecise, with no firm criteria (how long is "chronically" comatose?).

The President's Commission in 1981 suggested that whatever definition of brain death is finally accepted, we should cease talking about "brain death." The Commission believed this phrase falsely implied that there are two ways to be dead: "brain dead" and really dead. Sometimes journalists write statements such as, "Life-support was removed from the brain-dead patient, after which he died."[31]

The Commission's suggestion is unlikely to be accepted. There are too many standards of brain death to say that one simply *is* death. Second, if Veatch is correct that patients should be allowed to choose the standard under which they will be declared dead, the suggestion can never be followed. Some considerations of general utility may argue for adopting one single, national standard, but such adoption will not necessarily mirror what people think.

Families are unlikely to get much choice about standards of brain death. Recent changes in how hospitals are reimbursed (a fixed sum for each patient in a *DRG* or "Diagnostically Related Group") conflicts with allowing families such choices. No hospital can afford the luxury of allowing indigent families the choice of maximal care. The hospital has already been paid for the care of the comatose patient and loses money every day the patient stays in the hospital past the average time, e.g., in one VA hospital, one PVS patient lasted ten years and created a bill for millions of dollars. Few nursing homes are equipped to give medical care to clients who require hourly monitoring or one-on-one staff care. Virtually none will take PVS patients. Therefore, a hospital cannot transfer a PVS patient to a nursing home to cut its cost. This overall dilemma makes it tempting for physicians to say, "Your grandfather is dead; we want to remove the artificial support." But the more accurate statement is, "Here are the various standards of brain death. Your grandfather meets most of them, but not the most cautious ones. We would like to discontinue medical care because we believe he's already dead and because it would cost us a lot of money to continue this care indefinitely. But the choice is yours."

As America moved into the 1990s, two needs cried out for help. First, the U.S. Supreme Court needed to make a landmark decision about such cases. In 1989, this court announced that it would hear—for the first time—just such a case. The case involved a Missouri Supreme Court decision rejecting a family's decision to remove a feeding tube from a woman named Cruzan in PVS. Whether the court would make a narrow or broad decision in *Cruzan* remained to be seen. The New Jersey Supreme Court had repeatedly upheld various kinds of decisions letting terminal and comatose patients die. But other state supreme courts, notably New York and Missouri (in *Cruzan*) in 1988, forbade removal of feeding tubes for incompetent patients by decisions of their families. These courts argued that the ancient role of *parens patria* of the state—or guardian of the young, retarded, indigent, and impaired who lack the ability to defend their rights—dictated that medical care must, if it erred, err on the side of life.

Second, families needed help in caring for ventilator-dependent patients. Most people falsely believe that private medical insurance, Medicare, or Medicaid pays for nursing home care. Even if a family can afford years of nursing home costs running $50 to $100 a day, such homes will not voluntarily take ventilator-dependent patients (one home had to be forced to take Karen). The crunch comes because such patients can be transferred from hospitals once they are stabilized. Most such patients don't need the acute, exorbitant care of hospitals, yet they require more care than nursing homes provide. Some inconsistency between facility is needed. Daily costs of such a facility would be more than an expensive nursing home but less than a hospital. What happens now is that either the hospital keeps a patient it doesn't need (creating a huge bill for the family) or the patient goes to a nursing home and receives inadequate care.

This leaves us with the grim questions faced by pulmonary physicians today. Each year, they save thousands and thousands of ventilator-dependent patients (most of whom are conscious and not comatose), and given that virtually no families have insurance covering such inconsistency between care, where are the billions to pay for such care in a time of budget deficits? If such monies aren't forthcoming, what happens to families like the Quinlans, with comatose relatives, who can't afford nursing home care? What are hospitals supposed to do, given the legal and financial risks, with ventilator-dependent patients whom families and nursing homes won't accept for transfer? These are not happy questions, especially for families, doctors, nurses, and hospital administrators suddenly forced to face them. Medical ethicists aren't happy with them either, because they are sometimes asked to answer them, and because there are few simple answers.

FURTHER READING

President's Commission for the Study of Ethical Problems in Medicine and Biomedical and Behavioral Research, *Defining Death* (Superintendent of Documents, 1981).
Paul Ramsey, *Ethics at the Edges of Life: Medical and Legal Intersections* (Yale University Press, 1978).
Richard Zaner, ed. *Whole Brain and Neocortical Definitions of Death: A Critical Appraisal* (Reidel, 1986).

CHAPTER 2

Elizabeth Bouvia and Voluntary Death

This chapter discusses the case of Elizabeth Bouvia, a person afflicted with cerebral palsy who wanted to die, but who was forced to live. Ms. Bouvia was not suffering from a terminal disease but decided that she no longer wanted to continue living in her condition.

Ending life before the last possible moment is an issue today partly because more than 80 percent of people die in hospitals. At the turn of the century, only the poor and those without families did so. Moreover, before the Harrison Act of 1914, people could legally purchase heroin and opiates to keep themselves pain-free. Before World War II, most people died of sudden-onset, acute diseases, whereas today most people die slowly from stroke, diabetes, emphysema, cancer, and coronary artery disease. How people die, where they die, and around whom, of course, affects their attitudes to suicide.

HISTORICAL BACKGROUND

Voluntary Death in Ancient Societies

Ancient Greek aristocrats valued nobility, honor, and excellence, and striving for these grounded ancient Greek ethics. Noble Greeks valued lives which demonstrated such qualities, not simply having biological life.

One of the world's most famous death scenes occurred when Socrates drank a poison (hemlock) rather than suffer shame. Socrates' death was coerced but his attitude toward death exemplified ancient Greek stances. Socrates had already said, "The really important thing is not to live but to live well." He taught that studying philosophy (*philo* = friend of; *sophia* = wisdom) was a lifelong preparation for death. "True philosophers make dying their profession, and... to them of all men, death is least alarming." And, "So if you see one distressed at the prospect of dying, it will be proof that he is a lover not of wisdom but of the body."[1]

The background of Socrates' death scene is a fascinating topic and the trial of Socrates is one of the most famous stories in philosophy. The tension between democracy and aristocratic meritocracy created both. Complex legal and political events led to this scene, but we need not tell the whole story here.

At this death scene, Socrates' friend Cebes says it's easy not to fear death if one is convinced of life after death. Cebes seems to believe that the soul "may be dispersed and destroyed on the very day that the man himself dies [and] may be dissipated like breath or smoke, and vanish away, so that nothing is left of it anywhere." Moreover, "no one but a fool is entitled to face death with confidence, unless he can prove that the soul is absolutely immortal and indestructible."

Socrates replies that the soul may indeed be immortal, but if it is not, then death is like a sleep from which one never awakes. In the latter case, he says, there is nothing to fear because no one will exist who will feel pain or miss life. Throughout history, people have responded to Socrates' claim by retorting that not having a conscious self is exactly what they fear.

As this abstract discussion has been occurring, the hemlock has been working up Socrates' toes to his legs. (Hemlock is a poison which acts like nicotine in decreasing circulation at the extremities, giving subjects sensations of distal numbness, and eventually stopping the heart).

When the discussion is over, the state poisoner discovers that Socrates' thighs are numb and says that Socrates will die in minutes when the poison reaches his heart. As his followers began to cry, Socrates says, "Calm yourselves and try to be brave!" He dies minutes later, and Plato, the admiring follower who has been writing this account, writes, "Such...was the end of our comrade, who was, we may fairly say, of all those whom we knew in our time, the bravest and also the wisest and most upright man."

In later centuries, Roman Emperor Marcus Aurelius and the "slave philosopher" Epictetus celebrated suicide as more courageous than continued undignified existence in pain. Such Stoics defended the *argument for the open door:* "If the room is smoky, if only moderately, I will stay; if there is too much smoke, I will go. Remember this, keep a firm hand on it, the door is always open."[2] Seneca similarly wrote about old age, "if it begins to shake my mind, if it destroys my faculties one by one, if it leaves me not life but breath, I will depart the putrid or the tottering edifice."[3] In the 20th century, Jean-Paul Sartre revived the argument for the open door, emphasizing his Existentialist theme that choice is inescapable—even the choice to stay alive each day.[4]

Christian Views

The early Christians prohibited direct killing in all forms. Such prohibitions threatened Christian society's survival. The absolute pacifism of the church at this time, when it was lobbying emperors for toleration, undercut a Roman society threatened on all sides by warring peoples. As MacIntyre writes in a *A Short History of Ethics:*

> The paradox of Christian ethics is precisely that it has always tried to
> devise a code for society as a whole from pronouncements which were

addressed to individuals or small communities to separate themselves off from the rest of society. This is true both of the ethics of Jesus and of the ethics of St. Paul. Both Jesus and St. Paul preached an ethics devised for a short interim period before God finally inaugurated the Messianic kingdom and history was brought to its conclusion. We cannot, therefore, expect to find in what they say a basis for life in a continuing society.

St. Paul's dislike of marriage as other than expedient ("It is better to marry than burn") is not so inhumane as unhistorically minded secularists have made it out to be, if it is understood in terms of the pointlessness of satisfying desires and creating relationships which will hinder one from obtaining the rewards of eternal glory in the very near future...., [But] the crucial fact is that the messianic kingdom did not come, and that therefore the Christian church ever since has been preaching an ethics which could not find application in a world where history had not come to an end.[5]

Because of this vacuum in Jesus' ethical teachings, many key ideas of what is today called Christianity were formed in the 4th century, especially by Augustine, who attacked suicide as a "detestable and damnable wickedness." The worldly Ambrose had already defended Christians killing in war, and Augustine went even further by warring against the Donatists. Frederick Russell in *The Just War in the Middle Ages* says that through Augustine "the New Testament doctrines of love and purity of motive were accommodated to the savagery of the Old Testament and pacifism was defeated."[6]

Because the Bible contains no explicit condemnation of suicide (and even seems to accept those of Saul and Judas), Augustine used the Sixth Commandment (Exodus 20:13) to prohibit suicide. This commandment is known today in its King James translation, "Thou shalt not kill," but a more accurate translation from the Aramaic and Greek would be "Thou shalt not commit wrongful killing." In such a translation, the commandment offers less guidance because the question at hand is usually about which killings are "wrongful" and which are not. For example, a few pages after the Ten Commandments (at Exodus 23:23), God commands Moses to tell the Israelites to attack neighbors, such as the Hittites. Nor does God distinguish between enemy soldiers and civilians.

Margaret Battin's *Ethical Issues in Suicide* describes Augustine's position as follows:

Augustine draws a distinction between "private killing" and killing which is carried out at the orders of a divine or divinely constituted authority. Private killing, or killing undertaken "on one's authority," is never right....

However, according to Augustine, not all killing is private. God may command a killing, and when this is the case, full obedience is required. The command may take two forms: it may be a direct command from God, like the commandment to Abraham to sacrifice

Isaac, or it may be required by a just law. In these two cases, the
individual who performs the killing does not do it "on his own
authority" and is not morally accountable for it; he is "an instrument,"
a sword in the user's hand. This accounts for the permissibility of both
killing in war and in capital punishment, since both types of killing are
performed by persons acting under law. Augustine appears not to
permit killing in self-defense, though present-day Catholic moral
theology does permit it for persons not capable of attaining the "higher
way" of self-sacrifice.[7]

The obvious problem with Augustine's position is that no explanation is
given of how it is known that certain forms of killing by the state are divinely
ordered. Augustine was supremely self-confident and not known for intellectual humility. Critically acclaimed Christian historian Paul Johnson writes
of him: "He was a tremendous egoist: it is characteristic of him that his spiritual autobiography should have been written in the form of a gigantic address
to God."[8]

It is natural to ask here: so what if Jesus didn't talk about suicide? So
what if Augustine did ? What has that to do with modern Christianity? Don't
we know the general intent of Jesus' teachings and isn't that enough to know
the Christian view about suicide? Perhaps, but perhaps not. In its nearly 2000
years, Christian doctrine has been profoundly reconstructed. Each subsequent
theologian made confident claims, but each might not have grasped the whole
truth. (And what if the proper religious viewpoint is not a set of beliefs but a
process of searching for truth?)

Quakers have always rejected Augustine's position and followed the original pacifism of the early Church. Some devout Christians today oppose capital punishment. How it is known that suicide is sin but not killing in war?
Someone can, of course, just believe that what he or she has been taught is
God's will, but to do so is dangerous—especially in medical ethics. As Professor Paul Badham writes,

as Church Historian, I am very conscious of how Christians of previous
ages have vehemently denounced medical practices which today no
Christian would dream of questioning. For centuries Christians forbad
giving of medicine, the practice of surgery, the study of anatomy, or the
dissection of corpses for medical research. Later the practice first of
innoculation and then of vaccination faced fierce theological condemnation, as did the initial use of quinine against malaria. The introduction
of anesthesia, and above all the use of chloroform in childbirth, were
seen as directly challenging the divine edict that "in pain you shall
bring forth children," (Genesis 3:16) and hence were violently denounced from pulpits throughout Britain and the U.S.A.[9]

Presumably, if everything has a purpose, then there is a reason why
humans were made with critical intelligence and not with blind obedience. It
is not blasphemy to believe that people were given minds to think these things
out for themselves.

In the 13th century, Thomas Aquinas castigated suicide as the most dangerous of sins because it left no time for repentance.[10] Aquinas also said suicide was wrong because life was a gift from God and only God could take it back. Ever since, Thomists have argued this view vigorously. Aquinas also argued that suicide hurt the community by depriving it of talented people, as well as depriving children of their parents. Finally, Aquinas said, suicide was unnatural, going against the instinct of self-preservation.

Later Views

In the 16th century, Montaigne concluded his essay, "To Philosophize Is to Learn How to Die," with " If we have learned how to live properly and calmly, we will know how to die in the same manner."[11] In the 17th century, the philosopher Spinoza wrote, "A free man, that is to say, a man who lives according to the dictates of reason alone, is not led by the fear of death."[12] In the same century, the English poet John Donne wrote, "When the [terminal] disease would not reduce us, [God] sent a second and worse affliction, ignorant and torturing physicians."[13]

Scottish philosopher David Hume argued in the 18th century that suicide "is no transgression of our duty to God" and concluded, "The life of a man is of no greater importance to the universe than that of an oyster."[14] Similarly, in the 19th century, John Stuart Mill defended his *harm principle* that over his own life and body, a person could do whatever he wished so long as others were not harmed.

In the same century, medical views softened moralistic condemnations of suicide. Physicians imputed causes of suicide to heredity, chemical imbalance, or shape of head. About 1900, sociologist Emile Durkheim rejected the pathological view of suicide, and broadened suicide's definition to include indirect means.

American feminist Charlotte Perkins Gillman killed herself in 1935 and left a note saying she preferred "chloroform to cancer." In an essay published posthumously, she wrote: "The record of a previously noble life is precisely what makes it sheer insult to allow death in pitiful degradation. We may not wish to 'die with our boots on,' but we may well prefer to 'die with our brains on.'"[15]

Historically, society has generally been against suicide, and for this reason, this survey has over-represented the minority's view. In the main, suicide has been regarded as a disturbed, irrational, sinful act.

ELIZABETH BOUVIA

Elizabeth Bouvia was 25 years old in 1983 and was almost totally paralyzed, having never had the use of her legs. She had enough control over her right hand to operate a battery-powered wheelchair (and to smoke cigarettes) and enough control of facial muscles for chewing, swallowing, and speaking.

In September 1983, her father drove her from Oregon to Riverside General Hospital, where she admitted herself as a voluntary patient to the psychiatric ward. She was a California resident who had lived both in Riverside and in Oregon, and was eligible for Medi-Cal, a substantial supplement to Medicaid for indigent California residents. She was admitted for being suicidal when she declared that she wanted "just to be left alone and not bothered by friends or family or anyone else and to ultimately starve to death."

Her parents divorced when she was five years old and she lived with her mother for a few years after the divorce. Her mother placed her in a children's home when she was ten. Her life was never easy, as two physicians observe:

> For their 18th birthday, some children receive cars and gifts. When she turned 18, her father, a postal inspector, told her that he would no longer be able to care for her because of her disabilities. The chief of psychiatry at Riverside says that what she did next showed great drive and promise. She gathered her requisite amount of state aid and lived on her own in an apartment with a live-in nurse. Although she earlier had dropped out of high school, she completed her general equivalency degree and went on to graduate from San Diego State University with a bachelor's degree in 1981. She even entered a master's program at the university's School of Social Work but left in 1982 over a disagreement about her field work placement.
>
> For eight months, she worked as a volunteer in a San Diego placement program, but she has never been employed for salary or wages.
>
> During the last year [1983], Ms. Bouvia faced a series of devastating events. In August, 1982, she married an exconvict, Richard Bouvia, with whom she had been corresponding by mail. Together they conceived a child, but a few months later she suffered a miscarriage.
>
> Her husband's part-time job did not provide enough income for the two to live decently, so they called her father to ask for help. He declined to aid them, Richard Bouvia said. They next went to Richard Bouvia's sister in Iowa to ask for help. That did not work out for long, and soon they ended up back in Oregon, where Richard Bouvia still could not find work. At that point, he abandoned her, stating—according to pleadings in the case—that he "could not accept her disabilities, a miscarriage, and rejection by her parents."
>
> A few days later, Elizabeth Bouvia got a ride to Riverside General and wheeled herself into the emergency room, complaining that she wanted to commit suicide.[16]

Bouvia had decided that she would not eat and would starve herself to death. "Death is letting go of all burdens," she said. "It is being able to be free of my physical disability and mental struggle to live."[17] She may have had arthritis, which she said caused her great pain. She claimed to have previously attempted suicide at least once.

Her attending physician from September to late December was Donald Fisher, the chief of psychiatry at Riverside Hospital, who opposed her desire to die. Unlike most patients, Ms. Bouvia then contacted the ACLU and phoned a reporter.

ACLU's national policy in 1987 was not to require a physician to act against his conscience but to urge him to withdraw from requests for assisted death which he could not honor. As with defending the right of Nazis to free assembly, this decision created controversy within the ACLU. Physician Richard Scott of Beverly Hills, who was also a lawyer, took on Ms. Bouvia as a charity case.

A hearing was arranged before John Hews, a California probate judge, before whom psychiatrist Donald Fisher testified that he would not let Ms. Bouvia starve and would force-feed her. Convinced that she would eventually change her mind, Fisher said, "The court cannot order me to be a murderer nor to conspire with my staff and employees to murder Elizabeth."[18] Ms. Bouvia asked Judge Hews to enjoin the hospital from feeding her. At this point,

> The case escalated into a public debate. Disabled individuals held vigils at the hospital to convince her to change her mind. Bouvia's estranged husband hitchhiked to Riverside from Iowa, retained lawyers, and asked to be named her legal guardian. He charged the ACLU with using his wife as a "guinea pig." She filed for divorce. Columnist Jack Anderson's offer to raise funds for Bouvia's treatment was rebuffed. Richard Nixon sent a letter to Bouvia to "keep fighting." A meeting with President Reagan was discussed. Two neurosurgeons offered free surgery to help her gain the use of her arms. A convicted felon volunteered to shoot her.[19]

In December of 1983, Judge Hews permitted the hospital to force-feed Ms. Bouvia. Her lawyer said the judge accepted "the Chicken Little defense that the sky would fall if Ms. Bouvia wasn't force-fed."[20] Paradoxically, Judge Hews admitted Ms. Bouvia was "rational," "sincere," and "fully competent," but overruled her decision because of its "profound effect on the medical staff, nurses, and administration of the hospital," as well as its "devastating effect on other...physically handicapped persons."[21]

In saying this, Hews indicated that he was influenced by some organizations for the handicapped. Advocates for the Developmentally Disabled had held candlelight vigils outside Riverside Hospital and were afraid that if Ms. Bouvia died, other disabled people would too. A lawyer at the Law Institute for the Disabled said Ms. Bouvia symbolized a "social problem" of disabled people who had been told they couldn't be productive, and concluded, that, "She needs to learn to live with dignity."

Columnist Arthur Hoppe criticized such attitudes:

> I had the feeling that the judge, the doctor, and the hospital had found Elizabeth Bouvia guilty—guilty of not playing the game. It was as though the Easter Seal Child had looked into the camera and said being crippled was a lousy deal and certainly nothing to smile about.[22]

Because Ms. Bouvia was not terminally ill and could live another 15 to 20 years, Judge Hews continued his order permitting force feeding. He said, "There is no other reasonable option." Law professor George Annas bitterly disagreed:

> The judge's decision begs the question: Is there a reasonable option? In the adversary proceeding played out in California, no one seemed to search for reasonable options. The county, in fact, consistently took the most extreme position. It continually threatened to eject Ms. Bouvia from the hospital by force, and leave her out on the front sidewalk, hoping someone would pick her up and take her away. Almost from the beginning, the county and hospital made it clear that they did not care whether she lived or died but, because of their own fear of potential legal liability, would not let her die at Riverside Hospital.[23]

Ms. Bouvia appealed and, while she did, California physicians argued about the case. Habeeb Bacchus, whose patient Ms. Bouvia had become, dug in: "It is very simple. Physicians, if they err, should err on the side of saving life. When it comes to criminal charges, wrongful death is more of a crime than battery, so there you have it."[24] In the same context, Laurens White, who later became president of the California Medical Association, said that, "the most troublesome thing about this [case is that] Mrs. Bouvia's First Amendment rights may hit somebody else's medical ethics right between the eyes." He further said, "Refusal to take water and food is not suicide. Providing care while a patient is doing this is a tough thing, but I think she should have the right to do it. Forcing her to eat is battery." When asked about Fisher's force-feeding, White replied, "He's full of it... he's just completely off the wall about this."

When Ms. Bouvia was force-fed, she bit through the plastic tubing. Thereafter, four attendants held her down while the tubing was inserted through her nose into her stomach; she was tied down with her mouth forced open while a liquid diet was pumped in. Law professor George Annas here comments:

> I do not believe competent adults should ever be force-fed; but efforts at persuading the individual to change his or her mind, and offering oral nutrition should continue. If a court determines, however, that invasive force-feeding is required... then to avoid hospitals from becoming the most hideous torture chambers, some reasonable limit must be placed on this "treatment."[25]

What then happened has been interpreted differently (and in different moral tones) by different sources. Two physicians writing in the *Archives of Internal Medicine* wrote:

> The standoff continued until April 7, when Ms. Bouvia unexpectedly checked herself out of the hospital. The hospital bill for the 217 days, excluding physicians' fees, was more than $56,000, paid by Riverside County and by the State of California. Ms. Bouvia went to the Hospital del Mar at Playease de Tijuana, Mexico, known for amygdalin (Laetrile)

treatments for cancer. She believed the staff would help her die. Her new physicians, however, became convinced that she wanted to live. Two weeks later, Ms. Bouvia left the hospital, hired nurses, and moved to a motel. Three days later, with her friends, a reporter, and an intern from the Hospital del Mar at her side, she gave up her plan to starve herself to death and took solid food. Ms. Bouvia said that she wanted treatment, including surgery to reduce muscle spasms. As of August 1985, Ms. Bouvia's location and plans were not known. Her case was complicated further by the revelation that the newspaper reporter who covered the case most closely had a contract with Ms. Bouvia for a book, television, and movie rights to her story.[26]

This account emphasizes Ms. Bouvia's "unexpected" departure from the hospital, the high cost of her care, nonpayment of physicians' fees, the agreement of Mexican and American physicians in resisting her wishes, and a seemingly arbitrary decision to give up starvation. To this is added a final paragraph noting that the reporter covering the case hoped to make money by writing about the case.

Contrast the account of the same events by Annas, the law professor on Bouvia's side:

Two years ago this column dealt with Elizabeth Bouvia's unequal and doomed struggle.... After losing both in the hospital and in the courtroom, Ms. Bouvia fled to Mexico on April 7, 1984 to seek her death. She was soon persuaded that Mexican physicians and nurses would be no more sympathetic to her plan than those at Riverside, and so returned to California. Because of the brutal force-feeding she had endured at Riverside, she was afraid to return there. Since no other facility would admit her unless she agreed to eat, she resigned herself to eating and entered a "private care" location. There she remained, without incident, for more than a year.[27]

Consider another account of Bouvia by Derek Humphrey of the Hemlock Society:

Her troubles multiplied. The graduate school where she had been studying refused to re-admit her, and her brother was drowned in a boating accident. Not long after, Elizabeth had a miscarriage, and she learned her mother was dying of cancer.

Determined once again to be in charge of her fate, she asked her father to take her to the county hospital in Riverside, near Los Angeles (an area where she had friends), for an examination. She checked herself into the psychiatric ward and told physicians she wanted to die by starvation. Elizabeth specifically asked that, until she died, she be looked after normally and given pain killers when her arthritis was troublesome.[28]

Consider yet another view by Paul Longmore, a Ph.D. who thinks the Bouvia case and its reporting show social prejudice against the disabled:

The very agencies supposedly designed to enable severely physically handicapped adults like her to achieve independence...become yet another massive hurdle they must surmount, an enemy they must repeatedly battle but can never finally defeat.

[When she tried to go on internship] the SDSU School of Social Work refused to back her up. They wanted to place her at a center where she would only work with disabled people. She refused. Reportedly, one of her employers told her she was unemployable, and that, if they had known just how disabled she was, they would never have admitted her to the program....

The attorneys brought in three psychiatric professionals to provide an independent evaluation. None of them had any experience or expertise in dealing with persons with disabilities. In fact, Elizabeth Bouvia had never been examined by any psychiatric or medical professional qualified to understand her life experience....Her examiners prejudicially concluded that because of her *physical* condition she would never be able to achieve her life goals, that her [physical] disability was the reason she wanted to die, and that her decision for death was reasonable....[Judge Hews] too declared that Ms. Bouvia's physical disability was the sole reason she wished to die.[29]

The two physicians portray her as irresponsible. Annas and Humphrey portray her as a helpless heroine fighting a cold bureaucracy. Longmore sees her as a victim of a cold bureaucracy and of misguided, do-gooder lawyers. All of the four accounts above appeared in scholarly journals and books claiming objectivity. The physicians refer to her as "Bouvia," whereas Humphrey uses the warmer, "Elizabeth." Longmore only uses "Elizabeth Bouvia" or "Ms. Bouvia." The physicians say, "she got a ride" to Riverside, as if she hitchhiked to an arbitrary location; Humphrey writes that her father took her to a place where she had friends. Longmore emphasizes her desire to be independent: "she checked herself into the psychiatric unit...[and] announced her wish to die...." Humphrey emphasizes her physical pain and social trauma; Longmore emphasizes that focusing on her physical disability exemplified prejudice because it is society's problem not Bouvia's, that people discriminate. Humphrey writes from a viewpoint "inside" Elizabeth. The physicians write of her from the viewpoint of doctors inside a hospital who must accept patient "management problems."

On September 22, 1985, Ms. Bouvia entered Los Angeles County-USC Medical Center, where a morphine pump was installed to control pain for (what was diagnosed as) degenerative arthritis. After two months there, she was transferred to nearby High Desert Hospital, where another chapter of her story began.

Elizabeth Bouvia apparently ate voluntarily, but apparently High Desert decided she wasn't eating enough (she weighed 70 pounds at this time). The hospital began force-feeding her to achieve an ideal weight of 104–114 pounds, giving the rationale that, "Since she is occupying our space, she must accede to the same care which we afford every other patient admitted here, care designed to improve and not detract from changes of recovery and rehabilitation."[30] Several critics thought it odd to reason that if a patient "occupied" a hospital's "space," the patient had to do what the hospital said. That would make an interesting slogan for a hospital's advertising.

A consultant on nutrition had noted in Ms. Bouvia's chart that a gain of weight to 75 or 85 pounds "might be desirable." It is important to remember that Ms. Bouvia was paralyzed and had slight muscle mass, so her ideal body weight would be much lower than normal for her 5'0" height. This was important because she soon again petitioned the courts for relief from the forced feeding. At a new hearing, Judge Deering interpreted her low weight as evidence of starvation and "not motivated by a bona fide right to privacy but by a desire to terminate her life."[31] Although the right to privacy has been defined as the "right to be left alone," Deering said it did not include suicide-by-starvation. Any treatment necessary to preserve life could be forced on Ms. Bouvia. "Saving her life is paramount," he said.

The USC university hospital where Ms. Bouvia spent the previous months had neither force-fed her, increased her body weight, nor demanded that she socialize with patients. It also accepted her declaration that she would eat and live.

Bouvia again appealed and the three Justices of the Court of Appeals found in her favor. They said that she could refuse life-sustaining medical treatment. "A desire to terminate one's life is probably the ultimate exercise of one's right to privacy."[32] Moreover, they found "no substantive evidence to support the [lower] court's decision." Judge Deering had been impressed because Ms. Bouvia could live for decades more. The Appeals Court dismissed this. "This trial court mistakenly attached undue importance to the *amount of time* possibly available to [Ms. Bouvia], and failed to give equal weight and consideration for the *quality* of that life, an equal, if not more significant, consideration."

The Appeals Court concluded:

> This matter [Deering's decision against Bouvia] constitutes a perfect paradigm of the axiom: "Justice delayed is justice denied." Her mental and emotional feelings are equally entitled to respect. She has been subjected to the forced intrusion of an artificial mechanism into her body against her will. She has a right to refuse the increased dehumanizing aspect of her condition. . . . The right to refuse medical treatment is basic and fundamental. It is recognized as part of the right of privacy protected by both the state and federal constitutions. Its exercise requires no one's approval. It is not merely one vote subject to being overridden by medical opinion.

> [Precedents have said that when] a doctor performs treatment in the absence of informed consent, there is an actionable battery. The obvious corollary to this principle is that a competent adult patient has the legal right to refuse medical treatment. [Moreover] If the right of the patient

to self-determination as to his own medical treatment is to have any meaning at all, it must be paramount to the interests of the patient's hospital and doctors.... The right of a competent adult patient to refuse medical treatment is a constitutionally guaranteed right which must not be abridged.

The Court sympathized with Ms. Bouvia's plight:

...in Elizabeth Bouvia's view, the quality of her life has been diminished to the point of hopelessness, uselessness, unenjoyability, and frustration. She, as the patient, lying helplessly in bed, unable to care for herself, may consider her existence meaningless. She is not to be faulted for so concluding.... As in all matters, lines must be drawn at some point, somewhere, but that decision must ultimately belong to the one whose life is the issue.

As to the precedent of forced-feeding and what should be done in future cases, the Court said:

We do not believe it is the policy of this State that all and every life must be preserved against the will of the sufferer. It is incongruous, if not monstrous, for medical practitioners to assert their right to preserve a life that someone else must live, or more accurately, endure, for "15 or 20 years." We cannot conceive it to be the policy of this State to inflict such an ordeal upon anyone.

The Court also ended its decision with an important emphasis: "no criminal or civil liability attaches to honoring a competent, informed patient's refusal for medical service."

ETHICAL ISSUES IN THE BOUVIA CASE

Difficulty of Suicide

Sometimes people wonder why patients such as Elizabeth Bouvia don't simply go off somewhere and kill themselves, but it's not easy to commit suicide painlessly, certainly, and aesthetically, especially if patients are already very sick or disabled. Consider the attempted suicide of Robert McFarlane, former White House national security advisor, who took 30 to 40 tablets of 5–10 mg. Valium before the "Irangate" hearings. Some skeptics inferred that, because McFarlane didn't die, he didn't really want to kill himself. This commits the classic mistake of inferring ambivalent motives from a botched suicide. An equally plausible explanation is that most people don't know how to kill themselves. For example, it was revealed during the 1988 trial of Robert Rosier that this physician had first given his wife an inadequate amount of drugs to produce her death (see end of next chapter).

Suicide attempts among teenagers increased 300 percent between 1967 and 1982, but for every 50 attempts, only one succeeded.[33] The elderly are more knowledgeable, and one of three succeeds. Miami Beach has the highest suicide rate in America. Women try suicide more than men, but men are more successful. Men use violent means, such as guns; women use drugs.

Emergency room (ER) physicians confirm that most people don't know how to kill themselves. ER medicine is full of stories of bizarre survivals (often related with gallows humor).[34] A gunhand shakes an inch and creates a "drooling zombie." "Jumpers" survive the Golden Gate Bridge because drugs which give courage also relax muscles to soften the impact. One woman hit a parked car and neither died nor lost consciousness. Another elderly female jumper's skirt caught halfway down a skyscraper on a balcony, after which she fought off the fireman on the ladder. He got a medal; she got a straitjacket.

Valium and benzodiazepines are commonly used in suicide attempts but rarely cause death when used alone. Such drugs are often taken in insufficient quantities to produce death, and instead the unfortunate victim awakes with half of his or her IQ.

Results in most suicides are distasteful for family members. Drug overdoses, before they decrease respiration, relax bowel and bladder control. Jumping off buildings and using guns are obviously messy. Hanging is difficult to do correctly. The airway is frequently not broken and the victim, kicking in agony as he partially aspyhxiates, may not die. If he does, his family finds a dead man with loss of bowel-bladder control and an erect penis.

Other popular methods end up in the ER as often as the funeral home. Carbon monoxide poisoning may fail when a car stalls or runs out of gas, or the CO may not concentrate enough to produce death, so the person ends up in a permanent coma. Slitting wrists in a warm tub usually is neither easy nor certain because after unconsciousness but before death, blood may coagulate or an arm may move. Painful cuts must be very deep and in the right place. One ER physician says, "Most slashers just get a trophy: a claw hand."

Some suicidal people are unintentionally discovered, especially if their method takes hours, and wake up in ERs with N-G tubes down their throats. Syrup of ipecac is pumped down to produce vomiting, followed by injections of saline solution, followed by lavage, whereby the stomach is alternately flooded and suctioned. Granulated charcoal is forced in to absorb remaining poisons. These procedures are painful, messy, and unpleasant—especially when patients return to consciousness during them.

In 1975, British journalist Derek Humphrey, a cofounder of the American Hemlock Society, published *Jean's Way*, the story of how in 1975 he assisted his wife to "self-deliverance."[35] He did so 18 months after her diagnosis of breast cancer with distant bone metastases. In 1981 in America, Humphrey published *Let Me Die Before I Wake: Hemlock's Book for Self-Deliverance for the Dying*, which again gave detailed instructions about drugs and dosages.[36]

Humphrey and the Hemlock Society were criticized for publishing information which unstable mental patients might use too easily to kill themselves. Critics say the book contains dangerous knowledge, in that teenagers with transient, situational depression can know exactly what drug to take from the medicine cabinet to kill themselves. Critics point to the growing number of teenage suicides and say it's unwise to make such knowledge easily available. The Hemlock Society retorts that its books are not widely available and are unlikely to be read by unstable people. People can also kill with guns, which some people abuse, but we do not ban sale of guns, much less knowledge about guns.

Rationality of Choice

One ethical issue in this case was made famous by the play and movie *Whose Life Is It, Anyway?*—a movie which Elizabeth Bouvia had supposedly seen. The movie hero is a paralyzed sculptor, whose psychiatrist argued that his "obvious intelligence" undercut his rational arguments for suicide. Because the sculptor was intelligent and sane enough to put up an invincible case for suicide, he was too intelligent and sane to die. The sculptor can only prove his rationality by deciding to live.

Similarly, psychiatrist Nancy Mullen testified that Ms. Bouvia was incompetent to make medical decisions about her life and prospects. Dr. Mullen said she could conceive of no situation where someone could make a competent decision to take her own life.[37] Carol Gill, a clinical assistant professor of occupational therapy who used a wheelchair, criticized the ACLU for accepting the decision of "a handful of medical experts" that Ms. Bouvia was competent when she made the decision to starve herself.[38] Dr. Gill did not claim to have examined Ms. Bouvia before she concluded that Ms. Bouvia was incompetent.

This is called "begging the question." The "question" or point is whether a decision to die because of an unsatisfactory life is always irrational or due to mental illness. The question is "begged" when it is assumed to be true, rather than proved. Simply assuming that Ms. Bouvia's decision to die must be irrational begs the question against her.

This is not to say that Ms. Bouvia might not have in fact been suffering from clinical depression and that psychiatric tests might not have shown this. But the above people judging her decision were not her former therapists and were not professionals who had tested her. Instead, they were reacting to the kind of decision she made. Indeed, three psychiatrists had tested her and had found her competent.[39]

Autonomy

In the 19th century, John Stuart Mill in *On Liberty* defended the values of privacy and personal autonomy against the increasing powers of governments. Since then, individual rights have become limiting conditions of what governments can and cannot impose on citizens.

On Liberty saw the purpose of morality as not to further any particular vision of the good society but to create freedom of action in private life. Mill defended:

> ...one very simple principle, as entitled to govern absolutely the dealings of society with the individual in the way of compulsion and control, whether the means used is physical force in the form of legal penalties, or the moral coercion of public opinion. That principle is, that the sole end for which mankind are warranted, individually or collectively, in interfering with the liberty of action of any of their number, is self-protection. That the only purpose for which power can be rightfully exercised over any member of a civilized community, against his will, is to prevent harm to others. His own good, either physical or moral, is not a sufficient warrant. ... The only part of the conduct of any one, for which he is amenable to society, is that which concerns others. In the part which merely concerns himself, his independence is, of right, absolute. Over himself, over his own body and mind, the individual is sovereign.[40]

The key question is not so much whether Ms. Bouvia was absolutely sane but whether, when there is room for doubt, individuals or physicians control a person's decision to die. The principle of autonomy is important here, and specifically the principle that a person who has not been proved incompetent has the right to make decisions about her own life. Even if the principle allows results which are disliked in a specific case, its general application may create the greatest good. If the principle is not upheld, then there is not so much difference between a hospital forcing a competent patient to live on a psychiatric ward and involuntarily committing a competent woman to a psychiatric hospital (see Chapter 13 on Joyce Brown). But this is what Americans have criticized about Russian psychiatry.

Bouvia's detractors saw her as an unstable patient whose assisted death would have set a dangerous precedent. Because she did not kill herself, they felt vindicated. Is there not something odd about a patient who only wanted to kill herself *inside* a hospital and then, when she had the opportunity to do so outside the hospital in private, did not do so? So wasn't Ms. Bouvia something of a psychiatric patient after all?

Social Prejudice

American medical ethics often emphasizes the kind of personal autonomy championed by Mill above. While that is perhaps fine for young, healthy, adults, medical ethics encompasses more than autonomy. Paul Longmore, a ventilator-dependent quadriplegic who is a leading critic of voluntary death among the disabled, thinks Bouvia's case shows how a prejudiced system destroys independence and autonomy in the disabled and only leaves them with bogus decisions to die:

> Given the lumping together of people with disabilities with those who are terminally ill, the blurring of voluntary assisted suicide and forced

"mercy" killing, and the oppressive conditions of social devaluation and isolation, blocked opportunities , economic deprivation, and enforced social powerlessness, talk of their "rational" or "voluntary " suicide is simply Orwellian newspeak. The advocates of assisted suicide assume a nonexistent autonomy. They offer an illusory self-determination.[41]

Some critics of autonomy see Bouvia's case initially as a failure of community, as a failure of caring where Ms. Bouvia "slipped through the cracks" of an impersonal American system. How tragic she was, they say, fiercely alone even as a patient inside the hospital among others, and all the while asserting her right to tear herself away from life. Yet when caring people came forward to help her die in Mexico, she changed her mind, and such people showed her that her life could be worth living.

Moreover, to cast this case as a simple issue of whether a right to die exists, or a right to "assisted suicide" exists, is to miss the heart of the issue. What made Elizabeth Bouvia want to die was the cumulative effect of centuries of prejudice against the physically disabled. The new virulent form of this attitude is expressed in our culture's narcissistic idealization of youth, athleticism, sex, beauty, and fitness as the only values making life worthwhile.

So argues Longmore, who also attacks a spate of films giving disabled citizens the covert message that their only realistic choices are to be objects of charity, subjects of experimentation, or noble suicides. He cites the "social prejudice" in films ranging from *Annie Hall* to *Elephant Man*, and is especially contemptuous of *Whose Life Is It, Anyway?* which he claims depressed Elizabeth Bouvia after she watched it. Longmore believes that this film systematically ignores possibilities of sexual satisfaction, financial aid, and independence.

Longmore claims that Bouvia's problems resulted in part from failing to get the maximum sum owed her in a California county which (he claims) is well known for its stinginess in funding the disabled. He claims the hospital, where Bouvia was supposed to do her internship, refused to comply with Section 504 of the Civil Rights Act of 1983 (an Act important also in Baby Doe cases. See Chapter 7). This act prohibits discrimination against the handicapped and requires wheelchair access to all facilities. He emphasizes that Ms. Bouvia was strongly discouraged from seeking work or marriage by a system which reduces benefits for the disabled when employment or marriage occurs. California's In-Home Supportive Services program allowed Bouvia to manage her own life at home, but when she married, she became ineligible (her husband was expected to care for her at home). No wonder Bouvia then got divorced. No wonder she became discouraged about completing her training— for even in the unlikely event that she overcame discrimination and got a job, she would then lose her benefits.

Longmore concludes:

> This is a woman who aimed at something more significant than mere self-sufficiency. She struggled to attain self-determination, but she was repeatedly thwarted in her efforts by discriminatory actions on the part of the government, her teachers, her employers, her parents, and her

society. Contrary to the highly prejudiced view of the appeals court, what makes life with a major physical disability ignominious, embarrassing, humiliating, and dehumanizing is not the need for extensive physical assistance, but the dehumanizing social contempt toward those who require such aid.

A Duty to Live?

During the Enlightenment, the German philosopher Immanuel Kant, absolutely opposed suicide. His arguments are most clearly stated in his *Lectures on Ethics*. He argued that rights acts are those whose "maxim" or rule can be willed for all people to act on (his criterion of "universalizability,") and that we cannot will that all people have the right to suicide. Why? Because for Kant, the motive of suicide is self-interest, and morality is antithetical to self-interested motives. What is right for Kant is rarely coincident with self-interest.

Another formulation of Kantian ethics is that people should always be treated as "ends in themselves," never as "means" or things. To commit suicide is to treat oneself as a beast or thing—as just another amoral object which can be destroyed at will. "Man's freedom cannot subsist except on a condition which is immutable. This condition is that man not use his freedom against himself to his own destruction."[42]

Finally, Kant argues that a man "who does not respect his life even in principle cannot be restrained from the most dreadful vices." To respect the general principle that each life is sacred one must respect the sacredness of one's own life. Kant concludes, "Human beings are sentinels on earth and may not leave their posts until relieved by another beneficent hand. God is our owner; we are His property." To such religious arguments, we now turn.

Is Suicide Blasphemy?

Augustine and Aquinas held that suicide violated God's will. In contrast, David Hume, the 18th-century Scottish philosopher, historian, and essayist, argued that suicide "is no transgression of our duty to God." Especially for dying patients, voluntary death is not a sin: "A house which falls by its own weight, is not brought to ruin by his [God's] providence."[43] Hume argued deistically that God made the world work through the natural laws of causation studied by medicine and physics. Disease merely expressed such God-created laws.

Hume also attacked the argument that suicide is blasphemy. Some philosophers such as Kant said that God gave each person a place or "station" in the natural order which he must not give up. Hume replies that, "It is a kind of blasphemy to imagine that any created being can disturb the order of the world" [by taking his own life]. Any suicide is insignificant to the workings of the universe and it is blasphemy to think otherwise."

Hume also replied to Aquinas' argument that suicide harms the community:

> A man who retires from life does no harm to society: he only ceases to do good; which, if it is an injury, is of the lowest kind. All our obligations to do good to society seem to imply something reciprocal. I receive the benefits of society, and therefore ought to promote its interests; but when I withdraw myself altogether from society, can I be bound any longer? But [even] allowing that our obligations to do good were perpetual, they have certainly some bounds; I am not obliged to do a small good to society at the expense of a great harm to myself: when then should I prolong a miserable existence, because of some frivolous advantage which the public may perhaps receive from me?

On the other hand, Elizabeth Bouvia's case does not fit the typical case above. One could easily argue that forgoing medical treatment is not blasphemy when patients are terminally ill ("a house which falls under its own weight"). Importantly, Elizabeth Bouvia was *not* terminal, and so her wish to die could still be considered blasphemous.

Conceptual Problems about Dying

One question raised by Elizabeth Bouvia's case concerns what to call her intended action: "Suicide"? "Euthanasia"? "Assisted suicide"? "Voluntary death"? "Self-Deliverance"? "Free death"? Some distinguish between "direct" and "indirect" suicide. For most people, "suicide" connotes actions which are morally repugnant or caused by mental illness. As such, the word carries an inextricably negative condemnation. For this reason, supporters of Ms. Bouvia talk of her intended "self-deliverance," not of her suicide. An added complication is that "suicide" seems inappropriate when referring to medical patients suffering terminal diseases.

On the other hand, philosopher Margaret Battin, in *Ethical Issues in Suicide*, broadens "suicide" to cover the issues of whether it's morally permissible for a person: to choose to die, to determine that he shall die, to accept his death, or to kill himself.[44] Similarly, James Rachels in *The End of Life* broadens "suicide" to cover indirect means of taking one's life or of allowing one's death to occur.[45] These philosophers stress that if the intention is to end life, then it doesn't matter whether the means to that end is indirect or direct, because the motive and result are the same.

Nevertheless, it seems reasonable to accept philosopher Tom Beauchamp's view that a terminal cancer patient does not commit suicide by forgoing chemotherapy.[46] Court decisions in *Saikewicz, Conroy, Colyer,* and *Bouvia* agreed that withdrawal of treatment is not legally suicide. One practical point is that if a death is classified as suicide, many life insurance companies refuse to pay benefits. Moreover, many state laws forbid any person, physician, or hospital, from "assisting in suicide." In the Bouvia case, the hospital was explicitly relieved of any potential liability under laws prohibiting suicide assistance.

Thus, a semantic problem exists in describing the Bouvia case: if we say she was "suicidal," we beg one connotation against her. We also cannot correctly say her case was about "euthanasia," because this word has connotations of other people making that judgment or other people bringing about a death. Both terms are misleading when applied to the Bouvia case.

Perhaps the least confusing phrase to apply to Ms. Bouvia is "voluntary death." This will probably please no one but it seems to be the most neutral term. "Suicide" seems too cold, hard, and psychopathological. The phrase "voluntary death" at least implies consent in a way that "euthanasia" does not. If a patient had a terminal illness, then "voluntary patient death" would be even better, implying that concern about approaching death and illness were major factors in the decision.

Assisted Voluntary Death and Degrees of Active Euthanasia

Supporters of Ms. Bouvia said that if she had been wealthy and had hired a private physician, she could have starved herself so that her death could have been reported as a natural death. Because she was poor, she had to depend on the kindness of strangers.

Drs. Bacchus and Fischer may have seen such assistance as part of a slide to active killing and especially to accepting "active euthanasia." A continuum exists in medical assistance in voluntary death. Is keeping Ms. Bouvia pain-free while she starves to death over several weeks actively participating in her death? Is it different from giving her a lethal injection? How "active" must the participation of a physician be in a patient's death to count as "active euthanasia?" As "killing?"

These are important questions for two reasons. First, active euthanasia is often assumed to differ morally from "passive" euthanasia (allowing to die). Second, active euthanasia is legally considered murder, passive euthanasia is not.

This issue of assisting in voluntary death has become pressing with recent developments in Holland which have decriminalized "mercy killings." Because the Dutch situation makes this issue acute, discussion of this issue is deferred to the next chapter.

UPDATE

In the spring of 1988, physician-lawyer Richard Scott received a fee award from the State of California under its innovative private attorney general doctrine, which reimburses lawyers who bring suits for indigent patients which result in decisions addressing important issues of civil rights. Such awards show that the courts will compensate attorneys for what would otherwise be *pro bono* (free, for the public good) work, and hence, increase the future like-lihood of patients such as Ms. Bouvia having legal representation.

As of early 1989, Elizabeth Bouvia was still alive. Rumors abounded of books and movies in the process of being made about her case. For the most part, she lived a life of seclusion, removed from all media contact.

FURTHER READING

Derek Humphrey & Ann Wickett, *The Right to Die: Understanding Euthanasia,* (Harper & Row, 1986).

Margaret Pabst Battin, *Ethical Issues in Suicide* (Prentice-Hall, 1982.)

David Hume, "On Suicide" (1755), in *Collected Essays of David Hume* (Liberty Classics, 1986.)

James Rachels, *The End of Life* (Oxford University Press, 1986. 182.)

Tom Regan, ed. *Matters of Life and Death* 2nd ed. (Random House, 1986.)

CHAPTER 3

Mercy Killing in Holland

This chapter begins by discussing first, the Hippocratic Oath's opposition to mercy killing and then, the Nazi "euthanasia" program. The chapter's central "case" is contemporary mercy killing in Holland.

In the last chapter, problems surrounding terms such as "suicide" were discussed. "Euthanasia" and "mercy killing" suffer from similar problems, but, for now, the two terms will be used as synonyms. Later, they will be carefully analyzed.

Mercy killing or euthanasia may not be as rare as is commonly believed. The world learned in 1987 that King George V of England, the grandfather of Queen Elizabeth II, did not die naturally in 1936, as had been believed for decades. The 71-year-old king was instead, while dying at night, injected with a fatal dose of morphine and cocaine so that his death would be reported by the prestigious morning *Times* and not by the sensationalistic afternoon papers. The king had been slowly dying for months and was supposedly only hours from death when the Royal Physician complied with his wishes. Whether this was a good reason for assisting in death is controversial, but it was at least a royal one.

In 1988, the *Journal of the American Medical Association* produced a sensation by publishing a letter of a resident who had been a victim of mercy killing, a young woman named "Debbie."[1] His actions were severely criticized because Debbie was not his patient. He came to her one night, tired and cranky, after being awakened by a nurse's call that Debbie was in great pain. When he saw her, the resident said she said to him, "Let's get this over with." The resident interpreted this to mean she wanted to die, and he said he gave her a lethal injection.

Four physicians known for their interest in medical ethics wrote a letter in response to the "Debbie" case. They invoked the example of mercy-killing by physicians in Holland and argued:

> We must say also to each of our fellow physicians that we will not
> tolerate killing of patients and that we shall take disciplinary action
> against doctors who kill. And we must say to the broader community

that if it insists on tolerating or legalizing active euthanasia, it will have to find nonphysicians to do its killing.[2]

One year later, the *New England Journal of Medicine* published a special article by twelve physicians who advocated the opposite position. Many of these physicians were also leaders in medical ethics.[3] These physicians argued for open discussion of the issues with patients and ten of the physicians believed that it was "not immoral" for physicians to assist in the suicide of "hopelessly ill" terminal patients.

HISTORICAL BACKGROUND

The Prohibition of Euthanasia in the Hippocratic Oath

The time of Socrates in ancient Greece saw the beginnings of the Hippocratic Oath, which is often taken to be the origin of medical ethics and which forbids killing by physicians. This common view of Hippocrates was shattered in 1931 by the historian of medicine, Ludwig Edelstein. According to Edelstein, Hippocrates was a follower of the mystic Pythagoras, who gave civilization his theorem, who worshipped numbers as divine, and who believed that all life was sacred. According to Edelstein, Hippocrates was not at all representative of ancient Greek physicians.

Let us consider what the original Oath actually makes physicians promise. Here is the complete text in Edelstein's translation:

> I swear by Apollo Physician and Asclepius and Hygeia and Panaceia and all the gods and goddesses, making them my witnesses, that I will fulfill according to my ability and judgment this oath and this covenant:
>
> To hold him who has taught me this art as equal to my parents and to live my life in partnership with him, and if he is in need of money, to give him a share of mine, and to regard his offspring as equal to my brothers in male lineage, and to teach his art—if they desire to learn it—without fee and covenant; to give a share of precepts and oral instruction and all the other learning to my sons and to the sons of him who has instructed me and the pupils who have signed the covenant and have taken this oath according to the medical law, but to no one else.
>
> I will apply dietetic measures for the benefit of the sick according to my ability and judgment; I will keep them from harm and injustice.
>
> I will neither give a deadly drug to anybody if asked for it, nor will I make a suggestion to this effect. Similarly I will not give to a woman an abortive remedy. In purity and holiness I will guard my life and my art.
>
> I will not use the knife, nor even on sufferers of stone, but will withdraw in favor of such men as are engaged in this work.

Whatever houses I visit, I will come for the benefit of the sick, remaining free of all intentional injustice, of all mischief and in particular of sexual relations with both female and male persons, be they free or slaves.

What I may see or hear in the course of the treatment or even outside of the treatment in regard to the life of men, which on no account one must spread abroad, I will keep to myself holding such things shameful to be spoken about.

If I fulfill this oath and do not violate it, may it be granted to me to enjoy life and art, being honored with fame among all men for all time to come; if I transgress it and swear falsely, may the opposite of all this be my lot.[4]

This original small band of male physicians taking this oath in ancient times functioned like a guild. It had no place for women. Such followers of Hippocrates, and those who have taken the original Hippocratic Oath in modern times, have sworn to never perform abortions and never to kill patients who request death. The Oath also makes physicians swear not to do surgery.

Few medical schools today give the real Oath and if they use it at all, they change almost everything (especially the pagan curse at the end). When a physician or commentator says in public that such-and-such "violates the Hippocratic Oath," he or she erroneously assumes that medical students swore by such an Oath or that, if they did, the oath reflected values taught in medical school. In short, most people misunderstand the Hippocratic Oath, what it says, and its real place in modern medical ethics.

Ancient Greek physicians disagreed with Hippocrates and thought that life had certain natural limitations, after which life could end. The ancient Greeks had great respect for natural limits or *meson,* which infused their architecture, plays, science, and thinking. To attempt to go beyond *meson*—whether like a physician in going past the natural end of life, or like Alcibiades in acting like a god, was *hubris*—an arrogance which provoked the gods to strike one down.

As such, most ancient Greek physicians did not oppose letting patients die, or mercy killing. (It is doubtful that the distinction between active and passive death would have been important to such physicians.) Edelstein concludes, "That the Oath at first was not accepted by all ancient physicians is certain. Medical writings, from the time of Hippocrates to that of Galen, give evidence of the violation of almost every one of its injunctions."

One role of these physicians was to help patients die painlessly. Like the early Christian prohibition of abortion and infanticide, the prohibition of Pythagorean physicians against euthanasia was designed to set them apart from other physicians. It was not the way all of ancient medicine functioned, but the exception.

The Nazi "Euthanasia" Program

The debate about the ethics of euthanasia often invokes the Nazi euthanasia program. Under the name of "euthanasia," the Nazis in Germany killed 90,000 people. In their related program of the "Final Solution," the Nazis killed 6,000,000 Jews, 600,000 Poles, thousands of Gypsies, and their political opponents. They were killed because of "racial inferiority;" the victims of euthanasia, because of "mental or physical inferiority."

In an often-cited article from 1949, Leo Alexander, a New York psychiatrist and judge at the Nuremberg trials, argued that mass genocide of Jews, retardates, and other *lebensunwertes Leben* ("life unworthy of living") began when German physicians accepted the idea that some people were better off dead than living with low quality of life. According to this famous line of reasoning, from the moment when a mentally vegetative man was killed, medicine landed on a *slippery slope* ending in mass killings:

> The beginnings at first were a subtle shifting in emphasis in the basic
> attitude of the physicians. It started with the acceptance of the
> attitude, basic in the euthanasia movement, that there is such a thing
> as life not worthy to be lived. This attitude in its early stages
> concerned itself merely with the severely and chronically sick.
> Gradually, the sphere of those to be included in this category was
> enlarged to encompass the socially unproductive, the ideologically
> unwanted, the racially unwanted and finally all non-Germans. But it
> is important to realize that the infinitely small wedged-in lever from
> which this entire trend of mind received its impetus was the attitude
> of the nonrehabilitable sick.[5]

In 1986, Robert Jay Lifton, a New York psychiatrist, repeated Alexander's charge:

> The Nazis justified direct medical killing by use of the similar concept of
> "life unworthy of life" *lebensunwertes Leben*. While this concept predated
> the Nazis, it was carried to its ultimate racial and "therapeutic" extreme
> by them.
>
> Of the five identifiable steps by which the Nazis carried out the
> destruction of "life unworthy of life," coercive sterilization was the first.
> There followed the killing of "impaired" children in hospitals, and then
> the killing of "impaired" adults—mostly collected from mental
> hospitals—in centers especially equipped with carbon monoxide. The
> same killing centers were then used for the murders of "impaired"
> inmates of concentration camps. The final step was mass killing, mostly
> of Jews, in the extermination camp themselves.[6]

The work of Alexander and Lifton is often cited when people object that, if non-terminal patients such as Elizabeth Bouvia are allowed to die, much less if incompetent patients such as Karen Quinlan are allowed the same, we will slide down the slippery slope to doom. Columnist Cal Thomas and Surgeon General Everett Koop often cite the Nazi "euthanasia" program in this way.[7] Others emphasize that such changes began among physicians, especially among arrogant, elitist professors in medical schools.

Critics dispute Alexander's claim by saying, first, that the early years of the 20th century were blatantly racist, and that rather than being a subtle shift, Nazi racial murders were the expressions of then prevalent German racist attitudes. Second, the word "euthanasia" camouflaged mass murder: the Nazi "euthanasia" program was the Nazi *murder* program. All victims died involuntarily, and no documented case exists where a terminal patient was voluntarily killed.

This semantic sleight-of-hand by the Nazis confuses some people. If it continues, say opponents of Alexander and Lifton, it will be just one more evil caused by the Nazis. Elizabeth Bouvia's requested death could not be more different from murder. Supporters of mercy killing point out that if Bouvia were forced to live because of the Nazis' atrocities, it was just one more legacy of that "inversion of values" which haunts medical ethics today, e.g., when individual choice of a citizen under a democracy is overruled by citing the excesses of a totalitarian regime.

Alexander and Lifton specifically blame the degeneration of German medicine under the Nazis on physicians operating in secrecy. Critics say Alexander and Lifton confuse dictatorship with democracy, secrecy with public decisions. In Nazi Germany, a handful of physicians were ordered by a dictator to kill people and did so in secret. A few top administrators, not physicians, made up the list and the justifications. Euthanasia under the Nazis was no more an outgrowth of public medical practice than the arms-for-hostages deal of Oliver North was an outgrowth of public military practices.

Nevertheless, the Nazi slippery slope argument is difficult to refute. If Lifton and Alexander are right to blame secrecy, then American medicine may be more dangerous than Dutch. Because American physicians fear media attention and legal scrutiny, their decisions are made either in secret or privately with the family. Few physicians publicly argue for changing laws about mercy-killing and euthanasia. Moreover, Alexander and Lifton emphasize the German obsession with Aryan purity, which some historians say grew out of a German inferiority complex. Some critics detect similar narcissistic obsessions today in America about wealth, intelligence, health, and physical beauty.

On the other hand, Historian Lucy Dawidowicz, a famous scholar of the Nazis whose parents were killed by the Nazis, believes that the German "euthanasia" program has no relevance to modern debates about euthanasia.[8] For her, euthanasia of patients in modern hospitals and the Nazi "euthanasia" program are just not the same kinds of actions and raise entirely different kinds of issues.

The Modern Euthanasia Movement

In the early 1950s, theologian Joseph Fletcher rocked Christian ethics in several ways. He denied that any "real moral difference exists between self-administered euthanasia and the medically administered form when it is done at the patient's request."[9] Although widely attacked, Fletcher persevered for decades, arguing that the dying patient had become a "sedated, comatose, betubed object, manipulated and subconscious, if not subhuman." Fletcher later became famous in the 1960s for his book *Situation Ethics*, where he argued that consequences to real people should determine what is right or wrong, not abstract, historically handed down rules.

In 1969, psychiatrist Elisabeth Kübler-Ross' *On Death and Dying* outlined five stages of ideal dying (denial, anger, bargaining, depression, and acceptance) and shrilly criticized hospitals for ignoring the psychological needs of dying patients.[10] Her case histories of dying patients revealed their great sadness, anger, and abandonment. She sharply criticized fellow physicians for forcing patients to fight death until the very end. Her views were widely discussed and criticized, e.g., in an article in *Harper's* called "Turn On, Tune In, Drop Dead: You Haven't Lived Until You Died, Say the Apostles of Drop-Dead Chic."[11] Critics said there was something pathetic about a bright, healthy, suicidal 21-year-old contemplating "death with dignity."

In the early 1970s, physician Cicely Saunders founded St. Christopher's Hospice in London and claimed that painful deaths were always avoidable. Medical opinion on this claim has been divided, in part because of cultural differences between England and America. British physicians such as Saunders prescribe powerful "Brompton cocktails" (heroin, morphine, alcohol, and cocaine) for dying patients; American physicians do so less frequently. The British charge American physicians with greed in fighting cancer to the last breath, by using machines "simply because they're there," and with being stingy with pain-killers (calling them "pharmacological Calvinists"). American oncologists say the English give up too soon and produce patients who spend their last months in heavily drugged semi-consciousness.

Columnists Stewart Alsop in 1974 published a pivotal article in *Good Housekeeping*.[12] He described a 28-year-old fellow cancer patient and hospital roommate whose pain was uncontrolled and who "would begin to moan, or whimper very low.... Then he would begin to howl, like a dog.... [The pain medication] affected him no more than half an aspirin might affect a man who had just broken his arm."

Since then, the "War on Cancer" has had dismal results, despite the official literature. More people are supposedly "cured" today of cancer, but "cures" are semantically created by defining "cure" as survival past five years.[13] Moreover, five years of survival past diagnosis is more prevalent because new technology allows very early detection of cancer, often long before symptoms. Finally, the treatment of cancer patients, with radiation, surgery, and chemotherapy, has become one of the most dreaded symbols of the 20th century. For these reasons, more and more people with cancer today think of going "gentle into that dark night" and not raging with Dylan Thomas "against the dying of the light."

MERCY KILLING IN HOLLAND

Holland, the first country to liberalize mercy killing by physicians, was once actually occupied by the Nazis and was a country where physicians actively resisted the Nazi murder programs. The recent liberalization there of attitudes toward mercy killing signifies a new age in the history of medicine, and what happens in Holland may predict what will eventually happen in America. Religiously, Holland is a mixed country, with many Christian denominations. About 27 percent of its citizens claim no religious affiliation at all.

In the early 1980s, opinion polls repeatedly showed that about 75 percent of Dutch citizens would accept a law allowing physicians to mercy-kill competent, terminally ill patients at their request. In Holland, decriminalization of mercy killing began in 1971, when physician Geertruida Postma accepted her mother's repeated requests for death. Postma's mother suffered a cerebral hemorrhage, leaving her partially paralyzed, deaf, and with gross speech deficits. The elderly woman lived in a nursing home, where she needed to be tied into a chair to avoid falling. According to Geertruida Postma, her mother repeatedly begged for death: "When I watched my mother, a human wreck, hanging in that chair, I couldn't stand it anymore."[14] First she injected her mother with morphine to render her unconscious, and then killed her with an injection of curare. Dr. Postma then told the director of the nursing home, who called Dutch police.

Dr. Postma was found guilty of murder, but given only a suspended one-week sentence and a year's probation. Her lawyer argued that "rational suicide" assisted by a physician should be a legal defense. The judge rejected this, but did specify in great detail when physicians could mercy kill terminal patients who requested to die. The guidelines only allowed mercy killing for competent adults with terminal diseases.

A later case in 1973 established the legality of physicians complying with requests for mercy killing. This judge also made it clear that mercy killing could be done for diseases not immediately terminal but which involved inevitable physical and mental deterioration.

These developments sparked the Information Center for Voluntary Euthanasia, which functioned like America's Hemlock Society in trying to help terminal patients implement their choices about dying. Another Dutch group, the Foundation for Voluntary Euthanasia, worked for legal reform, like America's Society for the Right to Die. (Another American group, Concern for Dying, only educates citizens about euthanasia.)

Dutch medicine had long before rejected the traditional view in American medical ethics that mercy killing morally differed from withdrawing medical care. In 1973, the Royal Dutch Medical Association issued guidelines on mercy killing stating that: (1) only a physician may implement requests for mercy killing, (2) requests must be made by competent patients, (3) patients' decisions must be free of doubt, well-documented, and repeated, (4) the physician must consult another independent physician, and (5) a determination must be made that no one pressured patients into their decisions. Two other guidelines were vaguer: (6) the patient must be in "unbearable pain" and suffering without prospect of change, (7) no measures can be available—which patients will accept—that could improve their condition or render bearable their suffering.

In 1985, a Dutch commission proposed that mercy killing by physicians be a legal excuse to homicide, like self-defense or insanity. The proposal created emotional debate in Holland, in professional journals and the mass media. In 1986, opposition defeated the proposal. This opposition had been led by antiabortion groups and some Catholic bishops, who called the bill "a descent into barbarity."[15] Conservative religious groups produced a television show featuring old pictures of victims in concentration camps. These opponents said physicians would push the outer edges of mercy killing, generalizing to different but similar cases. They claimed that mercy killing by patient request was "murder" and that people are the creatures of God who did not have the right to end their own lives.

Two features of Holland's judicial system, which differ from American and English systems, should be noted. Trials are decided in Holland by judges without juries; moreover, Holland has professional judges appointed for life and who, because unelected, can make decisions unpopular with vocal opponents. Holland's five attorneys general (and the 200 public prosecutors they supervise) have more discretionary power than American district attorneys. What has happened is that the Dutch prosecutors—roughly equivalent in power to federal district attorneys—have agreed since 1985 not to prosecute physicians who perform euthanasia. Despite widespread reports to the contrary, Holland has officially neither decriminalized nor legalized active voluntary euthanasia. Its Supreme Court did issue a decision that physicians who follow all the guidelines will not be prosecuted for mercy killing, although an attempt to endorse mercy killing by a statute law failed in 1988.

ETHICAL ISSUES

Conceptual Issues

The word "euthanasia" has confused meanings. "Euthanasia" comes from the ancient Greek: *eu* (good) and *thanatos* (death), and may imply both *allowing* death to occur for merciful motives as well as *causing* death to occur for similar motives. It almost always is used to refer to causing or allowing death in another person, not oneself, so "self-euthanasia" is an oxymoron. However, some people do write of the Bouvia case as one about "euthanasia" or "voluntary euthanasia."

One important point is that the "eu" in "euthanasia" points to death being "good." This entitles us to ask, "good for whom?" Comparing the Quinlan and Bouvia cases shows the difference. In Ms. Bouvia's case, we know that she thought it would be good to die. Most often, people implicitly use the criterion of "a reasonable person," e.g., "No one would want to go on living like that." The problem is that such statements can be strong projections of the speaker's own feelings and not necessarily reflective of what any reasonable person would want. In Karen Quinlan's case, we did not know that she wanted to die. Instead, we merely have the testimony of the Quinlans that Karen would have wanted to die. This is a crucial difference.

The point is not whether the Quinlans were lying. Rather, the point is that, for many different reasons, when other people say that "death would be a good" for that patient, a much greater danger enters that errors may occur . Where physicians do not know patients well, where people stand to inherit money, where families squabble—errors may arise. In Chapter 7 (about Baby Doe cases), some families claim that, for some defective babies, death is better than continued existence. In these cases and Karen Quinlan's, guardians are saying that death would be good for incompetent others.

The phrase "mercy killing" is also problematic to some people. It assumes that a certain killing is merciful. Again, if a person requests such a killing and defines it for herself as merciful, then the phrase is correct. But with someone such as Karen Quinlan, the mercy may be more for the family than the patient. Of course, mercy for families is important, but we should not let this sidetrack us from the point, that "mercy killing" may misleadingly imply that killing an incompetent patient would be seen by that patient as merciful. This may not be so.

No Room for Mistakes

In his *One Life,* heart transplant surgeon Christiaan Barnard recalls a young woman with ovarian cancer who repeatedly begged him to kill her painlessly with morphine.[16] Knowing she was terminal and hearing her screams all night, Barnard decided her pain was so intense that he couldn't stand it. (When he decided to kill her, she had so much pain she couldn't even scream.) She lay in an inaudible semi-consciousness, beyond pain, only to awaken briefly to unbearable pain. Barnard loaded up a syringe with morphine to kill her, but at the last moment, changed his mind. The next morning, the woman felt better and soon achieved remission, living another few months.

Not all Dutch physicians agree with the new changes in Holland today. Dr. Karel Gunning led Dutch physicians opposed to physician-assisted euthanasia and claimed to know "quite a number of cases" where "we thought patients would die in 34 hours" but were mistaken and they "lived 30 more years."[17] He says a medical prognosis of a terminal condition is only "a guess" about the time of death. Oncologists retort that such remarks are unprofessional and ignorant. Moreover, Dr. Barnard later changed his mind, becoming an advocate for euthanasia.

Mercy

Peter Admiraal, an anesthesiologist and oncologist who practices in a large Catholic hospital, has emerged as a spokesperson for Dutch physicians favoring mercy killing. As of 1987, he assisted over a hundred patients to die (or, to put it differently, he has killed over a hundred terminal patients at their request). According to him, uncontrollable pain is rarely a reason for death because most pain can be controlled.

> But there is severe dehydration, uncontrolled itching and fatigue. These patients are completely exhausted. Some of them can't turn around in their beds. They become incontinent. All these factors make a kind of suffering from which they only want to escape.
>
> And of course you are suffering because you have a mind. You are thinking about what is happening to you. You have fears and anxiety and sorrow. In the end, it gives a complete loss of human dignity. You cannot stop that feeling with medical treatment.[18]

Admiraal also gives an example of a declining cancer patient who had constant, uncontrollable itching. Although not in acute pain, the patient found the itching to be intolerable.

Of course, a trade-off exists between maximal consciousness and maximal pain relief. When pain becomes very intense, only very potent painkillers such as "Brompton cocktails" can reduce it. The question then becomes whether to live out one's final days in a mostly unconscious state while the underlying disease ravages one's body, or to bear some pain and be conscious. This is not a wonderful choice.

The Role of Physicians

Many physicians paradoxically endorse mercy-killing but refuse to do it themselves. Nor do they think other physicians should kill. Notice that in the letter quoted at the beginning of this chapter, the four physician/medical ethicists suggest that if society favors mercy-killing, "it will have to find nonphysicians to do its killing." This person might be a special technician, medically trained and regulated by the state. Such a technician has been widely discussed as an alternative to physicians participating in capital punishment. This person could be called a "designated killer."

Physicians who support mercy-killing but who don't want physicians to kill commonly emphasize the importance of maintaining the role of the physician as a healer and preserver of life. One poll of American physicians showed 60 percent favoring euthanasia but less than half would perform it themselves.[19] To such physicians, taking life radically conflicts with the symbolic image of physicians. Such conflict, they say, destroys trust in physicians.

Perhaps more important than fear of death is fear of a painful death. If physicians would guarantee that a patient would not die in such a way, they would gain the trust of some patients.

Physicians have disagreed for years about whether physicians should be involved in capital punishment of convicted criminals. Some physicians vigorously support participation, often arguing that organs should first be removed for transplantation. One frequent objection to capital punishment is that sometimes techniques don't work the first time, resulting in lingering, painful deaths.

For any kind of killing, some physicians favor the creation of "designated killer" technicians. This would free physicians from the taint of killing, keeping their image pure and their hands clean. But is this workable? If designated killers are mere technicians, what prevents them from abusing their role? Wouldn't it be better for physicians, torn between saving life and honoring patient's wishes, to be reluctant killers? Wouldn't physicians know best what to do if something went wrong?

Discussing this problem in 1988, *New England Journal of Medicine* editor Marcia Angell called the idea of designated killers an "unsavory prospect."[20] She suggested that mercy killing may one day be the end point of a continuum of good patient care. She asks how can any physician excuse himself from "good patient care"? Dr. Angell concluded, "Perhaps, also, those who favor legalizing euthanasia but would not perform it should rethink their position."

Dr. Angell implies that it is hypocritical to favor mercy-killing but be unwilling to perform it. Is this true? There are at least two schools of thought. Some thinkers believe that if one favors, say, meat-eating, one should be willing to kill and prepare animals for eating oneself. Others conclude differently, seeing no reason why each person who favors a position must be willing to implement it. Must you be willing to kill a serial murderer to favor capital punishment? Critics say one must. Being face-to-face with one's victim creates basic moral qualms and such moral restraints are important to respect. In Stanley Milgram's studies on obedience, naive subjects under an experimenter's control were dramatically less willing to inflict injury as the victims became closer to subjects under study.[21] In contrast, as the consequences of actions became more remote, such as by pressing a switch which released a bomb on an unseen, unknown populace, it became easier to inflict injury. Such empirical studies do not justify or refute mercy-killing by physicians, but they do identify a widespread reluctance to personally inflict death.

Active vs. Passive Killing

One of the ethical issues in the Quinlan case was whether it was permissible to accelerate Karen's death in some active fashion, as opposed to merely withdrawing care, and whether doing so wouldn't be more humane than Karen's actual fate. Two years before the case began in 1973, the American Medical Association had declared as official policy:

> The intentional termination of the life of one human being by another—
> mercy killing—is contrary to that for which the medical profession
> stands and is contrary to the policy of the American Medical Association.

> The cessation of the employment of extraordinary means to prolong the
> life of the body when there is irrefutable evidence that biological death
> is imminent is the decision of the patient and/or immediate family.[22]

This statement implied that physicians could let terminal patients die, but could not kill them. Pope Pius XII, in 1957, similarly said that physicians may not kill terminal patients, but need not make "heroic" efforts to keep dying patients alive.

In 1975, philosopher James Rachels argued in a seminal article that the active/passive distinction had no moral significance, that in some cases active euthanasia was more humane than passive euthanasia, and that the traditional distinction led to decisions about death based on irrelevant factors.[23] If the motive was to bring about death, and if the eventual result was death, could there be an intrinsic moral difference between letting die and killing? The point cut two ways: letting a patient such as Karen Quinlan die was just as bad (or good) as killing her, and killing her was just as bad (or good) as letting her die. The states of being active or passive themselves had no intrinsic moral significance.

Rachels' attack on the distinction between mercy-killing and letting patients die was controversial. His critics argued that ceasing chemotherapy and respirators in patients was not the same as killing them. Medical ethicist Baruch Brody says:

> What is the difference between merely letting a patient die and killing
> that patient? Does it depend upon activity or passivity? Does it depend
> on an agent's intentions? I think that neither of these factors is relevant.
> What is relevant is the cause of death. A patient is killed when an
> action or inaction is the cause of death. When the cause of death is the
> underlying disease process, the patient is simply allowed to die.[24]

Other critics say mercy killing risks great harm, such as destroying trust in the physician/patient relationship. They also invoke the slippery slope metaphor, arguing that active killing of terminal adults would move society over time toward involuntary euthanasia—e.g., in the form of killing defective newborns (see Chapter 7 on Baby Jane Doe). They fear abuses, mistaken diagnoses where patients are killed needlessly, and erosion of resources directed at cures. They imply that opponents base their arguments on extreme cases, on which medical norms cannot rest. Besides, they argue, unusual cases can be handled in other ways, e.g., by juries letting mercy-killers go by reason of temporary insanity or by physicians engaging in civil disobedience.

Those agreeing with Rachels claim that the debate is merely semantic. Not acting can be considered "active," e.g., not giving antibiotics to Karen Quinlan in her final days. They emphasize that if killing is never allowed, what will occur is suffering, wasted energies, and financial hardship. What is more important, they say, suffering of real people or upholding an abstraction?

Philosopher Holly Goldman argues that death is only a harm or evil if continuation of a patient's life "would have been a benefit" to the patient.[25] If prolonging life would have been an evil for Karen Quinlan, then early death for her was a good. When such a death is a good, killing cannot be a harm and cannot be immoral. Killing and letting die, then, are not always cases of harming and allowing harm to occur.

Daniel Dinello believes that killing intrinsically differs from letting die.[26] Consider his thought-experiment: Angie needs a heart transplant which could come from Beth, who herself has failing kidneys. If killing is not worse than letting die, the following should be morally equal: (1) killing Angie and transplanting her kidneys to Beth, or (2) killing Beth and transplanting her heart to Angie. But Dinello claims these are not equal, so killing is not the same as allowing to die. Richard O'Neil argues that society prefers to let nature be a lottery of distributive medical justice by its processes of disease, rather than having men make such decisions.[27]

One odd argument about this issue came in 1989, when a criminal, Noel Pagan, in Maine, asked Judge Dana Childs to stop physicians from disconnecting the respirator of his victim, Mark Weaver. When Pagan had stabbed Weaver in the neck in 1985, lack of oxygen to Weaver's brain caused damage and his resulting persistent vegetative state. If Weaver "died," Pagan could be charged with homicide, not merely aggravated assault.

A Slippery Slope about Killing the Functionally Incompetent?

National columnist Nat Hentoff wrote in 1987 that during the *Quinlan* decision in 1976, champions of euthanasia argued that they wanted to do so only for patients who were in unbearable pain, near death, and who made voluntary, rational request.[28] Hentoff points out that Karen Quinlan met none of these conditions. He believes that not only will a slippery slope occur about euthanasia but that it already has: "People who thought about these things in 1976 could never have imagined how far down the deadly slippery slope we would slide in just 11 years."

In reply, it can be said that *Quinlan* was perhaps too radical and its criteria were too loose. Few decisions since then have gone past it toward the "pit" of the slippery slope, but instead, most decisions concerned cases further up the "slope." Nevertheless, the Baby Doe cases and their legal precedents are indeed further down the "slope"—if "slope" it is.

The most controversial ethical issue about euthanasia cases today concerns killing the functionally incompetent. The Quinlan case represents the typical, troublesome case because Karen was an incompetent patient who had no recorded "advance directive" and yet who was not brain dead. Conservatives say the slippery-slope objection must be answered about killing incompetent patients "for their own good," i.e., about killing mentally defective children, retarded adults, and demented, elderly patients. This is a difficult problem, requiring careful treatment. In Holland, voluntary mercy killing, in fact, moved quickly from killing by patient choice in hopeless cases involving great pain to killing by patient choice in hopeless cases where life was highly unaesthetic.[29] (In these cases, problems included loss of bowel and bladder control, paralysis with some memory loss, uncontrolled gross swelling, etc. Moreover, are not such unappealing states causes of as much suffering as physical pain?) However, the Dutch have *not* moved to killing mental incompetents, or comatose patients.

Both critics and defenders of euthanasia worry that different kinds of cases are too often run together. Honoring requests by competent, but terminally ill, individuals for death differ quite markedly from killing incompetent people. Clear thinking requires that different cases be analyzed separately.

Critics such as Hentoff also charge that champions of euthanasia too often invoke an idealized picture of the dying patient. The idealized patient is always highly intelligent and without family (Ken Harrison in the film *Whose Life Is It, Anyway?*) or in unbearable pain and without real family (Donald Cowart in the videotape *Please Let Me Die*). It is almost a tautology that terminal patients in unbearable pain should be allowed to die quickly and painlessly. Unfortunately, such easy cases are rare. Real cases are much messier, with family members at odds with each other, with ambiguous prognoses, with patients of varying levels of competence and incompetence, with trade-offs between pain and consciousness, and with various indignities and dysfunctions which may or may not be reversible.

Although no cases have been permitted, the Royal Dutch Medical Association has also accepted that children have a right to die even if parents oppose such a wish.[30] (The argument is that dying children do not understand why they have to live only to suffer and that prolonging life is too often done for the sake of the parents, not the child.) Moreover, Dutch physicians and judges have now gone beyond the original paradigms: under guidelines developed under Dutch case law, persons with paraplegia, multiple sclerosis, and major physical deterioration at advanced age may, if they wish, choose euthanasia. Although in all these cases, patients themselves must repeatedly request a physician's assistance in dying, the cases do break new ground for mercy killing.

Defenders of Dutch mercy killing retort that the slippery slope metaphor misleadingly implies that society cannot make small changes without creating moral nihilism, that physicians are eager to kill patients, that one's personal physicians cannot be trusted, and that if decriminalized euthanasia should create bad results, it could not be reversed.

Dutch opponents of mercy killing argue that physicians are already too arrogant and self-important. They argue that the handicapped will die early because they feel they should not continue to burden their relatives and children. To give doctors the power to kill, they say, will concentrate too much power in a profession which already does not control its members' excesses.

Decriminalizing Mercy Killing

James Rachels has proposed legalizing active euthanasia in a limited way by making mercy killing on request a legal excuse for homicide, much like the standard excuses of self-defense, accident, insanity, and coercion.[31] As with traditional excuses, there would be no question that the act was done or about how it was done (thus eliminating much of what courts consider in homicide cases). Instead, there would be only the burden of proof on the physician and family to show that the patient requested euthanasia and that he or she was, in fact, suffering from a terminal illness. This proposal would not legalize suicide. Its practical advantages are that it would remove many cases of euthanasia from the courts while holding out the possibility of redress by legal appeal in cases of abuse. In the actual workings of the law, district attorneys have much discretionary power to use in deciding which cases to prosecute.

Opponents argue that in practice it will be very difficult to distinguish mercy killing from homicide. A clever, deranged physician could use the excuse of mercy killing to mask murder. Moreover, opponents argue, whatever criteria of mercy killing are adopted will be difficult to enforce. Given the privacy of people's homes and physicians' acts inside hospitals, it will be difficult to distinguish killings which meet established criteria from those which do not. Finally, in withdrawing care from terminally ill patients, the underlying disease is allowed to kill. Should physicians be allowed to kill directly, the courts would have to take a much more active role to ensure that such great power was not abused. This means that lawyers and the adversarial process of the courts would encroach even more on the physician at the bedside of the dying patient.

Removing Food and Water: The American Scene

American medicine is far from Dutch mercy killing. The key issue today in American cases about euthanasia concerns the withdrawal of food and water from terminal, and/or comatose patients. This issue of the Quinlan case was fought out in the courts in the 1980s. Philosopher Daniel Callahan of the Hastings Institute argues that removing food and water from patients symbolically trespasses beyond natural limits:

> The feeding of the hungry, whether because they are poor or because they are physically unable to feed themselves, is the most fundamental of all human relationships. . . . It is a most dangerous business to tamper with, or adulterate, so enduring and central a moral emotion.[32]

Critics reply that Callahan begs the question and that "the hungry" should only be fed if they are persons. Corpses are not "fed" intravenously and maintained indefinitely. Such critics say such feeding is but one factor in human relationships, and it is simplistic to make it more important than all others— including such values as the patient's wishes, honor, love, human decency, costs, and compassion.

One defender of giving food and water argues that removing intravenous feeding is not removing medical care but is removing the ordinary care "that all human beings owe each other."[33] He believes that irreversibly comatose patients should be given the benefit of the doubt as persons and should always be given food and water.

Theologian James Childress and physician Joanne Lynn point out that, in opposing removal of all feeding, artificial feedings take two forms: a temporary, indwelling, nasal tube to improve hydration and electrolyte balance (through a N-G tube to a functioning GI tract), or a permanent IV-feeding line for a balanced diet (through one of the major veins of the chest).[34] The permanent chest tube is much more traumatic because it increases risk of infection, requires restraint of the patient, mandates hospital stay, jumps costs, and may cause iatrogenic problems.

The President's Commission said in 1983:

> Since permanently unconscious patients will never be aware of nutrition, the only benefit to the patient of providing such increasingly burdensome interventions is sustaining the body to allow for a remote possibility of recovery. The sensitivities of the family and of care-giving professionals ought to determine whether such interventions are made.[35]

In other words, if the patient is unlikely to recover, artificial feeding is unlikely to benefit him. Furthermore, while N-G tubes are usually well tolerated, they are not free from risks and sometimes are distressing to the patient. They may lead to pneumonia, cause discomfort, and require arm restraints so that patients will not dislodge the tube. The volume of fluid itself needed to carry nutrients is sometimes harmful.

Finally, dehydration may well not be distressing to dying patients. For unconscious patients who are unable to sense anything, withholding water may not result in more pain than the termination of any other medical treatment. On a related point, the Court in *Conroy* noted that patients near death who are not receiving nourishment may be more comfortable than other patients.

In an influential article in 1983, Margaret Battin emphasized how most patients who signed Living Wills didn't get "the natural death" they expected.[36] Patients do not understand that their court-given right to refuse medical care, if exercised, often condemns them to deaths by dehydration, vomiting, organ failure, or suffocation, not easy "Socratic" deaths. Battin supported mercy-killing and assisted suicide, arguing that patients have the right not only to informed consent but also to *informed refusal* in trying to achieve, if not the expected good death, then their least bad death.

In 1986, the AMA changed its 1973 position on withdrawing care, declaring that physicians could "ethically withdraw" feeding and hydration from irreversibly comatose patients.[37] The Council said that death need not be imminent for such withdrawal, provided that the condition is "irreversible," and that physicians should consider both the expressed wishes of the patient and the wishes of the family.

Critics say the Council's phrase, "irreversibly comatose," is too vague because the phrase covers everything from partial unconsciousness to death.

Neurologists especially object to the Council's use of "comatose" in an incorrect sense and want more precise phrases such as "permanently unconscious." Others reply that "permanently unconscious" is still not very precise.

In a survey commissioned by the AMA in 1986, 70 percent of Americans said they would want food and water discontinued if they were in irreversible comas. However, only 46 percent would make such decisions for a relative.

Finally, as explained at the end of the Quinlan chapter, state supreme courts in the late 1980s disagreed about the constitutional legality of withdrawing food from a comatose relative by the family. Supreme Courts in New Jersey, Massachusetts, Florida, and North Dakota have permitted relatives to discontinue respirators and feeding tubes on standards of either substituted judgment (a relative's judgment substituting for that of the patient) or best interests of the patient (as judged by relatives or physicians). However, similar courts in New York and Missouri declared that the best interest of the comatose patient was not to allow relatives the choice to remove feeding tubes. The U.S. Supreme Court needs to decide what will be the law of the land, which it may do in its 1990 *Cruzan* decision.

UPDATE

The Gilbert and Rosier Cases in Florida

Emily and Roswell Gilbert had been married over fifty year in 1978 when they moved to a luxury high-rise condominium in Fort Lauderdale, Florida.[38] Shortly thereafter, Emily developed osteoporosis, a crippling, extremely painful disease in which the spinal column rapidly deteriorates. At the same time, she developed Alzheimer's disease, a progressive neurological disease which eventually leaves its victims without self-control, memory, or intact personalities. Roswell nursed his deteriorating wife for seven years. During this time, neighbors say that he never lost his temper with his wife and cared for her assiduously—changing her soiled sheets, dressing her, feeding her, and applying her makeup. Unfortunately, the retired engineer refused to bring up these facts at his trial or to seek the jury's sympathy. ("He came across as coldhearted," one juror said.)

In the seventy-two hours before the killing, Emily had injured one of her vertebrae and was in great pain, but refused to go to a hospital; when Roswell tried to force her, she cursed him for the first time. The next day, she interrupted a building association meeting to find him. When she did, neighbors said she screamed, "I want to die. Somebody help me." Two days later, Roswell shot Emily—in the head, twice (to make sure she was dead).

The jury convicted Gilbert in 1985 of "murder one." Under Florida law, the judge had to give him a minimum sentence of 25 years. As of 1988, Roswell's appeals had been unsuccessful and no governor has pardoned him.

In April 1985, 42-year-old Patricia Rosier living in Fort Myers, Florida, was told she had lung cancer.[39] Seven months later, her cancer had spread to her brain and by January 1986, oncologists said there was little hope. Patricia decided to kill herself and asked her husband, a pathologist, to help. Peter was very depressed by his wife's cancer and after his insurance company granted him disability, had given up medicine at age 45. He even considered dying with his wife.

She swallowed 20 tablets of a barbiturate on January 15 after a last dinner with her two adult children and husband. Although she lost consciousness, she did not die, because her husband had only given her the minimal lethal dosage. Having a strong heart, she simply went into a coma.

No longer being a physician, Peter needed other physicians to prescribe more drugs. Over the next few hours, he convinced two physicians to prescribe them and he injected his wife with 6 milligrams of morphine and then gave her another 80 mg. by suppository, but Mrs. Rosier was still alive after these administrations.

Peter and his wife's stepfather and brothers went outside and sat around the swimming pool, trying to figure out what to do. Finally, the stepfather Vincent Delman became frustrated, said "enough is enough," and gently suffocated Patricia. Peter Rosier became unstable after his wife's death and on television admitted giving his wife something to use to kill herself. He wrote a book describing his actions in detail and tried to get 20 publishers to accept it. He wanted television stations to make a movie of her death. The documents he produced for these projects, as well as his admission on television, were used to prosecute him.

He was tried for murder after Vincent Delman agreed to testify against him, after being (mistakenly) offered immunity from prosecution. Neither defense nor prosecuting attorney disputed the above facts, which Rosier admitted in court. On December 3, 1988, a jury acquitted Rosier.

The Gilbert and Rosier cases differ in that Rosier's jury had no doubt that Patricia Rosier truly wanted to die, whereas Gilbert's jury was not given enough evidence to erase all doubts.

Holland: Once Again

In the introduction to the chapter, a letter from four physicians was quoted in the "Debbie" case. In that letter, the following sentence occurs: "In the Netherlands, where the barriers to physician killing are gone, there are now many well-documented cases of such cryptic and uninvited killing by doctors." This sentence is misleading. Yes, some physicians and nurses killed people outside of the guidelines, but they were prosecuted. These half-dozen cases do not count as "many." Nor could a killing be "cryptic" and simultaneously "well-documented." Because no patient like Karen Quinlan can be killed, and because the rules must be followed, it is incorrect to say that the "barriers" to killing by Dutch physicians "are gone." It is possible to read a lot of such misunderstandings today about euthanasia in Holland.

Performing euthanasia appears to have been accepted as an occasional duty by Dutch physicians. It has been spread out, with one study discovering that the average general practitioner would have two patients every three years to request euthanasia, of which one would be performed. Another study found that nearly 80 percent of general practitioners in Holland had experience with euthanasia.[40] The preferred method appears to be injection of morphine followed, after deep unconsciousness, with curare.

Physicians in Holland are not entirely happy with the present legal status. To say to such physicians, "You will probably not go to jail for something which is officially a crime but which you have an obligation to perform" occasionally is not totally comforting. Dutch physicians hoped for a new law telling them when they could practice euthanasia and not be prosecuted. They did not get this. One Dutch physician who failed to document a patient's request for euthanasia received a one-year prison sentence, and three nurses who (on their own initiative) killed comatose patients received similar longer sentences. None of those convicted had followed the official guidelines.

By 1990, the topics of assisted suicide and mercy killing had moved from never being discussed in medical journals and newspapers to being a frequent topic. The Hemlock Society initiated a proposal in California to legalize physician-assisted, voluntary death in terminally ill patients, but was defeated (although probably not because of public opposition but because of poor organization).

Future events are difficult to predict. The Netherlands may be seen as a laboratory of medical ethics where an experiment is occurring about mercy killing. It will eventually show whether mercy killing humanizes death or leads down to the pit, along the infamous slippery slope.[41]

More than anything else, mounting deaths to relatively young people from AIDS drove a reconsideration of the ethics of mercy-killing. By 1989, over a hundred thousand people had AIDS, with a million more predicted by the year 2000 (see Chapter 16). People with AIDS frequently suffered severe neurological impairment and many suffocated to death, a horrible way to die. Coupled with lack of a cure, such deaths from AIDS forced many physicians to wonder whether merely withdrawing care—to allow a lingering, wasting-away death—was really all that a good doctor could do.

FURTHER READING

Robert Jay Lifton, *The Nazi Doctors* (Basic Books, 1986).

Derek Humphrey & Ann Wickett, *The Right to Die: Understanding Euthanasia* (Harper & Row, 1986).

James Rachels, *The End of Life: Euthanasia and Morality* (Oxford University Press, 1986).

Courtney S. Campbell & Bette-Jane Crigger, eds., "Mercy, Murder, & Morality: Perspectives on Euthanasia," Special Supplement, *Hastings Center Report* 19:1 (January/February 1989).

PART 2

CLASSIC CASES ABOUT THE BEGINNINGS OF LIFE

CHAPTER 4

Baby Louise Brown's In Vitro Fertilization

This chapter discusses the ethical controversies surrounding the "test-tube" conception of Louise Brown in 1978. Such conception, less emotionally called *in vitro* fertilization (abbreviated IVF), refers to fertilization "under glass" in a Petri dish or anywhere else outside the womb. As some wit said about IVF, people already knew a way to have sex without making babies, and then they found a way to make babies without having sex.

LOUISE BROWN: THE FIRST BABY CONCEIVED IN VITRO

Lesley Brown, the mother of the first child conceived in vitro, grew up unhappily without much of a family. Her father left when she was born, and her mother placed her at an early age in a state home. She grew up in Bristol, a port on England's western coast with large unemployment and high illiteracy. Like many British teenagers in 1963, Lesley dropped out of high school and took a factory job. A few months later when she met her future husband, John Brown, she had been laid off. A few months later, the two were living together. Lesley got a new job in a cheese factory while John worked driving a truck.

John was seven years older than Lesley. When his first wife left him, he had to take care of their daughter Sharon. John was reluctant to remarry, although Lesley wanted children. When both decided to have children, John said he would "do the right thing" if Lesley became pregnant. After some rocky times, they married, although Lesley never became pregnant.

Some people believe that conception takes place when a sperm fertilizes an egg in a woman's vagina or uterus. In fact, sperm move up the vagina, through the uterus, and into the small Fallopian tubes, which carry an egg each month from the ovaries to the uterus. The tubes are the size of the thin lead sticks in a mechanical pencil. Inside the upper third of the tubes, conception occurs when the first sperm penetrates the egg. Then the fertilized egg (now called a "zygote" or "pre-embryo") goes down the last two-thirds of the tube. Three days later, it tries to implant on the uterine wall. In about 30–40 percent of pregnancies, the embryos abort.[1]

In Lesley Brown's case, an egg had fertilized in her Fallopian tubes years before and had started to grow there. This was an ectopic pregnancy. Unable to move, the egg had finally disintegrated and damaged her Fallopian tubes.

Not knowing of Lesley's problem, the Browns tried to conceive for years. They tried adoption but babies were scarce. An obstetrician injected dye through Lesley's Fallopian tubes and discovered the damage. A subsequent operation to open them failed. Lesley was told afterwards that conception was unlikely.

Like most infertile women, Lesley worried "that I might have done something that had caused the trouble with my fallopian tubes."[2] She felt depressed when other women talked about their children. She saw a future of "years of just weighing and packing cheese and coming back to a quiet, empty flat." After nine years of trying to conceive a child, Lesley said she wouldn't blame John if he abandoned her for a fertile woman. John said her infertility didn't matter.

MEDICAL BACKGROUND

Infertility

According to a 1982 government survey, about one in six American couples is infertile.[3] A more accurate figure is that one married couple in twelve cannot conceive a child after one year of trying. Such infertility stems from many factors, some of which are increased maternal age at first attempt to conceive, damage from pelvic inflammatory disease, previous abortions, and abnormal uteruses. Although infertility is often blamed on women, males account for 50 percent of it.

Adoption is increasingly a rare opportunity. Two million American couples every year seek 22,000 Caucasian babies available for adoption.[4] Between 1971, before abortion's legalization, and 1982, the number of babies available for adoption dropped by over 30,000, from 82,800 to 50,700. Adoption of babies from overseas doubled from roughly 5,000 in 1981 to 10,000 in 1986. Of these, over 6,000 came from South Korea; others came from South America and Mexico.

John and Lesley Brown tried for nine years to have children. Twenty years ago, infertile couples like the Browns had to resign themselves to being "barren." Today, other options are possible. Physicians first rule out underlying disease and counselors explore possible sexual dysfunction. The woman's basal body temperature is taken daily to predict the exact day (and even hour) of ovulation. Couples are told that timely sex is needed, not lots of it (because frequent sex lessens sperm per ejaculate and a man needs 24 hours to maximize his sperm count). After sex, the woman may lie on her back for an hour with her legs up to pool sperm in her uterus.

If these techniques don't work, tests are done to see if the woman is releasing mature eggs from her ovaries, to see if the man's sperm is able to reach the egg, and to see if the uterus lining is hormonally prepared to let the embryo implant.

In rare cases, couples may even have sex next door to a physician's office. One woman, after nine years, became pregnant using such techniques, but she says,

> The whole experience is very degrading. . . . Your whole private life is open, you even carry around jars of sperm. The doctors tell you when to have sex and when not to. And then after sex, everyone comes into the examining room to take a peek and see how successful you were.[5]

Next, X-rays are taken to detect blockages in the Fallopian tubes. If the tubes are healthy, artificial insemination by husband (AIH) will be tried. Because the man may not have been producing enough sperm during each ejaculation, his sperm will be concentrated after masturbation. The concentrate is then placed well up the uterus.

If the Fallopian tubes are damaged, surgeons may try to remove blockages by microsurgery, which can repair damaged Fallopian tubes in a small percentage of cases. Before 1978, when the tubes could not be surgically opened, nothing else could be done.

History of IVF

Obstetrician Patrick Steptoe and physiologist Robert Edwards helped the Browns conceive their daughter, Louise Brown. When the Browns arrived on a cold winter day in Manchester, in the north of industrial England, they went out to the nearby smaller, bleak city of Oldham, where Steptoe practiced. It was not the kind of place where medical breakthroughs were expected:

> Early the following morning, we walked up the hill that led to Oldham General Hospital. It was winter in a strange, bleak town and no one was about. We passed open spaces, with buildings flattened by bulldozers or bombs, and great empty mills, still standing, with their windows smashed, leaving dark, gaping holes like wounds.[6]

Newsweek described the same hospital as a "cluster of Victorian buildings that were originally a Dickensian workhouse."[7]

Physiologist Robert Edwards came from a working-class family. After military service, he went back to college in his early twenties, but did not excel. At 26, he found himself broke in Edinburgh with not much of an academic future. He was accepted in a course in genetics, which in the early 1950s was just beginning as a robust specialty. While earning a doctorate in animal genetics at the University of Edinburgh, he worked at the "Mouse

House" trying to fertilize mouse eggs. He later received an appointment at Cambridge University

Obstetrician Patrick Steptoe frequently encountered infertile couples: "There were men who, fearful that they were sterile, became impotent. There were women who, desperate, tried folk remedies, prayed long hours in a darkened room, or visited special shrines."[8] Steptoe perfected an instrument called a *laparoscope* to remove eggs for fertilization outside the Fallopian tubes. It used extremely thin tubes equipped with tiny lights.

With Lesley Brown, Steptoe slipped a laparoscope through a small slit at her "bikini line" and guided it into her ovaries, where he searched among the hundreds of eggs for the one being primed for ovulation. Searching for it was difficult, and when he found it, Steptoe inserted another thin tube and suctioned it out. Without Steptoe's perfection of this technique, IVF would have been impossible.

Robert Edwards' contributions were remarkable because he worked in such crude facilities (even in 1980, his lab at Cambridge lacked piped hot water). He not only had to make important new discoveries but also had to discover that several important beliefs about fertilization—taken to be facts by scientists— were really false. The first incorrect belief was that gonadotrophic hormones couldn't make a mammal's ovary release eggs. Edwards discovered that hormonal interactions were so extremely delicate that precise timings and interactions made all the difference to successful conception. Once he knew this, he studied preovulatory mice eggs dividing their chromosomes in preparation for fertilization, discovering that this process occurred in a precise, uniform way, such that the time between hormonal application and ovulation could be predicted to the hour:

> The chromosomes then moved like soldiers through a prepared drill.
> First they marched to the center of the egg, then out to the periphery.
> Next they slowly separated into two equal halves as they glided along a
> spindle. As if to inaudible military music, one half marched out of the
> egg for ever and into a small body known as the first polar body. The
> other half remained in the egg. The purpose of their maneuvers was to
> prepare the egg for fertilization and the precision of it all, as we peered
> through the microscope, was breathtaking.[9]

The ovaries normally release the hormones progesterone and estrogen, which thicken the uterine lining to receive a fertilized egg. If no egg appears, these hormones decrease. Edwards gave infertile women carefully balanced mixtures of these hormones.

Human sperm also must be "capacitated" for conception by removing chemicals from the head, chemicals which inhibit the sperm from penetrating the egg. In 1965, most scientists believed that such capacitation required exposure to uterine secretions. But one night that year, Edwards collected his own semen and added it haphazardly to a ripe human egg in a dish. The next morning, when he came back to his lab to see if anything had happened, he looked through his microscope and saw the characteristic cell division of human embryology. A human zygote had been created. Although he soon stopped the process, and although he couldn't repeat his accidental success when he later repeatedly tried to do so, he had overcome yet another "fact" about what could not be done. A human life had started to form outside a woman's womb.

Edwards didn't announce his discovery, probably because he couldn't repeat it. Also, it was precisely such casual creation of human life that worried critics of in vitro fertilization.

LESLEY BROWN'S BABY

An egg was removed by laparoscope from Lesley's ovaries after several attempts. Then John Brown's semen was introduced to her egg in a Petri dish containing the "magic culture fluid" of salt, potassium chloride, glucose, and a bit of protein. Examination by microscope revealed that a sperm had penetrated the ovum; the resulting embryo was cultured for two-and-a-half days. The embryo was then mixed with a supportive fluid, put in a syringe resembling a turkey baster, and squeezed through Lesley's dilated cervix into her uterus.

Many women before Lesley Brown had eggs successfully fertilized in vitro; fewer had eggs successfully implanted with a resulting pregnancy. Of those few who had become pregnant, each had lost her embryo after a few months.

In late 1977, Steptoe gave Lesley a Christmas present by telling her she was pregnant. Now the long wait began to see if she would lose her fetus like the others. Months passed and amniocentesis at five months showed a normal pregnancy.

Later, Lesley developed minor problems during pregnancy (the baby was slightly small) and Lesley had a mild case of toxemia (a metabolic disturbance caused by absorption of bacteria at the laparoscopy site). Her last month of pregnancy was spent at Oldham Hospital, which was then under a siege by the media.

Because of the need for secrecy, Lesley's cesarean operation occurred at night. Only a few people were present. A BBC film team in Oldham was still negotiating with the hospital when Steptoe announced that the birth would occur in minutes. By this time, Lesley had begun to realize how special her child was going to be. She left her room in darkness, nurses holding flashlights as she walked. "Dozens of policemen and security officers lined every corridor as I walked along. It felt as if I was moving in a dream."[10]

Lesley delivered on July 25, 1978, slightly before midnight. After amniocentesis, Steptoe had known the baby was female, but the Browns had chosen not to know. The Browns called their baby Louise Joy Brown. She weighed 5 pounds 12 ounces and was entirely normal, described as "beautiful, with a marvelous complexion, not red and wrinkly at all."[11]

The next day, London's newspapers broke the story, running huge banner headlines such as: "IT'S A GIRL!," "THE LOVELY LOUISE!" "BABY OF THE CENTURY!" and "JOY TO THE WORLD!" Even the staid *New York Times* gave the story frontpage coverage for three days. Immediately after the birth, John Brown said, "For a person who's been told he and his wife can never have children, the pregnancy was 'like a miracle.' I felt 12 feet high."[12]

ETHICAL ISSUES

Media Ethics

From the beginning, the press equated any new means of overcoming infertility with "genetic manipulation" and worried about creation of mindless slaves and supermen. In *Who Shall Play God?* in 1977, Jeremy Rifkin had already begun a decade of profitable opposition to all new reproductive techniques, lumping them all together under the rubric of "genetic engineering," which he defined as the "artificial manipulation of life."[13] (In contrast, John Brown saw in vitro fertilization merely as "helping Nature along a bit.") Rifkin was not alone, and the chief editor at the London *Times* equated in vitro fertilization with state-controlled eugenics.

Aldous Huxley's *Brave New World* was constantly cited. Using biological examples, Huxley in 1932 had worried about governmental control of individuals. Ironically, *Brave New World* was cited to justify the kind of result which it decried, namely, a world where couples lacked reproductive choice. Countless articles and television reports appeared about "genetic manipulation." None appeared about media manipulation of scientific discoveries to puffed-up "Andromeda Strain" stories.

The story of the behavior of the media during the last months of Lesley's pregnancy is interesting. Months into Lesley Brown's pregnancy, word had leaked out that a "test tube" baby was being born in Oldham. When someone at the hospital let it out that the birth was imminent, six reporters for America's *National Enquirer* left Florida and within 24 hours were at Oldham Hospital trying to buy worldwide rights. A bidding war started among similar English tabloids. Everybody wanted the name of the couple and their background, but Steptoe cloaked them with anonymity, both not wanting to upset Lesley and wanting to get the Browns a trust fund for their baby (reported to have been $600,000 for their exclusive story).

Despite the enormous interest, Steptoe and Edwards refused to be interviewed by reporters. (Edwards felt he had been harmed by British television, which discussed his work in a documentary that opened with pictures of an exploding atomic bomb.) This silence of Steptoe and Edwards frustrated reporters, who took certain liberties. *Newsweek* said: "Steptoe, 65, is a flamboyant and somewhat mysterious figure; he declines to discuss his origins (reported to be in Eastern Europe)."[14] Actually, Steptoe was born in Witney (near staid Oxford), educated in London at King's College and St. George's Medical School, and lived the life of an overworked obstetrician at a county hospital in an industrial English city. The "flamboyant" physician was married and had two children.

Other sensationalistic stories in the media were not entirely harmless. Edwards in previous years had worked on infertility at the National Institute for Medical Research in London by experimenting with surgically excised ovaries, which he bathed in hormones in attempts to get them to release eggs. After the alarmist television show, the Institute suspended his funding to avoid controversy. Edwards claims his scientific supervisor, who had herself frozen sperm, flatly told him his work was "unethical."[15] When asked "Why?" he claims she would only say, "Because it is." Edwards then departed for Cambridge University, where he worked thereafter, partially because of a Ford Foundation grant to study population control and fertility. In 1974, the Foundation ceased funding Edwards' work—officially because his work didn't promote population control—but also because his work offended some people.

Lack of interviews with Edwards and Steptoe prompted some reporters to guess at facts. *Newsweek* wrote: "[Edwards commuted] often in the company of a rabbit that was serving as traveling receptacle for an egg under study."[16] But Edwards himself writes:

> We transferred some fertilized human eggs into rabbits to see if they would grow there, but they didn't. This brief episode with rabbits led to all sorts or rumours in the press and elsewhere, and to a description of me taking hundreds of embryos to Cambridge, and of Patrick driving his Mercedes through Oldham with a rabbit in the seat next to him![17]

That the story would be big in England was without question. Daily headlines heralded rumors ("TEST-TUBE BABY ALMOST DIES"). Mrs. Brown was urged not to watch television or read newspapers, and because of telescopic lenses, she could not go near the windows.

As the birth approached, the integrity of some journalists vanished. One American reporter distinguished himself by telephoning a fake bomb threat to the hospital, hoping it would force Lesley outside. In the panicked evacuation, one pregnant woman went into labor. Undoubtedly, the reporter's paper at some time during the same year carried an editorial denouncing terrorism.

Another reporter disguised himself as a priest and approached John Brown, offering to comfort Lesley if he could be admitted. Throngs of Japanese photographers constantly photographed all women leaving Oldham Hospital on the off chance that one might be Lesley Brown. The *National Enquirer* made a $100,000 bribe to an administrator for details about the birth.

The press incorrectly called Lesley's baby a "test tube baby," implying that it had been created without human egg or sperm. This led many people to think that something bizarre had occurred. When Lesley Brown later took her baby outside, neighbors looked inside the carriage and expected to see something abnormal. Such was the media-driven impression of in vitro fertilization.

Condemnation of IVF

Louise Brown's birth was not greeted with jubilation by all medical researchers. Criticism took two, contradictory fronts: either the work was dangerous or the work was trivial. Nobel prize winner James Watson predicted that dangerous events would follow the birth of Baby Louise.[18] On the other hand, one fertility program's director characterized Steptoe's achievement as merely "a cookbook thing." A slightly different line said either IVF was impossible to accomplish (and hence, had not really occurred), or it was mundane (the birth being a "cheap stunt").

There was some sour grapes here because institutions with enormous research budgets had been surpassed by a self-described "county doc" in a small English city hospital with abysmal research conditions (one critic said Steptoe worked in a "cottage industry"). Others such as Richard Blandau, a famous fertility researcher, said Steptoe "had violated medical ethics by selling his story to the *National Enquirer*, instead of publishing his story in a medical journal" (actually, the Browns sold their story, not Steptoe), and had "given false hope to millions of women" by not revealing how many failures occurred before Louise Brown (which was true, but the point was that IVF could be done, not how probable it was).[19]

Given past claims, Blandau's skepticism was understandable. In the 1940s, physician John Rock had claimed successful IVF but had been unable to prove it. In the 1950s Italian researcher Petrucci claimed to have fertilized a human egg in vitro, grown it for 29 days, and destroyed it because it was growing "monstrous."[20] Although Petrucci's story fueled later "monster" worries, he never provided any evidence for his claim .

Unless Steptoe could prove Lesley's Fallopian tubes were irreparably damage, all too many critics were ready to say an egg could have "sneaked down" her Fallopian tubes and been fertilized. This readiness explains why Steptoe performed a cesarean operation on Lesley and filmed her damaged tubes, proving that no egg of hers could have been inadvertently fertilized.

Is IVF Intrinsically Wrong?

The Vatican condemned in vitro fertilization in 1978 after Louise Brown's birth. A New York priest feared mankind had slipped from "doctoring the patient to doctoring the race." After nine years of study, the Vatican in 1987 issued its Instructions reiterating its 1978 condemnation, equating IVF with "domination" and "manipulation of nature."[21] One bishop said: "The Christian morality has insisted on the importance of protecting the process by which human life is transmitted. The fact that science now has the ability to alter this process significantly does not mean that, morally speaking, it has the right to do so."[22]

Some people feel that infertility is God's punishment for the past sins. Abortion and sexually-associated diseases contribute to infertility. From these facts, some people (including those affected) conclude that the infertile are being punished for earlier behavior. In contrast, science sees infertile as due to problems of mechanics (blocked tubes) and chemistry (hormones).

The official, modern Vatican view is that intercourse between husband and wife is necessary for moral conception. Because IVF lacks coitus, it is condemned. Many Catholics and Christians reject this condemnation. They see nothing immoral with helping infertile couples have the children they want.

Ironically, such free-thinking Christians may be more in agreement with historical Church doctrine than is the modern Vatican. Christian theology for fifteen hundred years accepted the views of 4th-century Augustine, who taught that intercourse (and the desire for it) was evil. Marriage for Augustine was the only place where such desires could permissibly take place and even then, only to have children. Because of Augustine, Christianity held that original sin expressed itself in the desire for, and act of, coitus and was thereby transferred to a new generation.

So Augustine might have welcomed IVF. A man might sin only once in his life by masturbation, collect his sperm, freeze it, and have his wife artificially inseminated for each child desired. The marriage need never be consummated. The woman could remain virginal. Every birth to the couple could be a conception without sexual intercourse.

In modern times, theologian Joseph Fletcher defends IVF as permissible for Christians. Fletcher, who was cited previously for his views on euthanasia, favors any way of helping infertile couples have children:

> It is depressing, not comforting, to realize that most people are accidents. Their conception was at best unintended, at worst unwanted. There are those who are so bemused and befuddled by fatalist mystique about nature with a capital N (or "God's will") that they want us to accept passively whatever comes along. Talk of "not tinkering" and "not playing God" and snide remarks to "artificial" and "technological" policies is a vote against both humanness and humaneness.[23]

For Fletcher, each kind of case should be considered on its own merits to see if it helps or hurts humanity, and society must not be locked into antiquated, religious prohibitions which take no account of consequences to people. Religion is best when it is pro-people, not when it worships abstract "Thou Shall Not's:"

> The real choice is between accidental or random reproduction and rationally willed or chosen reproduction...laboratory reproduction is radically human compared to conception by ordinary heterosexual intercourse. It is willed, chosen, purposed and controlled, and surely

> those are among the traits that distinguish Homo sapiens from others in
> the animal genus, from the primates down.[24]

The difference between Fletcher (and most Christians) and the Vatican illustrates the difficulty of saying that any one view is "the" Christian position on any issue in medical ethics. When Lesley Brown was several months pregnant, Robert Edwards attended a special symposium at Washington's Kennedy Institute for Bioethics at the insistence of Sargent Shriver. The symposium on the ethics of IVF was attended by senators, national columnists, and scientists. As Edwards later described it, conservative theologian Paul Ramsey there severely criticized Edwards' IVF work.

> He had to be seen and heard to be believed. I had to endure a
> denunciation of our work as if from some nineteenth-century pulpit.
> It was delivered with a Gale 8 force, and written in a similar vein a
> year later in the *Journal of the American Medical Association.* He
> doubted that our patients had their fully understanding consent. We
> ignored the sanctity of life. We carried out immoral experiments on
> the unborn. Our work was, he thundered, "unethical medical
> experimentation on possible future human beings and therefore it is
> subject to absolute moral prohibition." I was as much surprised as
> made wrathful by this impertinent scorching attack. He abused
> everything I stood for.[25]

Ramsey, a conservative theologian at Yale, was an eloquent critic of IVF. He equated it with genetic manipulation and he believed it was wrong not because of consequences to the child, to parents, or even to society. He assumed that the zygote was a person from conception. He then argued that it would be wrong in itself because it was "unconsented to experimentation" on the zygote.[26] Because the zygote could never consent, and because experimentation without consent was immoral, such zygotic experimentation was immoral.

"Irrational Desires"

When the Browns heard of Steptoe's infertility work, they were willing to try experimental procedures. Like many infertile couples, pregnancy for them became an obsession. Although advised by their obstetrician in Bristol that IVF had little chance of success and that the costs would be great, the Browns plunged ahead. They were ready to sell their house, spend their savings, and move while John took a leave of absence from work.

In other cases, women have spent months lying virtually motionless in order to maximize chances of carrying an IVF fetus to term. Other couples live in poverty for years to finance IVF attempts.

Some people criticize such intense desires. Such criticisms are of two kinds: criticisms of personal ethics which are seen as irrational, sexist, or pathological, and criticisms of a public policy which encourages people to act on such desires. The latter judgment obviously depends on the first.

Philosopher Michael Bayles argues that people wanting their own genetic children have "irrational desires." He thinks they confuse the pleasures of begetting, bearing, and raising children. Because these three activities have always gone together, they are strongly associated. While the pleasures of creating children may be great, Bayles says, they could be had by donating sperm or ova to the infertile. The pleasures of raising children can be had through adoption, and women can experience the pleasures of bearing children as surrogate mothers. The desirable experiences intrinsic to begetting are "minimal:"

> Moreover, if the genetic relation were important, it would imply that adoptive parents cannot have as valuable experiences of child rearing as natural parents, which seems false. In short, due to cultural conditioning, most people think that rearing their genetic offspring is better than rearing children who are not genetically theirs, but any difference seems to stem solely from this belief.[27]

Sociologists emphasize that these matters deeply affect the lives of many women and children. They know that many men want their "own" babies and refuse to consider marrying a woman who has had children by another man. This is one reason, among many others, why so many women today are heads of households and raise their children alone. In the definition of parenthood, most sociologists emphasize the role of parenting more than the biological relation, and they often argue that if people thought of parenting more as raising a child, rather than as creating one, society would be better off.

This issue arises also with "blended families," which are composed when two divorced parents remarry and each brings children to create an entirely new family. Success in such families hinges on each parent's not feeling that certain children are his or her "real" children and others are not.

Bayles' position is most important in public policy. If desiring genetic offspring under certain circumstances is irrational, public policy should not encourage it. Many people believe that smoking is irrational and that public policy should discourage it, e.g., by heavily taxing tobacco and by restricting its use in public places. Similarly, if desiring one's own children is irrational, IVF should not be subsidized by federal or private medical insurance. If people want to act irrationally and finance such actions from personal funds, fine, but they should not ask others to help pay, just as nonsmokers are not required by law to subsidize the costs of cigarettes.

Critics of IVF also argue that any public policy which encourages IVF will harm orphans who would otherwise be adopted. Edwards and Steptoe were criticized for encouraging births in an overpopulated world. (China and India subsequently developed successful IVF programs.) The intimation here is that all orphans should be adopted before in vitro fertilization is subsidized. A more intrusive policy would simply forbid all IVF until all adoptable babies are taken.

The first problem with such a policy is that there are not enough adoptable babies for all infertile couples. The second problem is that there are not enough of the *right kind* of adoptable babies. Many babies of color and hand-icapped babies are rarely adopted. If the infertile want a baby so much, shouldn't they take one of these? Isn't IVF encouraging people to be racist and discouraging adoption of the physically and mentally disabled?

In reply, it may be observed that some couples will only change their expectations for their own child, not an adopted child. Is that irrational? It's not if parents who have their own kids have better experiences than those who adopt. But is that true? Defenders of IVF say, "It just wouldn't be plea-surable for *us* to raise an adopted child, but it might for others." To which Bayles would reply, "That's irrational."

Bayles thinks that most people are mistaken about the pleasures of child-raising. Take away the expectation that raising adopted kids is only a second-rate experience, and the pleasures of two sets of kids would be much the same. If two babies were switched in nurseries, the parents would treat the other child just the same. A great deal of the unique pleasures of a parent's raising his own kids may simply be the *belief* that the parent is the progenitor. The actual difference in pleasures—deriving from appreciating similarities of looks, personality, bodily build, and intelligence—might be very small.

Finally, isn't it unfair to single out infertile couples? Why not require all couples to adopt unwanted children? If adoption is to be encouraged, why not give everyone large tax credits for adopting unwanted children? More funda-mentally, shouldn't some areas of personal life be immune from moral criticism? Must the personal always be political? Decisions about whether to have children, about how many, about adoption, and about acceptable risks in having children are among the most intimate a couple makes. If government has a right to in-terfere with procreative decisions of infertile couples, doesn't it also have the right to tell any other couple when not to conceive or even when to abort?

Harm to Baby Louise

Many critics predicted that the first baby fertilized in vitro might be harmed or be defective. Obstetrician John Marlow emphasized that seriously defective babies could be created, and that "the potential is there for serious anomalies should an unqualified scientist mishandle an embryo."[28] Obstetrician John Marshall of Los Angeles similarly said, "What if we got…a cyclops? Who is responsible? The parents? Is the government obligated to take care of it?"[29] Biochemist and physician Leon Kass argued strenuously that babies created by artificial fertilization might be deformed. "It doesn't matter how many times the baby is tested while in the mother's womb," he averred, "they will never be certain the baby won't be born without defect."[30] Nobel prize winner James Watson feared that deformed babies would be born, who then would either be subject to infanticide or raised by the State in custodial homes.[31]

Edwards' colleague and Nobel prize winner, Max Perutz, said: "I agree entirely with Dr. Watson that this is far too great a risk. Even if only a single abnormal baby is born and has to be kept alive as an invalid for the rest of its life, Dr. Edwards would have a terrible guilt upon his shoulders. The idea that this might happen on a larger scale—a new thalidomide catastrophe—is horrifying."[32]

Author Jeremy Rifkin revved up the baby-might-be-a-monster fear. "What are the psychological implications of growing up as a specimen, sheltered not by a warm womb but by steel and glass, belonging to no one but the lab technician who joined together sperm and egg? In a world already populated with people with identity crises, what's the personal identity of a test-tube baby?"[33]

Daniel Callahan of the Hastings Institute (a medical ethics research institute) argued that the first case was "probably unethical" because Baby Louise couldn't be guaranteed to be normal, but thought it was ethical to proceed after her healthy birth.[34] He added that many medical breakthroughs are "unethical," because we cannot know that the first patient will not be harmed (e.g., medicine helped Baby Louise but not Baby Fae—see Chapter 12).

Many of these critics missed a sense that no reasonable approach to life can avoid all risks. Moreover, there is a psychological but illogical tendency to magnify the evil of an unlikely bad event. Even if the harm is very bad, a very small risk of a very bad result is still a very small risk.[35] An anencephalic baby is a very bad result, but the risk of such a baby doesn't prevent people from having kids. Moreover, a significant part of differences in ethics concerns attitudes to risk. In this case, all the consequences are borne by the infertile parents. Unless a baby fertilized in vitro would be in such horrible pain that it would be better if she had never existed at all, then her life is not worse than not existing. Thus, if prospective parents know that babies conceived in vitro might be defective, and if, for defective babies, their life is better than no life, who is harmed by allowing parents to conceive this way?

Harm to Possible People and the Paradox of Existence

A philosophically interesting question is whether *possible* children can be harmed by IVF conception. Theologian Hans Tiefel writes, "No one has the moral right to endanger a child while there is yet the option of whether the child shall come into existence."[36] Tiefel assumes IVF subjects a baby to risks beyond those of normal conception.

In comparison, suppose a woman intentionally runs a greater risk in conceiving her baby and it turns out defective. Suppose a mother smokes and drinks during pregnancy, resulting in a retarded boy. When confronted with her behavior, she replies, "If I had to give up smoking and drinking during pregnancy, I would have aborted him. So he can't complain. If it wasn't for my smoking and drinking, he wouldn't exist. And existing retarded is better than not existing at all." (Similar cases involving drug-dependent mothers are discussed at the end of Chapter 6.)

This dilemma will be called the Paradox of Existence. It refers to the paradox that it never seems worse to live with "low quality of life" than not to exist at all. The paradox emerges when we feel that the fetus born to the smoking-drinking mother was harmed. How is it possible to harm a fetus which might not have been born? That is the Paradox of Existence.

There are many approaches to solving this problem. One way is to distinguish between different meanings of "harm."[37] Like the concept of good (or goods), the concept of harm has a variety of meanings and covers a range of behaviors. Most abstractly, two ways of thinking about harm can be distinguished. In the first, both a baseline and a temporal component are necessary, such that a change occurs which makes a being worse off. In this "baseline" concept, harm requires an *adverse change* in a being's condition. In this concept, if a being doesn't yet exist, it can't be harmed, because it has no baseline from which it can change.

In the second concept, harm to a being compares a present condition to what the being otherwise would have been. In this "maximal potential" concept, a being can be harmed by being brought into existence if—in doing so—it is less fulfilled than it could have been. (Consider the old Yiddish joke: first speaker—"Life is so terrible! Better to have never existed." Second speaker—"True, but only one in a thousand is so lucky.") In this "maximal potential" concept, the event which causes the difference is usually identified as the cause of harm, e.g., in the above joke where life itself is considered a harm, birth is the event.

According to the baseline concept of harm, a being cannot be harmed by being created by IVF, because otherwise it would not have existed. According to the maximal-potential concept of harm, once a being exists as an embryo or fetus, it can be harmed by a mother's smoking.

The second concept of harm underlines the belief that the mothers should do everything possible to have the best babies. Anything less than maximal effort is blameworthy because a fetus is harmed. Such a "maximal potential" concept of harm implies a "maximal mothering" obligation, i.e., implies that it's wrong for a mother to take risks with a future person's intelligence or health because doing so may harm him or her.

Harm to Infertile Parents

Critics also argued that attempts at IVF could harm infertile parents. In the early days, critics say Steptoe's chances of helping an infertile woman conceive were only one in a hundred. Tiefel argues:

> Even if the meager success rate is explained to couples and they
> consent to the odds, there are moral limits to surgical risk, time,
> resources, and stress on human relationships. The fact that prospective
> parents say that they will do anything to have a baby of their own is
> not necessarily a moral justification.

These statements only make sense if "moral" implies some standard beyond possible harm to actual and possible humans. Tiefel argues that physicians cannot simply accede to parents' desires for children because,

> This is ethical relativism, where individual choice or preference settles
> moral issues. Medicine should avoid such quicksand, for shifting
> individual preferences offer no solid support for the objective values
> undergirding medicine and research. If one lets go of objective and
> universal values to defer to dubious patient choice, one also relinquishes
> the heart of medicine, whose life is the objective value of healing and
> doing no harm.

Some physicians share Tiefel's views that the correct relationship between people and medicine is not that medicine exists to help people implement choices about disease, but that medicine exists to heal people, regardless of what they choose. For Tiefel, what people choose is "ethical relativism," whereas healing is an "objective and universal value" crucial to the "heart of medicine." This is a very important distinction and defines a most sharply drawn division among some physicians as to what medicine is for.

This is a good example of how abstract moral language must be carefully analyzed in concrete terms. Normally, people unthinkingly agree to Tiefel's statement that "healing" is an objective value of medicine. Yet notice that in this context, Tiefel uses healing to oppose helping to cure infertility. Couples who choose IVF to overcome infertility are guilty of "ethical relativism."

Returning to the problem of harm to prospective parents from IVF, there is a real issue here today. The success of Louise Brown unrealistically raised expectations among the infertile. The overall success rate (as of 1988) is less than 10 percent. One often hears of successes, rarely of the 90 percent of failures. Competition among the two hundred clinics, and lack of federal standards to measure success, has resulted in inflated statistics. Success is defined not by conceptions per number of applicants to a program, but only by conceptions per number of women whose eggs actually implant. According to a study by the Office of Technology Assessment, which severely criticized the lack of regulation of IVF programs, at least half of America's IVF clinics have never sent home a successful IVF pregnancy. Women over 40 are successful only 5 percent of the time. For even the best clinics, the rate of successful pregnancies brought to term is probably less than 10 percent. Clinics charge $4500 to $6500 per attempt, and some IVF clinics are close to perpetrating fraud on their desperate customers.

Harm to Society

US News & World Report conceptualized Louise Brown's birth as a "disturbing" and "ominous" event, showing how "science wields its growing power to decide who shall be born, how and to whom."[38] Its unstated assumption was that "science" would decide who is born, not infertile parents. The slippery slope metaphor was widely employed by critics such as James Watson, who concluded that an international effort was needed to "de-emphasize" research "which would circumvent normal sexual reproduction," and Leon Kass, for whom IVF was the first step toward the unthinkable:

> At least one good humanitarian reason can be found to justify each
> step. The first step serves as a precedent for the second and the second
> for the third, not just technologically but also in moral argument.
> Perhaps a wise society would say to infertile couples: "We understand
> your sorrow, but it might be better not to go ahead and do this."[39]

Paul Ramsey's *Fabricated Man* (1970) implied that if physicians could find a tiny egg and fertilize it, why couldn't they alter its genes?[40] If they could, he predicted, they would. And if they would, it would be wrong. Ramsey was known for his literary eloquence and he came up with some memorable phrases, each implying vague, disturbing harm to society, such as "test tube babies," "dial-a-baby," and "playing God." Ramsey was especially good at generating neologisms for rhetorical effect, such as "mercenary gestation," a "supermarket of embryos," a "spare-parts man" (from a cloned twin kept unconscious and grown for such purposes), "celebrity seed" (sperm banks), and "human species suicide" (eliminating genetic diseases).

Both Ramsey and Watson severely attacked cloning ("carbon copy people"). Of course, in vitro fertilization had nothing to do with cloning. In vitro fertilization is *sexual* reproduction, cloning is *asexual* reproduction. In vitro fertilization matches two different sets of 23 chromosomes to create a unique individual with 46; cloning reproduces the 46 chromosomes of the donor. Nobel Prize winner James Watson warned of the dangers of cloning and foresaw scenarios from *The Boys from Brazil* with secret projects creating teams of identical assassins.

Another kind of criticism of IVF predicts global harm to women in society. Philosopher Mary Ann Warren suspects in 1988 that many NRTs (New Reproductive Technologies) are really devices of men to control women.[41] Although she would not ban NRTs (and prohibit other women from using them), she argues that, "every government body with responsibility for the regulation of the NRTs, every ethical oversight committee, and every public agency which funds reproductive research [should] be at least 50 percent composed of women." Moreover, she emphasizes "what may be the most important feminist objection to IVF," namely, the lack of attention to the "social causes" of female infertility. She says we must look to the macroscopic level, not just at individual, infertile females. Since PID (pelvic inflammatory disease) causes such infertility and is associated with "hormone-based contraceptives," she supports use of condoms to decrease PID. Moreover, "Heterosexual intercourse is much more likely to transmit infection than either oral sex or masturbation (mutual or solitary)." She asserts that such "normal" sexual practice is not the "inalterable result of human biology" but merely a "social institution." Therefore, heterosexual sex (especially without condoms) "must be included among the social causes of infertility." Rather than focus on NRT's, she argues that society should focus on preventing infertility in the first place.

Informed Consent

Some wonder whether Lesley gave informed consent to being the mother of the first baby fertilized in vitro. England at the time, unlike America, had no law covering informed consent. Still, many people felt the procedure could only be ethical if Lesley understood the risks and consented. Lesley understood she was merely to have an "implant." Steptoe says he explained IVF thoroughly to both Browns. In retrospect, it seems clear that Lesley didn't really understand what was to happen.

Some feminists say women desperate to have children will consent to anything and cannot really dissent. For Lesley Brown and other infertile women, consent does not seem to have been an ethical issue. Physician Kay Honea, a leader in infertility work, says only cancer patients are more willing than the infertile to try anything to overcome their problem.[42] This indicates that the problem here is not consent but "irrational desires."

IVF and Distributive Justice

Distributive justice concerns how society allocates burdens (such as taxes) and benefits (such as heart transplants). IVF is a benefit to the many infertile people who want children. In America, most insurance plans cover no IVF expenses, although most cover related costs such as sonograms.

Given costs of $4500 to $6500 per attempt, infertile couples argue that others should subsidize IVF. Bills in Texas and Virginia directed insurance companies to "consider" such coverage. Three such arguments have been advanced. First, infertile couples claim a human right to procreate. Such a right entails an obligation on others at least not to interfere with couples attempting to procreate (e.g., involuntary sterilization) and possibly a positive obligation to assist with the costs—especially if such costs can be spread over many people at very little cost to each.

Second, infertility is claimed to be an incapacitating "disease." Defined broadly, "health" isn't just the absence of disease but maximal functioning. As such, infertility treatments aren't merely cosmetic but are like other medical treatments for dysfunction. So defined, a woman isn't "healthy" unless she can conceive. Circumventing damaged Fallopian tubes, it is argued, is no more cosmetic than using physical therapy to circumvent limbs damaged by stroke. Furthermore, insurance often pays for very expensive microsurgery to repair Fallopian tubes—surgery which only works in a small percentage of cases. Whatever justifies such surgery also justifies (the much less expensive procedures of) IVF.

Third, not subsidizing costs makes IVF only the prerogative of the affluent. If having one's own children is a fundamental good—and many people think it is—then such a fundamental good should be widely available. Philosopher John Rawls' theory of justice argues that a just society minimizes the "natural inequalities of fate" and helps redress them by using public funds to help the unfortunate.[43] Unjust societies allow such natural inequalities to be magnified. If infertility is one such "natural inequality," then a just society will aid the infertile.

Restricting IVF by Marital Status and Sexual Preference

An additional issue in considering public finance of IVF is how many people might benefit from IVF. Australian philosopher Peter Singer argues that IVF should not be restricted in any way.[44] To the argument that new reproductive help should only be available to married couples (which entails only hetero-sexuals because homosexuals cannot legally marry), he retorts that this would be the only kind of medical treatment in which being married is required. Assuming that only heterosexuals are good parents begs the question against homosexuals; empirical evidence is needed to prove such a claim. Even if some such claim could be empirically supported, it wouldn't prove that any particular couple was incompetent. Finally, Singer argues that no restrictions are now placed on unmarried, fertile heterosexual couples, who may use medical help to conceive. Gay males are not prevented from becoming sperm donors or lesbians from becoming mothers (through artificial insemination), so "it would be unjust if a particular self-defining group" was denied access to any treatment available to others.

Against this position, one could argue first, that there is a big difference between "forbidding" a couple from obtaining a benefit (owning a house, going to college, having a baby) and providing that benefit. America presently allows legal abortions, but federal funds do not pay for abortions for indigent women. Similarly, the government could permit people to purchase IVF, but not fund IVF for the indigent.

IVF is an expensive new technique, potentially usable by millions. If medical insurance paid for this procedure, it would be insurance not against a medical tragedy but against a personal tragedy in the lives of people who highly value having children. Medical costs are very high in America, and a large reason for this cost is that when everyone pays for medical care, no one is motivated to forgo treatment. Thus, IVF might not be subsidized in a society which only gave people equal opportunities, not equal outcomes.

Finally, although infertility is more distressing than a passing flu, it isn't like diseases such as lupus, cancer, cystic fibrosis, or congenital arthritis, i.e., infertile people can still work and flourish. Perhaps the question of whether society should subsidize IVF depends on whether or not a particular society is having problems with overpopulation or underpopulation. France currently highly subsidizes native Frenchwomen having babies, but such a policy would be insane in an overpopulated society.

Ethical Status of Human Pre-Embryos Fertilized In Vitro

Giving extra hormones stimulates extra egg production during a monthly cycle (superovulation) and allows fertilization of more than one egg. To maximize chances of one pre-embryo implanting, three pre-embryos are implanted. (More than three further increases the chances of conception but also increases the chances of twins—a risk many of the infertile take, as witnessed by the dramatic recent increase in twins). After laparoscopy, a half-dozen eggs are often fertilized, with three implanted and the rest frozen for future attempts.

What is the ethical status of such pre-embryos? In 1981, a famous case dramatized this issue.[45] Mario and Elsa Rios, an American couple worth millions, traveled to Melbourne, Australia, where several eggs of Elsa's were fertilized in vitro with sperm from an anonymous male. Three pre-embryos were produced from Elsa's eggs. One was implanted in Elsa. The other two were frozen for future implantation in case the first attempt failed, which occurred ten days later. Unwilling to immediately make a second attempt, the Rios returned to the United States and then to South America. In the spring of 1983, they were killed in a plane crash. The case made headlines when the world learned that their frozen pre-embryos still existed in doubtful legal status. Neither the Rios nor the infertility clinic had provided for this contingency.

Several ethical questions arose. Could the pre-embryos simply be destroyed? If they were implanted in surrogate mothers, could they later sue for inheritances in American courts? Should the anonymous sperm donor be contacted to ask his wishes?

Writing on this issue, David Ozar points out that although pre-embryos may not be persons, they are neither just rocks.[46] After all, given the right support, each has the potential to develop into a full person. Each at least deserves "respect" (i.e., it should not be eaten). Ozar assumes that a pre-embryo is more than the property of owners, that it is both unique and potentially a person. Ozar points out that the Supreme Court's *Roe vs. Wade* decision cited a "compelling" interest in protecting potential personhood at *viability* (see Chapter 6), and points out that in its subsequent decision in *Danforth*, it defined viability as "that stage of fetal development when the life of the unborn child may be continued indefinitely outside of the womb by natural or artificial life-support systems." Ergo, frozen zygotes are technically viable under an idiosyncratic view of Supreme Court decisions.

In the Rios case, the Waller Committee was convened and recommended destruction of the pre-embryos. It concluded that removal of life support for the pre-embryos was like removing life support from terminal patients. The Australian Parliament took a different course and required preservation of the pre-embryos until some couple "adopted" each one.

Peter Singer argued that the destruction of pre-embryos in a case like the Rios is no different than the destruction of an individual egg or individual sperm.[47] Suppose a sperm and an egg are on two sides of an IVF slide. Case 1: just before joining of sperm and egg, the IVF couple changed their minds; hence, the contents of both slides are washed down the drain. Case 2: same as case 1, but one minute after joining. Case 3: same as case 1, but technicians discover blockage in the drain, such that sperm and egg may have united; if not retrieved immediately, the pre-embryo dies of exposure. Singer argues that the three cases do not morally differ and that none of the pre-embryos has a right to exist.

Is a Human Embryo a Person?

Some people believe personhood begins at the instant of conception. They believe that interuterine devices (IUDs) kill persons because they prevent implantation of zygotes or pre-embryos. Similarly, they believe it is murder to do a D and C (dilation and curettage) to terminate pregnancy—a procedure which involves dilation of the cervix and scraping of the uterine lining to dislodge an implanted pre-embryo (also called a fertilized ovum).

A 1988 medical study discovered that about one-third of fertilized ova fail to implant and are naturally aborted. Roman Catholic physician M. V. Viola wrote in 1968, "A significant number of fertilized ova (some estimate one in three) never implant in the uterus under normal conditions. If in fact these are lost souls, the Church should be consistent and make efforts to administer baptism to them."[48]

Opponents say a human pre-embryo has neither intelligence, consciousness, nor human form. Such a pre-embryo, they say, is not a person, only a *potential* person. An acorn is not an oak tree. If someone without permission cuts down his neighbor's large oak tree, the owner can sue for substantial damages, but not for destruction of an acorn.

Suppose someone says, fine, a pre-embryo is only a potential person, but the woman still has an obligation to gestate such a potential person. To many people, this is a reductio ad absurdum argument (an argument which shows that a logical implication of an idea is absurd, casting doubt upon the idea itself). A woman who starts giving birth before her teens and continues regularly may easily produce a dozen or more children. We here have what Derek Parfit calls the "Repugnant Conclusion:" if each newly created person is valuable, then we ought to create the greatest total of persons and continue doing so as long as each new person adds slightly to the total happiness.[49] Given overpopulation, does this make sense?

The personhood-begins-at-conception argument usually occurs in arguments against abortion. But pre-embryo freezing nicely separates the issue of pre-embryonic personhood from the emotional issue of abortion. Such separation illustrates the philosophical difficulty of claiming that a frozen pre-embryo has a "right to life" when this right is not claimed *against* anyone. No particular woman has a duty to have these pre-embryos implanted and to raise the resulting children.

EMBRYONIC RESEARCH

In 1974, Congress created an Ethics Advisory Board (EAB) to advise it on experimentation with human pre-embryos fertilized in vitro. Like a similar committee in England, the EAB recommended limited experimentation on such pre-embryos. However, EAB's recommendation was never accepted by the Secretary of Health Education and Welfare (then Joseph Califano) and no congressman since has been willing to champion the issue.

In 1979, obstetricians Howard and Georgeanna Jones established America's first IVF clinic at Eastern Virginia Medical School (EVMS). In October 1979, opponents of IVF jammed into the Norfolk Public Health Department auditorium for a debate on the intended IVF program at EVMS and charged that the IVF program would inevitably lead to destruction of "tiny human beings" and "mass production of artificially designed humans."[50] Although the program went forward because EVMS is private and is not subject to federal rules, the fury generated by opponents resulted in a de facto continuation of the ban on experimentation with human pre-embryos.

Australia took a different, more tolerant, approach to such experimentation, an approach which allowed it to leap ahead of other countries in fertility research. (IVF Australia is now franchised across America, with clinics from New York to Birmingham.) In 1980, an Australian team led by Carl Woods first duplicated IVF and soon achieved better fertilization rates. Ironically, a dispute about medical ethics arose when Steptoe and Edwards criticized Woods' team in *Nature* for selecting a 42-year-old woman as their first IVF candidate.[51] Woods replied that it was up to the 42-year-old woman to determine acceptable risks of a defective baby, not the physician. The baby was born without defects.

In 1983, Woods' team surpassed Steptoe and Edwards by achieving the first birth from a donated ovum. After the publicity about Baby Louise, the new mother wished to be anonymous. The egg was one of five donated by a 29-year-old woman attempting IVF because of blocked tubes.

UPDATE

By 1988, at least three thousand babies had been conceived in vitro worldwide—three thousand wanted children who would otherwise not have existed and who were born to thousands of couples who would otherwise be childless. A thousand of these were born in America. Over two hundred IVF clinics operated in the United States, from those run by universities to commercial clinics like IVF Australia. While the odds of successful in vitro fertilization were very low in 1978, by 1988 they had risen to an overall rate of between 5 percent and 10 percent.

As mentioned previously, not everything was rosy. Many IVF clinics give out misleading information. One unscrupulous physician gave HcG hormone to nonpregnant female clients, which caused their bodies to imitate the signs of pregnancy, and later told them that they had "miscarried." Some clinics charged as much as $7000 per attempt. A few couples went through this several times. One couple paid over $100,000.[52] As a whole, IVF clinics seemed to be a major industry whose own ethics and self-regulation were not protecting desperate couples from abuse.

James Watson, who had made alarmist predictions about IVF, cloning, and genetic manipulation, was named head of a project announced in 1988 to map the human genome. It would be a first step to any real effort to do genetic therapy. A decade after his alarmist views, the irony of his appointment was lost on most people.

Patrick Steptoe died at age 74, in 1988. His death came a few days before Robert Edwards was given one of the highest awards in the English scientific community, being made a Fellow of the Royal Society. Steptoe's death was but four months before Louise Brown's tenth birthday.

Louise Brown grew up in Whitchurch, a suburb of Bristol. She is blue-eyed, blonde-haired, healthy, and strong-willed. When she was five, she often dawdled on the way home from school at the candy stores. At ten, she often played outdoors too late. On June 14, 1982, her mother became the first woman to have two children fertilized in vitro, giving birth to daughter Natalie Jane. On July 25, 1988, Louise Brown celebrated her tenth birthday at a party with other kids. She is good at writing stories and poems. Her adoring father describes her as "friendly and full of life." He was worried that she might become a "spoilt brat," but now says that she is quite normal. On the event of her tenth birthday, Louise said, "I just like to play, and I like doing English."[53]

FURTHER READING

John & Lesley Brown, *Our Miracle Called Louise* (Paddington Press, 1979).

Patrick Steptoe & Robert Edwards, *A Matter of Life: The Story of a Medical Breakthrough* (William Morrow, 1980).

Joseph Fletcher, *Ethics of Genetic Control: Ending Reproductive Roulette* (Doubleday Anchor, 1984).

Hans Tiefel, "In Vitro Fertilization: A Conservative View," *Journal of the American Medical Association*, 247:23 (June 18, 1982).

Mary Anne Warren, "IVF and Women's Interests: An Analysis of Feminist Concerns," *Bioethics*, 2:1 (January 1988).

Peter Singer (with Deane Wells) "In Vitro Fertilisation: The Major Issues," *Journal of Medical Ethics*, 9 (1983), pp. 192–195; plus "Response" to "Comment" by G. D. Mitchell.

David Ozar, "The Case against Thawing Unused Frozen Embryos," *Hastings Center Report*, 15(4): 7-12, (August 1985).

CHAPTER 5

The Baby M Case

This chapter discusses ethical issues in the "Baby M" case involving Mary Beth Whitehead's "surrogate motherhood" for William Stern. Before the Baby M decision in 1988, no state supreme court had ruled on the legality of surrogate contracts. Surrogate means "substitute," so that a surrogate mother is a woman who bears a child for another.

"Surrogate mother" implies that the gestational woman is the real mother, not the woman who actually raises the child, and begs the question of the best definition of motherhood. The phrase will not be used again in this chapter, which instead will use the term "surrogate" alone, to refer to a woman who bears a child for someone else.

HISTORICAL BACKGROUND

The Old Testament says that Sarai (Sarah) bore her husband Abram (Abraham) no children and told Abram to "go unto" her handmaiden Hagar, so that "I may obtain children by her" (Genesis 16, 1–4). The child was named Ishmael, but this arrangement caused problems when Sarai became jealous of Hagar. Jacob's wife Rachel also used her maid Billah to create a son (Genesis 30, 1–5). Under Hebrew and Babylonian law, use of such surrogates was acceptable to create heirs.

Today various "third party" help is available to infertile couples. Artificial Insemination by Husband (AIH) has been used since 1790, but did not become popular until the 1960s. Artificial Insemination by Donor (AID) may be used, where the donor is a friend or is anonymous at a "sperm bank." In vitro fertilization (IVF) was discussed in the previous chapter.

Although frequently discussed as a "new reproductive technology" for infertility, surrogacy is really a new *social* arrangement, not a new technology. A woman today may partially beget a child by contributing an egg, bear a child of another woman's egg fertilized in vitro, or rear a child conceived by or borne by another woman. Hence, it is theoretically possible that a surrogate could bear an embryo of one couple for adoption by a second. This theoretical possibility illustrates just how complicated these social arrangements could be.

The only major study to date found that women become surrogates for mixed motives: for the money, to enjoy being pregnant again, and to atone for past acts.[1] The typical applicant has been a 25-year-old white woman with two children and a high school education. Of these, 20 percent were divorced, 25 percent had never married, and about half were Catholic and half were Protestant.

There were two odd cases of surrogacy in America before the Baby M case. In one, a Tennessee woman blackmailed the adoptive parents for more money and took illegal drugs during her pregnancy. In 1982, the 46-year-old accountant Alexander Malahoff signed a surrogate contract for $10,000 with Mrs. Judy Stiver, who bore him a son born lacking most of the brain. Malahoff asked for blood and tissue tests to prove his paternity.

Malahoff and the Stivers were guests on a live *Donahue Show,* where the result was revealed that, not Malahoff, but Judy's husband was the true father. As tense minutes ticked off, the Stivers huddled and Donahue nervously ad-libbed. Finally, Judy Stiver said that no one had told her not to have sex with her husband before the insemination. She then announced she would keep the baby. "I'm excited," she said as the show ended.

THE BABY M CASE

William and Elizabeth Stern were each 41 years old in March 1987 and each had a doctorate (he in biochemistry, she in genetics). William had lost most of his relatives in the Holocaust and wanted a child with half his genes. He earned around $43,500 a year. Elizabeth Stern had also completed medical school and was a beginning assistant professor of pediatrics earning $48,000 a year. As a pediatrician, she could later earn about $70,000 a year—less if she worked part-time, much more if she became a partner in a successful pediatric practice.

In 1972 and 1978, Elizabeth experienced numbness in her extremities, leg weakness, and optic neuritis, which in 1980 a neuro-ophthamologist said "probably" indicated multiple sclerosis (MS). Peer counselors with MS said pregnancy would exacerbate onset of symptoms, which could include blindness, deafness, incontinence, and paralysis. A friend of the Sterns with MS had become paralyzed after she bore a child, and this event convinced Elizabeth not to chance pregnancy.

Richard Whitehead for four years had worked as a sanitation worker, making $28,000 a year. During the previous thirteen years, he had worked at seven different jobs. He had served a year in Vietnam. Married twelve years to Mary Beth, he characterized himself as an alcoholic who could control his problem.

Mary Beth Whitehead dropped out of high school at age 16. She then worked in a pizza parlor, where she met Richard, a veteran just back from Vietnam and 8 years her senior. Six months later, she married him. The

Whiteheads had two children. When the trial began in January 1987, Richard was 37 years old, Mary Beth was 29, Ryan was 10, and Tuesday was 9.

Because of financial difficulties, the Whiteheads moved 12 times between their 1973 marriage and 1981, frequently living with other family members. In 1978, they separated, and Mrs. Whitehead received public assistance. During this time when she needed money, she worked for three months as a go-go dancer.

A year before Mrs. Whitehead first sought to be a surrogate, the Whiteheads had filed for bankruptcy. At the time, both mortgages on their home were in default. A few months later, Mrs. Whitehead answered an advertisement to be a surrogate for $10,000. Her family's financial difficulties made the money seem like the answer to their problems. Besides, she said, being pregnant wasn't bad and a child was "the most loving gift" a woman could give to another couple.

The Pregnancy

In 1984, Mary Beth Whitehead applied to the Surrogate Mother Program in New York, a surrogate agency with rigid screening procedures, which rejected her.[2] She then enrolled at the Infertility Center of New York (ICNY), an agency which only rejected applicants for reasons of health or age. Her husband Richard opposed her decision but ultimately went along.

In an interview, Mary Beth said she would have strong feelings against giving up the child but would do so. The interviewer noted that such feelings should be explored more before fertilization was attempted. They were not.

Over the next eight months, Mary Beth tried to become pregnant with a client at ICNY who was *not* William Stern. Before attempts at insemination were tried, Mary Beth and Richard were asked to go over the Surrogate Parenting Agreement for several hours with an independent lawyer. After this process, they made several minor changes.

The contract stipulated that Mrs. Whitehead would undergo both a psychiatric evaluation and a second-trimester amniocentesis. The contract also said she would abort if defects were found. The contract stated that if the baby was born handicapped, the adoptive parents would accept the child, and that Mrs. Whitehead would not "form or attempt to form a parent-child relationship" with the baby.

Surrogate agencies work in different ways. Infertility Associates International of Washington, D.C. forbade surrogates from meeting adoptive couples. At ICNY, everyone met frequently, and some couples observed births in delivery rooms.

In August 1984, William Stern entered into an agreement with ICNY. The Sterns chose Mary Beth Whitehead from several candidates because she looked like Elizabeth. In January of 1985, the Whiteheads and Sterns met to look each other over, fully 2 years before the case finally came to trial and 15 months before the baby's birth. In February, Mary Beth signed a contract with William Stern which was similar to the one she had formerly signed.

William Stern regularly drove from New Jersey to New York, where artificial insemination occurred nine times. Elizabeth Stern sometimes accompanied him. Sometime in August of 1985, Mary Beth Whitehead knew she was
pregnant. During the subsequent "honeymoon" period, everything went
smoothly with the four calling each other "Betsy," "Bill," "Rick," and "Mary
Beth." Mary Beth said that she would give up the child and only wanted an
annual picture and letter.

Six months later, relations between the couples turned sour as Mary Beth
began to think of the third-trimester baby as "her" child and as the Sterns
began to think of the baby as "their" child. Mary Beth refused to take a prescribed drug. The Sterns saw taking the drug as following good medical practice; Mary Beth saw it as risky to the baby (Mary Beth neither drank nor smoke
during the pregnancy from similar concerns and as stipulated in the contract).

Another conflict arose when Mary Beth's obstetrician, whom she had
selected at random from the Yellow Pages, recommended against amniocentesis (he felt it was an unnecessary expense for such a slight risk). Mr. Stern
insisted on amniocentesis in compliance with the contract. Mary Beth had the
procedure, but retaliated by not revealing the fetus' sex.

In the last months of the pregnancy, Mary Beth's blood pressure rose,
and the Sterns tried to get her to lower it by various means. Mary Beth claimed
they tried to take over her life.

During this time, Mary Beth and Richard began to talk to Ryan and
Tuesday about how they didn't want to "sell" their "sister." A month before
birth, Mary Beth delayed signing the paternity papers which would give the
baby to the Sterns, although she eventually did so.

The Birth

The baby (called "Baby M" by the trial court) was born on Thursday, March
27, 1986, in Monmouth Medical Center in Long Branch, New Jersey. The
Whiteheads concealed their surrogate agreement from the staff and acted as
if Baby M was a normal family birth. Richard Whitehead's name went on the
birth certificate as the father, and the baby was named Sara Elizabeth
Whitehead. Not knowing about William Stern's intended role, nurses did not
permit him to hold the baby.

Mary Beth testified that at birth she bonded intensely with the baby:
"Seeing her, holding her. She was my child. It overpowered me. I had no
control. I had to keep her."[3] Moreover, she felt the baby looked like her, and
this increased her feeling of wanting to keep the baby.

The next day, Mary Beth told the Sterns she was having trouble giving
up the baby and felt suicidal about doing so. Several days after the birth,
she took the baby home. There, she agreed to meet the Sterns to relinquish
the baby. At that time and place, the Sterns expressed gratitude. When
pressed by the Sterns, Mary Beth reluctantly let them take the baby and
leave.

Later that night, Mary Beth became distraught and in the middle of the night woke up her husband to ask, "Oh God, what did I do?"[4] Still upset the next morning, she went to the Sterns' home and asked to visit the baby. The Sterns let her do so. Mary Beth then told them that she felt terrible about giving up the baby and claimed she had almost tried to kill herself the night before by taking an overdose of Valium. She asked to take the baby home for a week until her feelings stabilized. Believing her suicidal, the Sterns reluctantly agreed.

The next day, Mary Beth said she was going to visit an aunt and would be unreachable, but instead took the five-day-old child to her parents' home in Florida. A few day later, she called the Sterns and said she needed more time to think, claiming that Richard had threatened to leave if she kept the baby, but not revealing that she and the baby were in Florida.

When Mary Beth returned to New Jersey, the Sterns visited the Whiteheads' home, and Mary Beth said she wanted to keep the baby permanently. She said that if the Sterns went to court, she would take the baby out of the country. When Mr. Stern asked to hold the baby, she refused and threatened to call the police.

A week later, the Whiteheads listed their house for sale, intending to move to Florida without telling the Sterns. To prevent their departure, Hackensack family court judge Harvey Sorkow froze their assets on May 5 and signed a "show cause" order directing them to surrender the baby. With this order, Bill Stern accompanied local police to the Whiteheads' home, where the Whiteheads delayed complying with the order by phoning their lawyer. During some confusion, Mary Beth took the baby to a bedroom at the rear of the house and passed it to Richard outside. Unable to find the baby, the police and Bill Stern eventually left. The next day, all the Whiteheads and the baby moved to Florida. Their location remained unknown to the Sterns until they recovered Baby M.

During the next three months, the Whiteheads left Ryan and Tuesday with Mary Beth's parents in Florida and lived in different motels as the Sterns' private detective tracked them. Around July 15, Mary Beth called William Stern, who secretly recorded the call. The tape recording of this call was introduced into the trial proceedings—amazingly!—at the instigation of the Whiteheads' lawyer to show Mary Beth's anguished mental state during this time. The introduction of the tape was—amazingly!—vigorously opposed by the Sterns' lawyer. Yet the introduction of the tape would be the key event shifting public opinion *from* Mary Beth Whitehead *to* the Sterns.

In the following transcript, "WS" indicates William Stern and "MBW" indicates Mary Beth Whitehead. (Perhaps because he knows he is taping the call, William Stern seems calm, rational, and sympathetic, whereas Mary Beth seems distraught.)

WS: Mary Beth, what can we do?
MBW: Bill, I'll tell you right now if you don't do something, I am going to do something that I am going to be very sorry for —

ws: What do you mean, you're going to do something you're going to be sorry for?

mbw: [getting upset] I'm telling you right now, Bill, you think you got all the cards. You think you could do this to people. You took my house. I mean we don't even have a car anymore. I can't even afford the car payments. You took everything away from me.

ws: I, I—

mbw: Because I couldn't give up my child?

ws: Mary Beth—

mbw: Because I couldn't give up my flesh and blood, you have the right to do what you did?

ws: I didn't freeze your assets; the judge froze your assets.

mbw: Oh, but oh, come on, Bill, your lawyer did it, and you knew about it.

ws: [matter-of-factly] The judge froze your assets. He wants, he wants you in court.

mbw: [accusatory] Uh-huh, sure, Bill, and how about the baby's sake, and how about Ryan and Tuesday? You're ruining a lot of people's lives.

ws: Aren't—don't you think you're ruining their lives, too?

mbw:: I have?

ws: Yes.

mbw: Yes. I have. So maybe I should just, me and Sara, vanish off the face of the earth.

ws: No, you shouldn't face—vanish off the face of the earth.

mbw: Well, that's what you're forcing me to do. . . .

ws: I want my daughter back.

mbw: And I want her, too, so what do we do, cut her in half? [angry]

ws: No, no, we don't cut her in half. [resigned]

mbw: You want me, you want me to kill myself and the baby?

ws: No, that's why I gave her to you in the first place, because I didn't want you to kill yourself. . . .

mbw: . . .I didn't anticipate any of this. You know that. I'm telling you from the bottom of my heart. I never anticipated any of it. Bill, please, stop it. Please do something to stop this.

ws: What can I do to stop it, Mary Beth?

mbw: Bill, I'll let you see her. You can have her on weekends. As soon as she gets a little older, you can have her a couple of weeks. Please stop this.

ws: [anguished] Oh, God!. . .

mbw: . . .So you want to go to court and get hurt more?

ws: Well, that's a chance I have to take. I can't live with myself letting her go.

mbw: What do you mean, letting her go? I told you you could see her. We would, we could be decent about it.

ws: Hah—you mean I would just get her—

mbw: You can't live with that?

ws: I can live with you visiting. I can live with that, but I can't live with her having a split identity between us. That—that'll hurt her.

mbw: What's the difference if I visit or you visit?

ws: The difference is—

mbw: Who do you think she's going to want more? Her own mother? And I've been breast-feeding her for four months. Don't you think she's bonded to me?

ws: I don't know what she's done, Mary Beth.

mbw: She's bonded to me, Bill. I sleep in the same bed with her. She won't even sleep by herself. You tell me, what are you going to do when you get this kid that's screaming and carrying on for her mother?

ws: I'll be her father. I'll be a father to her. I am her father....

mbw: I took care of myself the whole nine months. I didn't take any drugs. I didn't drink alcohol. I ate good. And that's the only reason that she's healthy, Bill. The only—because of me, because of me...I gave her life. I did. I had the right during the whole pregnancy to terminate, didn't I, Bill?

ws: It was your body.

mbw: That's right. It was my body, and now you're telling me I have no right....

mbw: You don't want her; you've made, you've made your point quite clear.

ws: No, I want my daughter back.

mbw: Forget it, Bill. I'll tell you right now I'd rather see me and her dead before you get her.

ws: Don't Mary Beth, please don't do—

mbw: I'm going to do it, Bill.

ws: Mary—

mbw: I'm going to do it; you've pushed me to it. Now you're telling me I can't—my children can't get their house back? I've done this to everybody's life.

ws: Wait!—

mbw: ...I gave her life. I can take her life away. If that's what you want, that's what I'll do.

ws: No! Mary Beth. No! Mary Beth. Wait! Wait!

mbw: That's what I'm going to do, Bill.

ws: Please—

mbw: You've pushed me.

ws: Please don't—I want—don't want to see you hurt. I don't want to see my daughter hurt. I really—

mbw: My daughter, too. Why don't you quit doing that, Bill, OK?

ws: O.K., O.K., all right—

mbw: It's our daughter. Why don't you say it, "our daughter"?

ws: All right, our daughter. O.K., Mary Beth, our daughter.[5]

In later portions of the tape, Mary Beth says that if Bill Stern doesn't drop his suit, she will accuse him of sexually abusing her daughter. Later, she said she really hadn't meant her threats and had made them in panic at the prospect of losing her baby. She thought people would understand that women say things they don't mean when they get emotional.

Two weeks later, Mary Beth was hospitalized for a kidney problem. Baby M was left at her grandparents' home. The private detective relayed this information to authorities, who took Baby M and returned her to New Jersey. Judge Sorkow awarded temporary custody of the baby to the Sterns.

Mary Beth's mother called a newspaper, which sent reporters to Mary Beth's hospital room, where she gave her side of the story. The Whiteheads returned to New Jersey and were referred for family counseling by Judge Sorkow. They kept only one appointment, for undisclosed reasons.

The Trial

A trial to determine first, the legality of surrogate contracts, and second, custody of Baby M, began in January 1987 before family court judge Harvey Sorkow in Hackensack, New Jersey. During the trial, Mrs. Whitehead claimed the baby might not be William Stern's because she and her husband had sex during the insemination process—contrary to stipulations in the contract. The judge ordered an HLA antigen test, which was legal in New Jersey, which showed a 98 percent chance that Mr. Stern was the genetic source. Mrs. Whitehead later revealed that her husband had undergone a vasectomy just after Tuesday was born.

William Stern testified that if he lost, it would be better for the baby not to see the Sterns anymore, saying that having two sets of parents would not be healthy. Mary Beth said that if she lost, she would still want to see the baby.

Almost a dozen psychologists, psychiatrists, and psychiatric social workers interviewed all parties, including the famous child psychologist Lee Salk. Most concluded that the best interests of the baby were never again to see Mary Beth. They said Mary Beth could not separate her own needs from the baby's.

During the trial, an issue arose over Mary Beth's involvement of Ryan and Tuesday in the events, with seemingly no attempt to shield them from possible harm. One version of this involvement is that Mary Beth's lawyer made her use this strategy to make it more difficult for Judge Sorkow to deny Mary Beth custody, i.e., to make it seem that the two children would be harmed by losing their "sister."

The other version is that Mary Beth manipulated her children to get custody. She placed a crib in Tuesday's room for the baby, who was described to her as the "sister" who was "sold." She petitioned the court to let Tuesday and Ryan visit the baby. She twice came to court with Tuesday, whose crying was soon displayed in newspaper photographs. She sought to have Tuesday testify about how much she missed the baby. (Judge Sorkow denied the motion, trying to keep the Whitehead children out of the case.) Mary Beth also let Tuesday be interviewed for television, during which Tuesday was said to often look at her mother for direction.

During the trial, the main character witness for Mary Beth was her former neighbor, Susan Herherhan. By this point, Judge Sorkow must have been convinced that Mary Beth was a chronic liar: she had technically committed fraud in not listing some assets when declaring bankruptcy, she had concealed her husband's vasectomy, she had illegally fled twice to Florida with Baby M, she had threatened Baby M's life and a vicious suit against Bill Stern—and then said she hadn't meant it—and she had manipulated (or let her lawyer manipulate) her children to win custody of the baby. The final straw probably came for Sorkow when he discovered that Susan Herherhan had forged a letter to him and signed Mary Beth's name (when Sorkow asked Mary Beth about the letter, she didn't know what he was talking about). Herherhan admitted she had lied (perjured herself) in former testimony before Sorkow. It seemed to Sorkow like a tangled web of lies within lies.

Judge Sorkow's Ruling

Judge Sorkow was well aware that his decision broke new legal ground.[6] Lower court judges rarely set even temporary precedents, so his 120-page opinion was exhaustive and written with an eye to the higher courts. He found the custody dispute between the two parents clear-cut and his opinion had few kind words about the Whiteheads. He clearly thought Mary Beth Whitehead was a manipulative woman who emotionally abused her children and who constantly lied to get her way.

He ruled that the contract was legal, gave permanent custody to the Sterns, terminated the Whiteheads' visiting rights, declared Mr. Stern the baby's father, ordered birth records changed, enjoined the Whiteheads from interfering with the Sterns, and awarded $10,000 to Mary Beth. He concluded that litigation needed to end for the good of "Melissa Stern," who needed to have her parentage fixed, be no longer manipulated, and have a "strong support system."

Judge Sorkow especially incensed supporters of Mary Beth Whitehead by immediately taking Elizabeth Stern into his chambers after his ruling and allowing her to adopt the baby. By making Elizabeth Stern the legal mother, he had denied that the woman who bore the baby was, in any legal sense, the mother. As such, Mary Beth was entitled to no visiting rights and was ordered not to see the baby again.

ETHICAL ISSUES

Media Bias

One of the interesting aspects of the Baby M case was its intense and biased media coverage. The case generated sensational interest comparable to the kidnapping of the Lindbergh child. When the case started, virtually every newspaper, television network, and magazine was against the Sterns. *Newsweek* and *Time* wrote articles very sympathetic to Mary Beth.[7]

Then, when testimony at the trial began, the media suddenly switched sides after the playback of the tape of the conversation between Mary Beth and Bill Stern. Suddenly, Mary Beth became the villain. A two-night television movie about this case accurately reflected this development, as the program completely switched sympathies from one night to the next (but alas, without explanation).

Such "taking sides" is understandable in a movie. It is less so in our best newspapers, magazines, and television networks. In Australia, a frenzied media contributed to injustice in the case of Lindy Chamberlain (a role played by Meryl Streep in *Cry in the Dark*), where an uncritical public let its opinions be formed by television reports. And television goes for ratings, not canons of evidence.

Could reporters have turned against Mary Beth because of her "hard jaw"? Because she wasn't like them? Was American reporting of the "Baby M" case our Lindy Chamberlain case?

Making a Mountain of a Molehill?

Before this case, hundreds of babies were born by surrogates. Of these, only about four cases had disputes and all were settled out of court. One surrogate agency's director said, "The Whitehead case is a real aberration. She's one of a half a dozen who have changed their minds, out of 800 to 1000 surrogates who have given birth."[8] A 99 percent success rate in any public policy is very good.

Moreover, custody fights are not unique to surrogate arrangements. Such disputes are not ideal, but marriage is not forbidden because of them. Why therefore should surrogacy be banned? Former New York City Family Court judge Nanette Dembitz agreed, saying the case shouldn't have been handled as a contract dispute at all, but "simply as a custody case."[9]

The two most famous surrogate mothers have been Mary Beth Whitehead and "Elizabeth Kane" (a pseudonym). Both ended their surrogacy wanting to keep their babies. Both became well-known.

In good thinking in ethics, it is a fallacy to put too much weight on one or two cases. Similarly, in medicine, this is the mistake of referring to "anecdotal" evidence. In statistics, it is the mistake of having "$N = 1$." In practical reasoning, it is called "hasty generalization."

Given that hundreds of babies were happily born to surrogates, and that less than 1 percent of their surrogates expressed regrets, surrogacy's supporters claim that it is a hasty generalization to ban surrogacy. The publicity received by Mary Beth Whitehead and Elizabeth Kane seems disproportionate to the experiences of most surrogate mothers.

"Irrational" (Machismo) Desires

A recurring criticism of critics of surrogacy is that it fulfills sexist male desires to have heirs. Former President of the National Organization for Women (NOW) President Eleanor Smeal disliked Elizabeth Stern's passivity and William Stern's dominant role.[10] She felt surrogacy was mainly for men, not for infertile couples. Such critics point to William Stern's intense concern with having a child with his genes. They say this is a typically male, irrational, desire. Although women can make more choices today, they say, men still control the parameters of many choices, and most men still want wives who can have babies.

This criticism is the "irrational desires" objection discussed in the preceding chapter. Suffice to point out here that if William (and Elizabeth) Stern's desire for a child is objectionable, then many other desires in private life will be objectionable. Critics of surrogacy retort that private life is one thing, making surrogacy legal is another. The latter is public policy, and such policy should not satisfy irrational desires.

On a related issue, Elizabeth Stern was criticized for using multiple sclerosis (MS) to avoid pregnancy.[11] The National MS Society thought MS women shouldn't avoid pregnancy unless so disabled that they couldn't care for their babies. It believed that Dr. Stern was in little danger from pregnancy.

Several experts testified that previous medical opinion had agreed with Dr. Stern's decision, but that such opinion had now changed.[12] However, they said, pregnancy still had a 5 to 40 percent risk of intensifying MS. They said her choice to avoid pregnancy was medically reasonable.

The National MS Society was saying that Mrs. Stern's desire to avoid pregnancy was irrational. Are attitudes toward taking such risks purely personal matters or subject to ethical criticism? The modern world has complex attitudes: we think a person a coward if he refuses to drive to work for fear of being killed, but we also think that, if he so chooses, he has the right to walk and not be forced to drive. But if such a person was a single-parent father and also forced his children to walk to shopping malls and back, we would say he needs counseling.

Measuring Motherhood

Can motherhood be measured? Experts in the trial said "yes" and concluded that Mary Beth Whitehead was clearly inferior to Elizabeth Stern. For them, it was no contest: a working-class mother versus an educated pediatrician. Many people rejected such measurement. Anyone can be a good mother, they said, and even if a child has less than ideal parents, it can still be a happy adult.

For some people, surrogacy violates the Norman Rockwell picture of Mom with peaches-and-cream complexion cooking at the hearth, with two happy kids near by. People today fear society and children will be hurt by single-parent families, surrogacy, and "blended" families. As theologian Richard McCormick said,

> Clearly, the notions of marriage and parenting must and do go beyond...biological beginnings. But these beginnings are the foundation upon which the rest, the complex network of kinship, bonding, and support, is built. If we untie this biological knot, what will happen to the institution that for so many centuries has taken shape around it?[13]

These worries sometimes get mixed in with other worries about generations of welfare families, teenage mothers, legal abortion, and "test tube babies." One critic worried that if commercial contracts for surrogacy were allowed, "our culture will become more fragmented, rootless, and alienated."[14] The ideal of motherhood, which many assume was a real norm at some previous time, seems under attack from too many directions.

A minority but opposing view is that the mystique of bearing a child has been exploited by traditional mothers for special attention. These traditional mothers saw surrogacy as a threat to their role and value as biological mothers. Philosopher Harriet Baber argued this in a paper written while she was seven months pregnant.[15]

Hence the debate over the psychological evaluation of Mrs. Whitehead was seen by many in broader terms. Viewed simply as evidence, the expert testimony overwhelmingly found against Mrs. Whitehead. One psychiatrist said Mrs. Whitehead had a mixed-type personality disorder, with impulsiveness, self-importance, exploitiveness, and lack of empathy.[16] Famous child psychologist Lee Salk said the Whiteheads lacked emotional stability, a peaceful home life, a capacity to respond to children's needs, a commitment to education, a reasonableness in daily judgments, and were not sufficiently hostile to drug-dependence.[17] A senior social worker found Mary Beth to be narcissistic and manipulative of her children: "Mrs. Whitehead appears unable to acknowledge Baby M as a person with an identity and needs separate from her own. Her need for having possession of this baby is overwhelming."[18] Moreover, "she feels threatened if her needs are not met. Mrs. Whitehead is capable of exploiting her children to achieve her goals."

But other people saw Mary Beth differently. What was so wrong with a mother totally committed to her baby? A courageous mother who would risk running afoul of the law by moving to Florida? Isn't that better than going off to work and dropping the kid off for ten hours at Cradle Rock? This was a mother who became a go-go dancer so her children's needs could be met. As philosopher Bonnie Steinbock sympathetically writes of Mary Beth: "Not surprisingly, she thought of Sara as her child, and she fought with every weapon at her disposal, honorable and dishonorable, to prevent her being taken away. She can hardly be blamed for doing so."[19]

Empathy with Mary Beth led some to attack the psychological experts who had found her so unfit. Physician Asa Ruskin wrote about Mary Beth, "Probably the most stressful and anxiety-provoking act in human existence is the separation of a woman from her newborn infant."[20] After such separation, he said, humans and animals experience panic, rage, and distress. He concluded, "Who can dare to judge the psychological acts and responses of a woman put to such a test?"

This controversy about motherhood often focused on *bonding*, a popular view that women have hormonally determined feelings about their baby. Phyllis Chesler, a psychology professor who writes books about popular topics, claimed in *Sacred Bond* that, "How can we deny that children bond with their mothers in utero, and that children suffer terribly in all kind of ways when this bond is prematurely or abruptly terminated?" and that "All the studies cited by experts such as Drs. Steven Nickman, Phyllis Silverman, Marshall Klaus, Rueven Pannor, and Betty Jean Lifton strongly suggest that being separated from one's birth mother constitutes a lasting trauma."[21] Chesler gives no further reference to these studies, which is unusual since this is the central claim of her book. Moreover, some of these people joined Chesler in an anti-surrogacy, pro-Mary Beth Whitehead support group.

In a review of the literature on bonding, philosopher Harriet Barber concluded there was little evidence in the social sciences proving bonding in primates. While there is evidence that infants need *some* maternal figure, there is no evidence of a psychological connection stemming from gestation or breast-feeding. One suspects that children who had wet nurses loved their rearing mothers. There is also no evidence that biological progenitors are better parents than adoptive couples.

Critics agree, saying that many of our important beliefs about motherhood and parenting are unproven. In that case, they say, we should be slow to experiment with radically new arrangements before we have sound evidence for changing.

To return to Mary Beth's capacities as a mother, law professor George Annas disliked the faulting of her by the courts and media:

> Judge Sorkow's opinion implicitly counsels: hire a mother for your child whom a judge is likely to view as unfit to raise it. Why aren't we all outraged at this suggestion and all the trashing of Baby M's mother?... [She] was successfully portrayed as an ogre for fleeing the police, and fighting the child's father with the only weapons she thought available to protect her daughter.[22]

Annas adds that Judge Sorkow "apparently decided to attempt to dehumanize the Whiteheads, to lionize the Sterns, and to pontificate on the devastation of infertility and the joys of parenthood."

A basic philosophical question underlying this case was, "What is a mother?" Surrogacy forces us to choose between identifying the "real" mother as: (1) the egg donor, (2) the gestator who carries the fetus to term, or the (3) rearing mother who raises the child.

In a time when most women work, and when almost all women feel some degree of guilt about not spending enough time with their infants, perhaps people compensate by wanting to make more important the biological bonds of gestation, "bonding" at birth, and "natural" maternal affection. Or perhaps our society has turned more conservative and reverted to traditional conceptions of sex roles and the family.

Related to the question, "What is a mother?" is the question, "What is a *good* mother?" This question in turn involves the larger question, "What is the ideal relationship between a wife, husband, and children?" This ideal is important because public policy should encourage and not undermine it.

Mary Beth saw her primary meaning in life as a mother in all the senses of creation, gestation, and rearing. She assumed she would be the person responsible for rearing the baby. Elizabeth Stern seems to have had a more modern, mixed view of motherhood, sharing duties with her husband and blending the duties of rearing a child with those of her career. Probably Elizabeth, not William Stern, wanted Elizabeth to stay at home with the baby. Had the contract gone through smoothly and without the subsequent publicity, the Sterns would have soon placed their child in day care, just like many other working couples, or would have hired someone to attend the child during their work day, whereas such options were inconceivable to Mary Beth. Then again, Mary Beth would need a man or government assistance to provide money for raising kids her way.

Family Disputes

More general critics claimed surrogacy undermined the family. Surrogacy supporters replied, "How can that be when a family is being created?" Critics replied, "Look at the Whiteheads! Look at the diversion of Mrs. Whitehead's attention from Ryan, Tuesday, and her husband. Look at their eventual divorce!" Law professor Herbert Krimmel chastized surrogates who began a life with the idea that they were not responsible for it, and implied that a similar attitude in men and women today was responsible for great misery.[23] Such irresponsibility, he concluded, should not be encouraged in law and public policy.

Feminist Barbara Katz Rothman opposed surrogacy because the man is "hiring himself an extra wife."[24] She seemed to say that William Stern had no claim on the baby because he did not bear it his body. Her critics replied that men never bear babies in their bodies, so that aspect of the case was not unique. Yet in ordinary life, men are held responsible for creating life, e.g., when they unintentionally get women pregnant and a child is brought to term. Indeed, a new federal law in 1989 makes it much harder for such males to avoid paying child-support.

Thus, if a man intended to create a pregnancy, as did William Stern, and he accepts legal responsibility at the beginning, he is held to be equally responsible for bringing up the child. If divorce occurs, he must either raise the child himself or provide half of its support. It seems unfair to say that a man like William Stern has no rights over the child but, nevertheless, has to pay child support until the child becomes an adult.

Feminists reply that men frequently ignore such obligations. Some recent studies showed that when men remarry, they decrease the legally required support of their children in the custody of their ex-wives, especially when such children go to college.

Feminist Objections

Most women who identified themselves publically as feminists sided with Mary Beth. Meryl Streep and Gloria Steinem sided with Mary Beth. Betty Friedan called surrogate agencies "surrogacy pimps." The feminist periodical *Off Our Backs* blasted Judge Sorkow in "Whitehead v. sperm" [sic]. Citing the Sterns, "six-figure annual salary," it saw the case as a "condemnation of motherhood and vindication of father-right:"

> The manner in which the trial was conducted has starkly revealed the
> class bias of reproductive health in the U.S., the pervasive negation of
> women's right to control reproductive control....The primary focus of
> the trial was a harsh concentrated attack on Whitehead's personality
> and emotional state and the stability of her home and marriage. The
> evidence presented at the trial brought out that Whitehead was a high
> school dropout and mother of two at age 19, was facing foreclosure on
> her house, that her husband had drinking problems, that she had spent
> three months as a barroom dancer in 1978 when she was 21, that she
> had been on welfare. In other words, she was facing the problems of a
> working-class mother.[25]

The periodical defended Mary Beth against the experts, noting that charges against women of being "emotionally unstable" and having personality disorders are typical of the "facetious charges made against mothers fighting for custody." It furthermore claimed the Sterns, not Mary Beth Whitehead, lacked empathy with the child. Philosopher Patricia Werhane objected that it was difficult to evaluate good parenting, that richer parents were not necessarily better, and that to characterize Mrs. Whitehead as "manipulative, impulsive, and exploitive" did not imply bad motherhood: "She sounds like many normal mothers, a person with cares and feelings."[26]

Underneath disputes about bonding and motherhood lay a deep and widespread tension in feminism and feminist ethics. This question concerned whether women are biologically superior parents or whether this belief is a culturally conditioned myth. Do women innately have any mothering traits simply as women? More important, which is more sexist: to think they have such traits or to deny that they do? As Rosemary Tong stated in a 1988 survey of feminist philosophy:

> After more reflection on patriarchy's construction of gender, however,
> many radical feminists concluded that androgyny was not really a

liberatory strategy for women; that is, that it was not desirable for women to "masculinize" themselves in any way, shape, or form. Some radical feminists asserted that "femininity" was not a problem in and of itself. Rather, the problem was the low value which patriarchy assigned to nurturance, emotion, gentleness, and the like. All we need to do is value the feminine at least as much as the masculine, and women will be liberated from the social forces that oppress them. Other radical feminists disagreed, insisting that "femininity" had to be a problem, since it had been constructed under patriarchy for patriarchal purposes.[27]

Some feminist scholars in the 1980s, such as Harvard education professor Carol Gilligan, attacked male norms in science, psychology, and ethics. They argued that women-centered norms such as caring and nurturing had been neglected in ethics.[28] One female expert who testified in the trial said Mary Beth exhibited the female ethics of family and relationships, not the male ethics of analysis and contracts.

In a similar vein, philosopher Patricia Werhane attacked surrogacy and the awarding of custody to the Sterns because the "court opted for middle class material values over the value of natural motherhood." She objected to overriding the values of natural parenting by comparing, in "cost/benefit terms," the value to the child of one set of parents rather than another.

Other feminists accused such feminist experts of being sexist themselves and of accepting reactionary notions. An example of this dispute was when philosopher Allison Jaggar argued for a universal "standpoint" to integrate feminist thought, but was promptly criticized by three postmodern feminists who objected that the notion of "one," "true" standpoint was a male philosophical myth and "phallogocentric."[29]

In the Baby M case, this theoretical division in feminism became divisive over interpreting the experience of breast-feeding. Mary Beth had breast-fed Baby M moments after birth and said this experience had bonded her to Baby M. One set of feminists rejected this "epiphenomenalist" view of women which held that women's mental moods and beliefs are by-products of their fluctuating physical states. Other feminists embraced such determinism and rejected "disembodied" male norms of epistemology.[30] They argued that all knowledge is "body-mediated." Because men and women have different bodily experiences, they differ in how they know the world. A pregnant woman has a different body, and hence, a different set of feelings, experiences, and beliefs, than when she was not pregnant. She is "connected" to the world and its inhabitants in a unique way.

Similar debates occur in medicine, where increased numbers of females have been predicted to "soften" its harshness. Whether this has happened is unclear. Some female patients express surprise at being treated no differently by female than male gynecologists. Medical education may be so demanding as to "harden" the "softest" female. When female residents want to work less than men because they are pregnant or have children, male physicians often angrily resist. It will be interesting to see which is harder to change: female "nature" or the system of medical education.

Surrogate Motherhood Dehumanizes

Columnist George Will said that "voluntary donation of wombs for gestation should be forbidden as dehumanizing."[31] He said the real villains were legalized abortion and scientists "who locate the essence of man in raw material subject to manipulation."

His critics retorted by asking how exactly Mary Beth Whitehead was "dehumanized" in contracting to bear a child? Did she not exercise rational thought, use the highly civilized arrangement of legal contracts, create a child very much wanted by its adoptive parents, and receive a very good fee for agreed-upon services? Are these not civilized arrangements of humans? What then is not humanistic about surrogacy? Simply its newness?

Moreover, his critics continued, what Will accuses surrogacy of, albeit in high-sounding language, is being *unnatural.* The Vatican saw it the same way: like in vitro fertilization (IVF), surrogacy was not intended by God as the natural means of motherhood, and was therefore immoral. Critics of both Will and the Vatican asked why helping people have children should be equated with "manipulation of the essence of man?"

Just Distribution of Surrogacy

If we allow surrogate gestation, Will continued, "there will be no grounds for denying the entitlement to unmarried people of whatever character." Edwin Newman feared that a new "right to parenthood" was implied by the Baby M case.[32]

Their critics said this was nonsense. It is worse than the illogic of saying that if we allow IVF, we must pay for it for anyone who wants it. In the case of a claimed entitlement to surrogacy, which no particular person has an obligation to fulfill and which necessarily requires another person to fulfill it, there is not much of an "entitlement."

Class Conflict and Exploitation of Surrogates

Critic Barbara Katz Rothman warned about dangers in surrogacy where fertilized eggs of rich women would be implanted in lower-class "breeder women." Margaret Atwood's futuristic novel *The Handmaid's Tale* was cited as an example, like *Brave New World,* of what could happen.

Many critics didn't want class conflict extended to procreation. As George Annas wrote:

> It was primarily the financial ability of the Sterns to hire an expert on family law and successfully obtain an *ex parte* [one-sided] order for temporary custody that determined the ultimate outcome of this case.

In this sense, reinforced by the economic bias of the mental health
experts and the judge, those critics who have labeled this custody
decision a classist opinion favoring the haves over the have nots are
correct. Justice seems to have been for sale along with Baby M.[33]

Was Mary Beth Whitehead a poor woman exploited by surrogacy? Judge
Sorkow disagreed in his opinion. (In his continued comments below, he assumes the reader understands that prospective adoptive parents may pay fees
up to $20,000 for "expenses" of private agencies which arrange the adoptions.)

To the contrary. It is the private adoption that has that great potential,
if not fact, for the exploitation of the mother. In the private adoption,
the woman is already pregnant. The biological father may be unknown
or at best uninterested in his obligations. The woman may want to keep
the child but cannot do so for financial reasons. There is a risk of illegal
consideration being paid to the mother. In surrogacy, none of these
"downside" elements appear. The arrangement is made when the
desire and intention to have family exists on the couple's part. The
surrogate has an opportunity to consult, take advice, and consider her
act and is not forced into the relationship. She is not yet pregnant.

In other words, if surrogacy is wrong because such mothers are exploited,
then so is commercial adoption at private agencies.

Judge Sorkow obviously begs the question of whether the financial need
of someone like Mary Beth Whitehead didn't indirectly coerce her into agreeing to surrogacy. In another case, one Mexican woman who was not a U.S.
citizen was paid only $2,000 for surrogacy for a California couple.

Clearly, exploitation is a possibility when any service is bought and sold.
When the service is a very intimate one, such as paying for sex or gestation,
strong feelings enter about what constitutes exploitation. At some point, however, charges of exploitation become silly, e.g., would payment of a million
dollars be "exploitive?"

Commercialization and "Baby Selling"

Issues of exploitation and class conflict can thus be distinguished from those
of commercialization per se. A person opposes exploitation because a surrogate is not paid *enough*; a person opposes commercialization because a surrogate is paid anything *at all*.

Columnist Ellen Goodman objected to commercializing procreation: "If
a mother can legally turn over the rights to her womb, then the ethic of the
marketplace has won. Pregnancy becomes a service industry and babies are a
product for sale."[34] Law professor Angela Holder said in a television interview, "A woman's relation to her baby isn't like a factory worker's to a product. Will you tell the kid, 'We paid $25,000 for you. How do you feel about the
biological mother who sold you?'"[35] ABC reporter Carole Simpson

said babies born of surrogate bearers were "conceived without love or sex, but for money."[36]

These people argued that commercialization *per se* is wrong, i.e., that any payment is wrong. Arguments for this usually appeal to the bad consequences of buying and selling life or to the different argument that such buying and selling of life is just intrinsically wrong.

Some say surrogacy is permissible, but not for money. They distinguish between *altruistic* surrogacy and *commercial* surrogacy, and would allow the former but not the latter. Yet some critics say altruistic surrogacy is more "exploitive" than paying women.

Similar arguments occur that subjects of nontherapeutic medical experimentation should never be paid because payment is coercive. Equally good arguments claim that since some subjects will be talked into volunteering anyway, it is immoral not to pay subjects. Similar arguments say it's paternalistic to say poor women are too stupid to refuse to take risks for money. Others object that the point has been missed that the *system* can create immoral "free" choices by its design, e.g., when poor women in the past were forced by extreme poverty to sell their breast-milk as wet nurses and deprive their own babies.

Defenders of the marketplace claim this is a hypocritical, knee-jerk reaction to commercialization. If women are banned from surrogacy, why not ban other sorts of services which women contract for? If we want only traditional mothers, why not forbid women from working as maids? Or as day-care workers, nannies, wet nurses, and governesses? Indeed, why not ban them from working at all?

Moreover, if the product was a food or telephones, not babies, the shortage of babies would be seen as a failure of the system. Russia forbids market contracts which mutually benefit buyer and seller, and as a result, shortages occur because of inefficiencies. America forbids procreation contracts and it is not surprising that similar shortages occur. So argues *New Republic's* editor, Michael Kinsley:

> The basic moral case for contract law, and indeed for capitalism itself, rests on the voluntary nature of exchange. Commercial trade is good for all parties involved, or else they wouldn't engage in it. And in the vast majority of commercial transactions—including the vast majority of surrogate-motherhood contracts—the deal goes through with no problem, suggesting that both do indeed consider themselves better off.[37]

Some people suggested banning commercial surrogacy but permitting altruistic surrogacy as a gift. Such donation is now encouraged of blood, a kidney, bone marrow, and organs. Such a status as a gift might make surrogacy more consistent with the traditional ideal of the altruistic nature of motherhood. In a famous book about altruistic versus commercial blood donation, Kenneth Titmus argued that altruism works better because voluntary givers had no motive to disguise any diseases, whereas sellers of blood did.[38]

Banning commercial surrogacy discourages baby brokers. The Sterns paid a $25,000 fee, but only $10,000 of it went to Mrs. Whitehead. After medical expenses were deducted, lawyer Noel Keane got the rest. His surrogate practice grossed $600,000 in 1986, a fact which to some is objectionable but which to others shows the desperate need for the services.

Philosopher Baruch Brody argues that focusing on the consequences of baby-selling misses the real point.[39] He critiques surrogacy from a *deontological* viewpoint in ethics—the kind of ethical theory emphasizing not consequences but duties (*deontos*). Deontologists emphasize that people have a duty not to use each other as "means" to other ends. For them, ethics is about rights and duties, not cost/benefit ratios.

Brody argues here by analogy. He says there are 30,000 women in Manila selling their bodies as prostitutes because of poverty and 60,000 Americans with end-stage renal disease who seek a kidney for a transplant. Why not let Americans buy kidneys from Filipinos for $50,000? There is no increase in morality or morbidity after selling a kidney and the benefited Americans would live longer and be happier. Moreover, the Filipino donors would make more by their sale than in ten years of work. Why not allow this, Brody asks, if the consequences are good for each side? Because, he answers, the practice is intrinsically wrong. Surrogacy is wrong for the same reason.

The Vatican in its 1987 Instructions on procreation took the same view as Brody and condemned surrogacy along with IVF as intrinsically wrong.[40] The Vatican held that every aspect of the creation of life should be kept between a husband and wife and rejected all involvement of third parties.

Critics of surrogacy reply that allowing economic exploitation in areas of life such as work and finance is bad enough, but it is intolerable to extend it to life itself. Our society often works by achieving a compromise of conflicting values, and the incentives of capitalism must be tempered by the humanizing values. Otherwise, why not allow the marketplace free rein and allow the selling of organs from live patients, of children into factories and prostitution, or even the selling of one person by another into slavery?

It is illegal to sell babies in most states. A Michigan court had already invalidated one surrogate contract because of such a law. But Judge Sorkow ruled that,

> The fact is, however, that the money to be paid to the surrogate is not
> being paid for the surrender of the child to the father. And that is just
> the point—at birth, mother and father have equal rights to the child
> absent any other agreement. The biological father pays the surrogate for
> her willingness to be impregnated and carry his child to term. At birth,
> the father does not purchase the child. It is his own biological,
> genetically-related child. He cannot purchase what is already his.

Law professor George Annas and many feminists specifically criticized the analogy Sorkow made between men being paid for donating sperm and women being paid for surrogacy. Annas and feminists both said that the proper analogy to men donating sperm was women donating eggs, not bearing fetuses. Donating sperm and bearing a fetus were not equal, proportional contributions to creating a baby.

Annas stressed that the essential contractual issue was whether the Sterns contracted for Mrs. Whitehead's child-bearing "services" or bought a product (a baby): "The sale of children should be specifically outlawed, as should the sale of human embryos." The leftist *Guardian* agreed, as did *Off Our Backs*. Angela Holder chimed in, "It's baby selling, pure and simple." Baby-buying and baby-selling are illegal.

It is interesting to note that laws against commercialization of procreation ("baby-selling") arose in previous times for different reasons. These laws originally protected unwed girls who were tempted to sell their children to childless couples. They weren't intended to prevent a woman from helping childless couples to have children.

Harm to the Child

Perhaps the most important consideration is whether surrogacy harms the created child. Britain's Warnock Committee, charged with recommending public policy on surrogacy, suggested that to protect such children, society should not encourage every couple to think it had the right to hire a surrogate, and that surrogates should be screened by impartial agencies.[41] The assumption here was that it was not good for the child to be created by undesirable parents and that such parents could be identified.

But this issue is not nearly as simple as it sounds and is rife with thorny philosophical dilemmas. The Paradox of Existence rears its ugly head here. Is it worse not to exist at all than to be borne by a surrogate mother to parents who want you? The judgment that it is seems difficult to justify.

Another solution to this problem is to argue that although babies can't be harmed by being brought into the world with surrogate mothers and adoptive parents, they can still be wronged.[42] On the other hand, shouldn't governmental public policy do what it can to encourage selection of good parents through regulations and screening? The price, then, of regulation is denial of parenthood to some couples.

On more practical grounds, a telling argument against commercial surrogacy is that it would be demeaning to the child later to learn, either purposely or by accident, that his or her conception was "bought." On a different point, one law professor emphasizes that some babies inevitably will be born defective (like the Malahoff baby), and that couples having children in normal ways are more ready to accept such babies than would be couples who contract for gestational services. Finally, when a child learns of its special origins, the knowledge may be traumatic. Some evidence suggests that learning that one was adopted, or conceived from an anonymous sperm donor whose genetic history one can never know, deeply bothers some adults.

Consent

Mrs. Whitehead's lawyer Harold Cassidy said surrogate mothers "cannot know, until after that child is born, their true feelings about bearing that child."[43] Psychologist Lee Salk agreed, "There are neurophysiological changes in pregnancy and surrogacy interrupts these. Any woman agreeing to bear a child under a surrogacy arrangement should have this explained to her and should be made to watch videotapes of mothers' reaction after birth."[44] Some women objected to such patronizing remarks and said they were insulting to surrogates who had already experienced childbirth.

Ellen Goodman wrote that surrogate mothers should be forbidden from signing contracts requiring them to give away their child, implying that bearing a child overpowers a woman's reason and memory. A minority of women who defended surrogacy strongly objected to Goodman's view: no matter that Mary Beth Whitehead had borne two previous children and knew what childbearing was like; no matter that 400 to 500 other surrogates had given up their babies; no matter that contracts about marriage and child custody often protect women. The "sad, human part of this drama is that neither the Whiteheads nor the Sterns could predict her [Mary Whitehead's] emotions," Goodman wrote. Yes, Goodman's female critics said sarcastically, women are like that, aren't they? Emotional creatures who shouldn't be surgeons, lawyers, or write syndicated columns?

Contract

Another issue was attitudes to contracts and the law. For the Sterns, contracts seemed almost sacrosanct—things to be studied minutely, carefully negotiated, and stuck by. In contrast, the Whiteheads seem to regard contracts as unimportant, especially when they conflicted with their basic values.

The contract signed by Bill Stern and Mrs. Whitehead was not recognized by statute, but many times previously in legal cases, contracts on the edge of the law were subsequently recognized as legal. Would this be such a case? The answer partly depended on reasons for and against using legal contracts in such arrangements.

Contract law is a much broader area than is understood by most Americans, who think they only encounter contracts when they buy a house or get married. In fact, much of American business is covered explicitly or implicitly by contracts, and contracts are a crucial part of daily law practice. Contracts occupy a semester course in law school.

In contract law, two redresses are available for violations: first, *compensation* for damages, or, second, *specific performance*, where the violating party is required to carry through on the contract's terms. Sorkow's compromise and his proposed "new rule of law" was that surrogates may change their minds and keep their babies up "until the time of conception." After that, if they changed their minds, they could keep their babies but could be sued for damages but not for specific performance, i.e., they could not be forced "by the male progenitor" to carry the child. To do so, among other things, would violate a woman's constitutional right to abortion before viability.

Some argued over the fairness of the contract. Wildly unfair contracts, such as selling oneself into slavery, are sometimes overruled. Some said the risks of the contract were all Mrs. Whitehead's. The Sterns denied this, replying that if the child turned out defective, Mr. Stern would be responsible. Moreover, he argued, he had paid $25,000 for an arrangement without a guaranteed result. *Off Our Backs* disagreed: "the biological mother's rights must be protected and not be considered disposable by virtue of a piece of paper." Others noted that the same "pieces of paper" protect mothers in making ex-husbands pay child support.

Juvenile or deranged people cannot enter into valid contracts. Contracts are also invalid where one party was fraudulent. *Off Our Backs* asked, "Was Whitehead led to believe that she could change her mind about giving up the child after conception? If she was, the contract could be declared invalid on the basis of fraud or misrepresentation under ordinary contract law." Sorkow's emphasis, that a contract is a promise to do something regardless of how one feels about it later, smelled too much to *Off Our Backs* of legalistic machismo.

Finally, Judge Sorkow unfortunately avoided the essential philosophical question about whether certain areas of life ought to be exempt from contracts. The ordinary legal idea, that a contract is a contract is a contract, holds over many areas of life concerning property and services, but the one area where it seems least persuasive is in the creation or cessation of life. It is precisely there that other considerations enter, considerations which must be balanced against the general usefulness to society of legally enforcing uncoerced contracts.

NEW JERSEY SUPREME COURT DECISION

In February 1988, the New Jersey Supreme Court reversed Judge Sorkow's decision in a unanimous 7–0 vote, decreeing that surrogate contracts were illegal.[45] It allowed Melissa Stern to remain in custody with the Sterns because the home life of the Sterns was more "secure" and "nurturing." However, the court allowed voluntary, unpaid surrogacy as legal so long as the mother could change her mind and keep the baby. The justices disallowed the legal adoption of Melissa by Elizabeth Stern. The court opinion said, "We thus restore the surrogate as the mother of the child. She is not only the natural mother but also the legal mother, and is not to be penalized one iota because of the surrogate contract."

The court found surrogate contracts to be baby-selling: "This is the sale of a child, or at the very least, the sale of a mother's right to her child, the only mitigating factor being that one of the purchasers is the father. The surrogate contract creates, it is based upon, principles that are directly contrary to our laws. It guarantees separation of a child from its mother; it looks to adoption, regardless of suitability, it totally ignores the child; it takes the child from the mother regardless of her wishes and her maternal fitness; and it does all this, it accomplishes all of its goals, through the use of money."

The court said the contract also violated "public policy" by assigning custody to a father without a custody hearing focusing on the best interests of the child, by guaranteeing separation of a child from its natural mother, and by giving William Stern greater rights than Mary Beth Whitehead. The court also agreed with some feminists: "The whole purpose and effect of the surrogate contract was to give the father exclusive rights to the child by destroying the rights of the mother."

It disagreed with Judge Sorkow's reasoning on every theoretical point. His 120-page opinion was dissected and left in shreds. Gleeful supporters of the Whiteheads said Sorkow had been treated as contemptuously as he had treated Mary Beth. Where Sorkow had held that surrogate contracts transcended limitations of existing law about adoption and custody, the high court held just the opposite and implied that even voluntary surrogacy would have to abide by ordinary laws of adoption and hearings about custody.

One law professor blasted the decision, saying the higher court had allowed the problems of the Baby M case to overrule first, "compassion" for "the real human need" of those who can only have children by hiring a surrogate; second, the women who would like to be surrogates; and third, the babies who would only be created through surrogacy.[46] He allowed that the surrogate should have the chance to keep the baby and give up the money, but "if she chooses to give up the baby at that time, her choice is at least as well informed as that of parents who give up their infant child for adoption."

UPDATE

After this decision and as the legal mother, Mary Beth returned to a lower court to obtain visiting rights. Three judges of the Superior Court allowed the baby to visit with Mary Beth one day a week up to six hours, thereafter growing to two days a week with an overnight stay, including two weeks with Mary Beth in the summer of 1989.[47] The baby would alternate holidays between the two families. The court concluded, "Melissa's best interests will be served by unsupervised, uninterrupted liberal visitation by her mother" and by allowing mother and daughter to "develop their own special relationship." The Sterns said the child's best interests would best be served by keeping the case out of court and said they would not appeal the custody decision.

When the Court's opinion appeared, Noel Keane's agency had achieved 200 successful, surrogate pregnancies with 47 "on the way" and another 150 couples matched and beginning insemination. In 1985, Britain banned commercial surrogacy. Michigan and Florida did so, also. However, the Michigan courts kept the door open for altruistic surrogacy, in which the adoptive couple could pay for medical expenses.

By 1989, and as much as is ever possible in America, a consensus emerged that commercial surrogacy should be discouraged by public policy and should not be legally enforceable. However, the consensus held that altruistic surrogacy, under some careful regulation, should be allowed. A New York task force concluded that undisputed altruistic surrogacy could be handled by existing laws covering artificial insemination, embryo implantation, and adoption.[48] Conservative Henry Hyde (R-Ill.) surprisingly combined with liberal Barbara Boxer (D-Calif.) to sponsor a bill to outlaw commercial surrogacy.[49]

In August of 1987, Mary Beth Whitehead separated from her husband Richard. Her lawyer's prepared statement said that "extraordinary stress placed upon her marriage and the public discussion of private matters rendered Mr. and Mrs. Whitehead's marriage an inevitable casualty of this unusual case." In October 1987, Mary Beth opposed surrogacy before a House subcommittee and on *Good Morning America:* "Your eyes are not open until you hold that baby in your arms and she becomes real." In November 1987, Mary Beth Whitehead announced that she was pregnant by Dean Gould, a New York City accountant, whom she had been seeing for several months. She married Gould after her divorce from Richard Whitehead became final, and in 1988 she gave birth to a new child, conceived the normal way and indisputably belonging to the new Gould family.

FURTHER READING

William Prior, ed. *Manufactured Motherhood: The Ethics of the New Reproductive Techniques,* in *Logos: Philosophic Issues in Christian Perspective:* 9, Philosophy Department, Santa Clara University, 1988.

On the Problem of Surrogate Parenthood: Analyzing the Baby M Case, (Edwin Mellen Press, 1987).

Bonnie Steinbock, "Surrogate Motherhood as Prenatal Adoption," *Law, Medicine & Health Care,* 16:1–2 (Spring 1988).

Phyllis Chesler, *Sacred Bond: The Legacy of Baby M* (Vintage, 1989).

New York State Task Force on Life and the Law, *Surrogate Parenting: Analysis and Recommendations for Public Policy* (1988).

CHAPTER 6

Abortion and the Trial of Kenneth Edelin

This chapter discusses the trial of physician Kenneth Edelin, who was charged with manslaughter in Boston in 1973 for performing an abortion. The chapter also discusses the ethical issues of abortion. The following definitions will help. In human embryology, the successful union of sperm and egg is called a "zygote" (or "fertilized ovum"). The zygote begins dividing, forming 2, 4, 8 cells, and so on. During these stages, it is called a "morula" and "blastula." Sometimes, a cell between 1 and 4 weeks is called a "pre-embryo." In between 4 and 8 weeks, the organism is called an "embryo." From 9 weeks until birth, it is called a "fetus." "Baby" refers to a newborn human being who exists outside the womb.

HISTORICAL BACKGROUND

Paul Badham, professor of church history at St. David's University in the United Kingdom, says this about Christianity's position on abortion:

> The Bible certainly teaches the value of human life, and forbids the murder of any human being (Psalm 8). But life, in biblical terms, commences only when the breath enters the nostrils and the man or woman becomes a "living being" (Genesis 2:7). . . . Consequently in biblical terms the fetus is not a person. This is brought out clearly in the laws relating to murder. For though the Ten Commandments in Exodus state clearly "you shall not murder," the text goes on, in the following chapter, to differentiate between causing the death of an adult human being and causing the death of an unborn fetus. For whereas "whoever hits a man and kills him shall to be put to death" (Exodus 21:12), ". . . if some men are fighting and hurt a pregnant woman so that she loses her child, but is not injured in any other way, the one who hurt her is to be fined." There is no suggestion in the Old Testament law, as there is in a comparable Assyrian one, that "he who struck her shall

114

compensate for her fetus with a life." Indeed, the biblical text does not even regard the loss of her fetus as causing the woman "harm," for it goes on to specify what should happen "if any harm follows." At no point is any consideration given to the notion that the fetus itself might have rights. And this absence of concern for the fetus is also implied by the imposition of the death penalty on women who conceive out of wedlock, without any consideration being given to the fact that this killed both the fetus and the woman (Deuteronomy 22:21, Leviticus 21:9, Genesis 38:24).

Turning to the issue of abortion as such, I am somewhat puzzled that biblical fundamentalists who oppose abortion so strongly, should pay so little heed to the silence of the Bible on this issue.... Whether this silence is significant or not, the fact ought to be faced that whatever views one may hold about abortion, no straightforward appeal can be made to the teaching of the Bible, for the Bible simply does not discuss it.[1]

As an organized religion, the Roman Catholic Church has always opposed abortion. But its view of what counts as an abortion has changed quite a bit over time.

In the 12th century, abortions began to be distinguished from homicides by differentiating "unformed" from "formed" fetuses. Thomas Aquinas said God "ensouled" the latter, if male, at 40 days, and if female, at 80 days. Killing early male, but not female, embryos, was sinful. Killing an embryo before 40 days was neither abortion nor murder.

Beginning with the mid-19th century, the Popes denounced abortions in increasingly absolutistic terms, partly because scientific evidence discredited the Thomistic view of ensoulment. During this time, religion felt very threatened by science. Pope Pius IX in 1870 reacted by declaring that his edicts (and those of other Popes) were "infallible," by encouraging the neglected worship of Mary, by supporting Creationism against geological explanations of the origins of the universe, and by emphasizing miracles, such as the one recognized shortly thereafter at Fatima.[2] During this time, when medical biology revealed the small beginnings of human life, the Catholic view began that personhood began at conception. Most conservative Protestant denominations followed suit.

During the previous 1300 years of Christian rule, abortion was rarely conceptualized as murder, even after the fetus "quickened" or kicked. During these centuries, personhood was not considered to begin at conception but at some later time, such as ensoulment, quickening, or viability. The view among some Christians that personhood begins at conception is less than 150 years old.

Exceptions were made for ectopic pregnancies (where the fetus implants outside the uterus in the Fallopian tubes) and for cancerous uteruses (where uterus and fetus had to be removed together). In both cases, the *doctrine of double effect* allowed physicians to save the mother because it said that an action having two effects, one good and the other evil, was morally permitted if (1) the action was good in itself or not evil, (2) if the good followed as immediately from the cause as the evil effect, (3) only the good effect was intended, and (4) there was a proportionately grave cause for performing the action as for allowing the evil effect.

This doctrine became famous in the early part of the 20th century as physicians struggled with abortions. What if a mother had a uterine perforation which could only be treated by endangering the life of the fetus? The doctrine held that the physician must, in his mind, primarily intend only the repair of the uterus and not the death of the fetus.

In 17th-century European common law, aborting a quickened fetus was not indictable. An English statute in 1803 made abortion a capital crime but continued to use quickening as the key marker, providing for lesser penalties before this point. America followed English common law from the 17th to 19th centuries, making abortion before quickening only a misdemeanor, or legal for therapeutic reasons if recommended by two physicians. Only after the Civil War in America did most states make abortion illegal, with stiff penalties and firm cutoff points.

Feminist historians consider medicine's opposition to abortion from 1870 to 1970 to reflect its paternalism and misogyny. Before the Civil War, most American babies were delivered by professional midwives, who competed with physicians. Thereafter male physicians played a key role in keeping women in their place: "Anti-abortion legislation was part of an antifeminist backlash to the growing movement for suffrage, voluntary motherhood, and other women's rights in the 19th century. The prevailing public prudery and antisexual moralism condemned feminism and considered sex for pleasure evil, with pregnancy as punishment."[3]

The Supreme Court, in 1973, in *Roe vs. Wade* reviewed the history of abortion and concluded:

> It is thus apparent that at common law, at the time of the adopting of
> our Constitution, and throughout the major portion of the 19th century,
> abortion was viewed with less disfavor than under most American
> statues currently in effect. Phrasing it another way, a woman enjoyed a
> substantially broader right to terminate a pregnancy than she does in
> most States today. At least with respect to the early stage of pregnancy,
> and very possibly without such a limitation, the opportunity to make
> this choice was present in this country well into the 19th century. Even
> later, the law continued for some time to treat less punitively an
> abortion procured in early pregnancy.[4]

A Pivotal Case: The 1962 Finkbine Baby

Sherri Finkbine was married in 1962 and living with four children in Phoenix, Arizona. During her fifth pregnancy, she took tranquilizers prescribed for her husband and later, after learning that she was pregnant, discovered that her husband had purchased thalidomide in Europe as a tranquilizer. Thalidomide was a teratogen ("monster former") and often produced babies missing arms or legs.

The Finkbines requested a therapeutic abortion for Mrs. Finkbine's health at a local hospital, even though their real desire was not to have a defective baby. The abortion was scheduled, but reporters picked up the story, prodding the district attorney to threaten to prosecute. Forced to go to Europe for their abortion at considerable expense, the Finkbines discovered that the aborted fetus was indeed a monster.

As a result of this case and others, several states legalized abortion in the early 1970s. The first was Colorado, followed by North Carolina, and then California, where Governor Ronald Reagan signed it into law. When *Roe vs. Wade* came in 1973, a popular groundswell among voters had built up, resulting in legalization of abortions in several states. Had *Roe vs. Wade* not prohibited all states from restricting abortions in the early stages, this momentum for legalization of abortion would have probably resulted in several other state legislatures legalizing abortion.

Abortions before Legalization in 1973

Before legalization, illegal abortions were often horrifying experiences. Physicians who did abortions often did so only for the money and sometimes treated their patients badly. Some disturbed physicians demanded that women have sex with them before they did abortions. Physicians at times lectured women on their "promiscuity" while performing abortions. Illegal abortions by physicians were very expensive and beyond the finances of poor women and of teenagers who wouldn't tell their parents. The procedures helped physicians more than they did women. As a result, anesthesia was sometimes not used and no prior explanation was given of what would happen and why. If anything bad happened, the woman had no legal recourse. She rarely knew the physician's name and was usually forbidden to try to contact him again.

Hundreds of thousands of illegal abortions were performed annually in the United States in the 1950s and, during those operations, perhaps a thousand women died. Desperate women came into emergency wards at the last possible moment and died of widespread abdominal infections—victims of botched or unsanitary abortions. Some women who recovered from such infections found themselves sterile or chronically ill. Poor women ran the greatest risks with illegal abortions. In 1969, 75 percent of the women who died from illegal abortions were women of color.[5] Ninety percent of all legal, private, abortions in that year were performed on white women.

After abortion was legalized in America in 1973, the number of legal abortions grew to 1.5 million per year, where it has hovered since.[6] The years since legalization provide a stable picture of who gets abortions. Less than 1 percent of women getting abortions are under 15, while older teenage girls make up about 30 percent. Women in their twenties get the majority (55 percent) of abortions. Women in their thirties get 14 percent of abortions. Married women have 20 percent of abortions. White women get 70 percent of abortions, black women, 30 percent. Blacks have 57 abortions per thousand; whites, 24 per thousand.

Legalization of Abortion (*Roe vs. Wade*, 1973)

The United States Supreme Court's *Roe vs. Wade* decision in 1973 concerned "Jane Roe," a single woman from Dallas, Texas, who in March 1970 wished for a safe, legal abortion from a physician. A Texas law criminalized abortions and Jane Roe challenged its constitutionality. She was joined in her suit by a physician named Hallford, who had two abortion prosecutions pending against him. (Jane Roe claimed she had become pregnant because of a gang rape, but in 1987 recanted her story. In 1989, she revealed that her name was Norma McCorvey.)

The Court had already decided in *Griswold vs. Connecticut* that the right to "privacy" (a misnomer for personal liberty) was implied by the Constitution and allowed couples to receive birth control pills. The Court decided in *Roe vs. Wade* that the same right grounded the right of women to have abortions.

This right was not unqualified. The Court balanced the increasing rights of the fetus, which grew with fetal age, with the rights of a woman to terminate a pregnancy. Emphasizing that people differed greatly in their religious and philosophical views about personhood in fetal development, the Supreme Court drew the line at *viability*. After viability, states could make abortions illegal; before then, they could not.

The Court said viability was when the fetus was "potentially able to live outside the mother's womb, albeit with artificial aid. Viability is usually placed at about seven months (28 weeks) but may occur earlier, even at 24 weeks." The Court summarized its trimester system, where viability divides the second and third trimesters, this way:

1. A state criminal abortion statue of the current Texas type, that excepts from criminality only a *life-saving* procedure on behalf of the mother, without regard to pregnancy stage and without recognition of the other interests involved, is violative of the Due Process Clause of the Fourteenth Amendment.
   (a). For the stage prior to approximately the end of the first trimester, the abortion decision and its effectuation must be left to the medical judgment of the pregnant woman's attending physician.
   (b). For the stage subsequent to approximately the end of the second trimester, the State, in promoting its interest in the health of the mother, may, if it chooses, regulate the abortion procedure in ways that are reasonably related to maternal health.
   (c). For the stage subsequent to viability, the State in promoting its interest in the potentiality of human life may, if it chooses, regulate, and even proscribe,

abortion except where it is necessary, in appropriate medical judgment, for the preservation of the life or health of the mother.

Note that a state "may" forbid abortion. It need not. A state could legalize abortion up to birth.

The above "trimester" system later became a point of much dissension of the U.S. Supreme Court. Various judges held it to be artificial and unworkable, a "Procrustean" bed, as Justice Rehnquist later called it.

Note, too, that preserving not only the life but also the health of the mother can justify third-term abortions. Antiabortionists charge that this loophole justifies almost any abortion, because two physicians can often be found who will say that the health of the mother is in danger from further pregnancy. Indeed the concept of "health" is vague and can be used this way. In the 1960s, some states—Alabama, for example, permitted—abortions for the health of the mother, and some physicians interpreted "health" quite broadly, performing third-trimester abortions virtually on request.

The EDELIN CASE

The Edelin case occurred in Boston, in October 1973. Just months before, in January, many of Boston's Catholics had disagreed with the Supreme Court's *Roe vs. Wade* decision.

A key event preceding the Edelin case was two experiments on aborted fetuses which had been performed just after *Roe vs. Wade* at Boston City Hospital, where Edelin was a resident. Some physicians reasoned this way: if aborted fetuses were going to die anyway, why not use them in experiments to help other fetuses? To study which drugs crossed the placenta (and to prevent cases like Sherri Finkbine's), physicians gave antibiotics to women undergoing abortions and examined the aborted fetuses. They found that clindamycin crossed into the fetus and concentrated in fetal liver. What this proved is that fetal syphilis, in mothers allergic to penicillin, can be treated by clindamycin.

The article about the study appeared in the *New England Journal of Medicine*. Copies of the article were sent to Boston's Catholics, who were infuriated.[7] A councilman held a hearing to investigate fetal experimentation at Boston City Hospital. Antiabortionists packing the auditorium heard Mildred Jefferson, an assistant professor of surgery at Boston University. She claimed, perhaps correctly, that some of the girls undergoing abortion were too young to legally consent to the study and had not given written consent. Lack of such consent left experimenters open to technical charges of "grave robbing" (illegally procuring human bodies for medical experimentation, reminiscent of Burke and Hare in Edinborough).

Mildred Jefferson was asked to testify at the City Council's hearing not only as an antiabortion physician but also as a black physician. Edelin was also a black physician. Although District Attorney Newman Flanagan denied it, many wondered if it was a coincidence that the first physician prosecuted for performing an abortion was black.

Nothing much resulted from the hearing other than allowing antiabortion feelings, which the Councilman had intensified, to be ventilated. The hearing concluded on September 18, 1973, 3 days before Alice Roe came to Boston City Hospital for a late-term abortion.

Kenneth Edelin at the time was 35 years old. The son of a postman, he grew up in a poor section of Washington, D.C. An undergraduate at Columbia, he took his M.D. from Meharry Medical College in 1967. He interned in Ohio, and then worked for 3 years as a U.S. Air Force physician (with captain's rank) in England. He began his residency at Boston City Hospital, in 1971, on July 1st. In a PBS documentary about the case, Bill Moyers called Boston City Hospital the "city hospital in the Boston ghetto." Edelin was in his third year, and chief resident in obstetrics, when "Alice Roe" appeared.

Alice was a 17-year-old, black, West Indian student. She remained anonymous throughout the case, so little is known about her. She was examined by Edelin's faculty supervisor, Hugh Holtrop, who estimated her to be 22 weeks pregnant. She was also examined by resident Enrique Giminez, a first-year resident from Mexico. Giminez later testified against Edelin and estimated Alice's fetus to be 24 weeks old. A third-year medical student agreed with Giminez's estimate.

To complicate matters, Dr. Holtrop obtained Alice's and her mother's permission for Alice's participation in another pre-abortion experiment to see if aminoglutethamide would increase the hormone output of the placenta. The substance was given to Alice intravenously, and her urine was analyzed over the next 24 hours. The study took one day, from October 1 to October 2.

As a third-year resident, Edelin carried out substantial work at Boston City, Boston's "St. Elsewhere" hospital. All attending obstetricians had private practices and spent little time at Boston City. Edelin was assigned to Alice Roe's abortion, even though the fetus was very late-term and even though Holtrop had admitted her. Holtrop later said he admitted her only because he was the only obstetrician on duty, but Edelin disagreed, claiming Alice was Holtrop's patient. Surgeon William Nolen, who wrote a book reviewing the case, believes that Holtrop dumped the case on Edelin.[8]

Edelin wanted to abort by injecting saline solution into the amniotic sac, but when he inserted a needle to sample the amniotic fluid, he drew blood. The blood indicated that Alice had an anterior placenta (one attached to the front wall of her uterus), and that injecting saline into the placenta, and from there into her bloodstream, was risky and could kill her.

The abortion was rescheduled for the following day, when a hysterotomy was performed. A hysterotomy is essentially abortion by caesarean surgery, cutting through the lower abdominal wall. Instead of resident Giminez, Edelin chose as his assistant, Steve Teich, a third-year medical student. Unasked, Giminez watched the hysterotomy anyway.

What happened next is controversial. Giminez testified that Edelin made the caesarean section, reached in, cut the placenta, and then allegedly waited a few minutes before removing the fetus. Other staff on the scene deny that he waited.

Babies spontaneously begin breathing when brought out of the uterus and cannot breathe inside. Edelin was charged with neglecting the baby by not removing it immediately, with the result that it suffocated. Some time later, Edelin removed the dead fetus from the uterus. Later, it was taken to the morgue. Hospital policy required aborted fetuses above 600 grams to be preserved in formalin. This policy later allowed the district attorney to have a "body," photographs of which were shown to the jury.

Edelin's Trial

A grand jury decided enough evidence existed to indict Edelin. Some legal strategists believe Edelin erred in testifying at the pretrial hearing and by not invoking his Fifth Amendment right against self-incrimination. Medical professor Hugh Holtrop did so and refused to testify. After the hearing, and after Holtrop was not also indicted, Edelin changed lawyers.

Edelin was charged with manslaughter of a black male child. Manslaughter can occur by commission or omission of acts. Edelin was charged with a "wanton, reckless" omission of an act which caused death. Massachusetts law defined "wanton, reckless" conduct as "the legal equivalent of intentional conduct" and as "disregard of the probable consequences to the rights of others." Trial judge McGuire said, "The essence of wanton or reckless conduct is the doing of an act or the omission to act where there is a duty to act, which commission or omission involves a high degree of likelihood that substantial harm will result to another."[9]

The principal participants in the trial were Newman Flanagan, the prosecuting district attorney, described as "dramatic, competent, and tough;" Edelin's trial lawyer, William Perkins Homans, Jr., a wellborn Boston lawyer who often defended unpopular causes; and, presiding, Judge McGuire.[10]

Massachusetts did not pass an abortion law until August, 1974, 22 months after *Roe vs. Wade*. In the absence of state law, *Roe vs. Wade* was—as the trial judge instructed the jury—"absolutely controlling." Since *Roe vs. Wade* equated viability with personhood, the jury had to determine the meaning of viability, even where the federal Supreme Court had not. If the fetus was not viable, no person was killed. If no person was killed, Edelin could not be guilty of manslaughter.

A study found that jurors likely to convict Edelin would be blue-collar Catholics over 50 years old, who had dropped out of Catholic high schools, and who regularly read conservative Catholic newspapers. After much wrangling between both lawyers, a mostly white jury of 3 women and 13 men was selected. Ten of these were Catholic. (Few women were selected because of historical sex discrimination in Massachusetts trials—a problem undergoing federal correction at the time.)

Resident Giminez testified that Edelin and "the whole group" looked up for "3 minutes" while Edelin did "nothing else" but stand "looking at the clock." Giminez implied that this inaction killed the fetus. Operating room nurse was asked if Edelin had stood watching a clock and replied, "No. I recall that in one of the operating rooms, the clock was not functioning." She also said Edelin's "back was to the clock." Operating room nurse Ellen Curtis testified that Edelin "never looked at any clock" and that "there was no clock on the wall" at that time.[11] The defense introduced records showing the clock had been removed that day for repairs.

Edelin said the clock was behind him and that he never stared at it. The procedure seemed long to Giminez because, at this midstage in pregnancy, the thick abdominal muscle wall was not stretched enough to be easily cut. Edelin said he made a Pfannenstiel ("bikini incision") rather than a vertical incision to be "safer" (perhaps, too, so the young girl would have less of a scar). Surgeon William Nolen said such an incision would take longer, especially by a resident who had never done one, but not 3 minutes.[12]

Discrepancies also arose about the size of Alice's fetus and various methods of estimating its size (the poor hospital didn't have an ultrasound machine). Resident Giminez estimated the fetus to be much older than did Edelin, Holtrop, or the medical student.

Defense attorney Homans angrily objected when Judge McGuire allowed Flanagan to introduce a picture of "the deceased" as evidence. Homans said the picture would tell laypersons nothing of fetal age or viability and would be "inflammatory." The judge allowed the picture and charged the jury not to view it "from any emotional point of view."

The media intensely followed the trial. Both sides of the abortion controversy supported their side. Pro-abortion groups supported Edelin, as did antiabortion physicians who hated prosecution of physicians more. Antiabortion groups saw District Attorney Flanagan as their knight. Edelin had stepped over the legal line, they said, and had to be punished. A few months later, Karen Quinlan's physicians took notice.

Flanagan summed up. First, the fetus was a person when the placenta was cut; second, Edelin's long wait constituted wanton, reckless conduct; and third, legal abortion was intended to end a pregnancy, not produce a dead fetus.

The judge instructed the jury that an unborn fetus was not a person and not the subject of a manslaughter indictment. Such an indictment could only refer to a person, who was defined by Massachusetts law as a being who had been born. Unborn fetuses could not be victims of manslaughter. Because birth was the key event, the judge instructed the jury, "you must be satisfied beyond a reasonable doubt...that the defendant caused the death of a person who had been alive outside the body of his or her mother." The jury had to decide: (1) was Alice Roe's fetus alive outside her mother's body? and (2) if so, did the fetus (now called a "baby") die from "wanton, reckless conduct" by Edelin?

The jury said "yes" to both questions, and convicted Edelin of manslaughter. Edelin was sentenced by Judge McGuire to 1 year probation. Had the conviction stuck, Edelin could have lost his medical license. The decision was appealed and the Massachusetts Supreme Court agreed to hear the case on direct review (without review by intermediate, appellate courts). Edelin received a vote of confidence by Boston City Hospital's board of trustees, who offered him a permanent position.

When the jury's verdict was announced, the media implied that a black man in an abortion case couldn't get a fair trial from white Catholics in Boston. Even William Buckley reportedly noted "that the case can be presented as the lynching of a black Marcus Welby by a bigoted community."[13] The foreman of the jury retorted furiously that the aborted fetus was black and that the jury had been concerned about *its* life. Medical journals strongly supported Edelin.

The Massachusetts Supreme Court Decision

In December 1976, the Massachusetts Supreme Judicial Court, which had agreed to hear the case on immediate appeal, overturned Edelin's conviction, declaring that no evidence of manslaughter had been presented at the trial. The court said, "In the comparative calm of appellate review, the essential proposition emerges that the defendant had no evil frame of mind, was actuated by no criminal purpose, and committed no wanton or reckless act in carrying out the medical procedures on Oct. 3, 1973."[14]

During the period between the lower-court trial and the supreme court decision, the U.S. Supreme Court said that "the determination of whether a particular fetus is viable is, and must be, a matter for the judgment of the responsible attending physician."

All but one of the appellate justices ordered Edelin acquitted because they believed no evidence had been introduced showing "wanton, reckless" conduct. The five justices opposed the usual procedure of ordering a new trial, which the sixth justice wanted. Even if evidence had been introduced on the above count, three justices would have reversed and acquitted anyway, because they believed that no evidence had been presented of live birth and also that the trial judge should not have allowed testimony about Edelin's "prenatal conduct." Another justice disagreed and said that the judge should have allowed more testimony about Edelin's prenatal conduct. Yet another dissenting justice thought the trial judge had failed to give the jury a standard of what Edelin might have "reasonably" been expected to know.

After the decision, Edelin was described as "jubilant" and said he felt "terrific" about the verdict, saying, "It's great to be able to smile again after two and a half years."[15] He claimed his reversal was a victory for all physicians, regardless of whether they performed abortions, and that it upheld the principle of nonprosecution of physicians who acted in good faith and who followed accepted medical standards.

Reactions to the Acquittal

On the evening of December 17, 1976, Walter Cronkite triumphantly announced that Edelin had been acquitted of "manslaughter by abortion."[16] William Nolen, a famous surgeon who spent much time investigating the case, concluded that the fetus had not been outside the womb, thus had not been technically "born," and thus was not a person. Hence, there could be no manslaughter and Edelin broke no law.

As a surgeon who is antiabortion, Nolen believed Edelin intended to kill a late-term fetus and that Edelin was surprised when he opened Alice to see that the fetus was viable. Nolen doesn't say Edelin suffocated the fetus, but he does say that whether a newborn has the will to live ("that spark") can only be known if it is taken out of the womb, slapped, and helped to breathe:

> What is disturbing in the Roe case is that, by his own admission, Edelin made no attempt to see if the child had that spark. As [witness and physician, Jeffrey] Gould said, the will to live isn't always immediately apparent; it becomes obvious only if "the physician will try to stimulate, will try to give a little bit of oxygen, and look for a favorable response."
>
> The Roe baby wasn't given this bit of provocation that might—just might—have shown it had the will to live. Why? The answer is distressingly simple. No one wanted the Roe baby to live.[17]

ETHICAL ISSUES IN THE EDELIN CASE

Viability

The most important ethical issue in this case concerned the ethics of abortion. One question concerned when the human fetus became a person with the right to life. The Supreme Court said in *Roe vs. Wade* that this began with "potential viability," but the concept of viability is vague. "Viability" designates ability to survive as an independent entity, but when is that? The Court, in 1973, said anywhere from 24 to 28 weeks, but left things otherwise indeterminate.

Flanagan seized on this vagueness during the trial. One physician testified that babies could live outside the womb as early as 12 weeks. But for how long? Only a few minutes, the physician testified, but maybe longer. Defense attorney Homans counterpunched by asking the physician how he defined viability, which turned out to be "capacity to survive [outside the womb] even for a second after birth." Time and time again, Homans questioned hostile, expert-witness physicians, successfully getting each to admit that he had never known a fetus under 24 weeks to survive.

Edelin's critics retorted that they knew exactly what was meant by viability, i.e., the ability to survive independently of the mother. Some fetuses, no matter how hard physicians try, will never live to 40 weeks. Others will. Neonatologists know which is which. Tests by ultrasound machine measure such things. The point to them was that Edelin never tried to find out if the fetus was viable and, at best, just assumed it wasn't.

Edelin's supporters privately replied that, of course, no one tried to determine viability. The whole point of abortion was to kill a fetus. The point is not to look inside, see if a fetus is "viable," and if it is, to save it. The intention is to kill it, regardless.

In all the books and documentaries made on this case, no one emphasized one fact which was obvious but which perhaps should be mentioned here. The day before the hysterotomy, Edelin had intended to abort the very same fetus by saline injection, a legal procedure. No matter how "viable" or large, if such a procedure had been carried out, the fetus would have died. The only thing which prevented this procedure from happening was the arbitrary fact that the fetus was turned around one way and not the other. It was not in the interior of the mother's body but near her skin. In both cases, the legally permitted intention and the legally permitted result, was death of the fetus. Because of this arbitrary fact, the abortion required a hysterotomy. Because of the hysterotomy, the fetus was seen to have been possibly viable. Because of the fetus' possible viability, Edelin was charged with manslaughter and a trial occurred. Had the fetus not been in the anterior position, Edelin would have done a normal, late second-trimester abortion and his name would never have become linked with a famous case in medical ethics.

The Argument from Marginal Cases

The objection, "Where do you draw the line?" figured in this case. It is basically the *argument from marginal cases,* one of the most popular ideas in ethics. This argument—in essence—denies that beings at the margins of the concept of personhood can be nonarbitrarily distinguished from those at the core. It is used in arguments about euthanasia, animal experimentation, and clinical genetics.

Its basic use is simple in this case. Fetal development is smooth and continuous; there are no quantum jumps of "ensoulment." No matter what week is emphasized, antiabortionists claim that it's arbitrary to make a particular point such as viability the marker of personhood, because a fetus has almost the same qualities the week before. Whatever time or marker is picked, someone can always plausibly ask: Why not a week before? Why not some other marker?

Is the argument from marginal cases true? Abortion's supporters say there is a fallacy here like the paradox of Zeno, which said that an arrow cannot go from X to Y because each point in between can be divided into an infinite number of smaller spaces, and no arrow can cross an infinite space. Similarly, there is no place to justifiably distinguish an embryo from a newborn baby because of the smooth continuity of fetal development. Opponents retort that it's a mistake to say there's no difference between an 8-day-old embryo and an 8-day-old newborn baby.

Some antiabortionists say that everything in the newborn was in the embryo in potential. If so, this throws us back to the discussion in the last chapter about the status of embryos.

Standards of Personhood

Some antiabortionists say something is awry here. At the other end of life, society finds it perfectly acceptable to say that life does and does not exist on various sides of a factual marker. For example, it says that comatose patients without brain-wave activity are no longer persons. If that is so, shouldn't society be consistent and say that fetuses, who can be determined to have brain-wave activity during the first trimester, are persons at that point? If not, why is brain-wave activity a marker of personhood at one end of life but not the other?

Some people dislike the brain-wave standard as a marker of nonpersonhood and prefer the more general standard of irreversibility of unconsciousness. Why is this? Most generally, it's because virtually all potential for normal life is gone when patients lapse into such long, deep comas. But again, if potential is the real reason, why, at the other end of life, is potential said by pro-choicers to be irrelevant?

Thomson's Limited, Pro-Abortion View

If a fetus in the Edelin case was a person, does it logically follow that killing it is always immoral? If a fetus has a right to life, isn't it always wrong to kill it? Philosopher Judith Jarvis Thomson says no.[18] Suppose you enter a hospital for an operation, wake up afterwards, and find yourself hooked up to a famous violinist, whose blood enters and leaves your body though tubes. Your kidneys are being used against your will to keep him alive.

Thomson says it's immoral to force you to keep the violinist alive, although it would be saintly if you did. The same applies to slavery. It might be that Scarlet will be poor and Tara will be lost if slavery is abolished, but morality does not require some to be slaves so that Scarlett might be happy.

In this analogy, Thomson has granted the antiabortionist the crucial premise that the fetus is a person with a right to life. But even then, she says, it does not follow that all abortions are immoral. Why? Because killings in self-defense are justified. The violinist cannot demand, as his right, that you keep him hooked up. Society, she argues, similarly cannot force a woman to remain "hooked up" to a fetus against her will, using her body for 9 months as a fetal incubator.

The most telling case for Thomson is rape. In no sense has a raped woman consented to conceiving a child, yet conception may occur. Just as the violinist has no claim for life support, so a rapist's fetus has no claim on the woman's body. Similar arguments apply to women who responsibly use contraception which fails them. Thomson's argument is important in the Alice Roe case because the case contained a hint of incest. One rumor was that Alice waited so long because she didn't want to accept, or didn't want her mother to know, what had happened. If Alice was in such a situation, then even if her fetus were a person, Thomson would allow her to abort. On the other hand, if Alice was merely irresponsible, Thomson's arguments would not apply.

Thomson thinks that live-born, aborted fetuses ought to be saved. Once the fetus is physically separated from the mother's body, her original argument no longer applies, i.e., abortion rights for Thomson do not entail a mother's right to a dead fetus. Her basic intuition is that independently existing persons have rights to life and control of their bodies. And, as medical ethicist Daniel Wikler argues, separation from a mother is as good a place as any to make the transition from fetus to person. It is certainly no more arbitrary than viability.[19]

Rights to Abortion and Rights to Dead Fetuses

It was remarked that Thomson believes that live-born fetuses ought to be saved and that Wikler believes that separation of a fetus from a mother is a good place to begin personhood. On these accounts, once a fetus draws a breath outside the mother's womb, that fetus is a person and efforts ought to be made to save its life. This criterion also agrees with the implication of Genesis 2:7 that God's gift of "the breath of life" establishes personhood.

If this position is correct, something seems odd about the Edelin case in that merely by being taken out of the womb, the fetus could have become a person and have had a right to life. This implication seems odd. So instead perhaps a distinction should be made between a right to an abortion and a right to a dead fetus. Edelin could have taken the fetus from Alice Roe, discharged her from the hospital in a few days, and made the baby a ward of the state of Massachusetts. He could have granted Alice's right to abortion, but recognized no right to have the abortion result in a dead fetus.

Feminist Views

Feminists say that differences about abortion are not about the metaphysics of fetal personhood but about worldviews. Such differences are about proper roles of women, about sex, about children, and about relations between men and women. The fact value gap arises here. If evaluative premises about fetal personhood are dependent on worldviews, then acceptance of such premises can be gained only to the extent that worldviews are subject to rational proof or disproof. Evaluative conclusions can only be validly derived from *evaluative*, and not factual, premises, and to think otherwise is to jump the fact value gap. Even if some people take brain-wave activity to establish personhood, it does not establish that such activity ought to be the standard

Feminist and *Village Voice* editor, Ellen Willis, says that the key question is whether women should be forced to bear children in a way in which men are not. If fetuses are persons who have the right to life at a mother's expense, then women always will be potential slaves of biological reproduction:

> With all the imperfections of our present-day attitudes, I'm still a lot
> better off in terms of the sexual choices I have than women of my
> mother's generation. I was a lot better off after the sixties than I was
> before them. What sexual freedom I now have has been very hard-won.
> I wouldn't give it up for anything. . . . There is a larger crisis, one that
> has to do with the tensions between feminism and the backlash against
> it. On the one hand, society is encouraging sexual freedom; on the
> other hand, it's punishing people for indulging in it and not emotion-
> ally preparing them for it. Both women in general and teenagers in
> particular are caught in the middle.[20]

In contrast to Willis, antiabortionists urge "responsibility"—meaning either abstinence or responsible birth control. Whether "responsibility" can work
is controversial. A 1986 NIH study of never-married women in their twenties
discovered that 80 percent had had sex, that one-third had lived with a man,
and that of sexually active women, one-sixth did not use contraceptives.[21]
These 8.1 million American women in 1983 had 400,000 births and 660,000
abortions. For women such as Phyllis Schafley, these figures show that more
responsibility is needed, especially in this day of AIDS. For others, they show
that responsibility isn't working.

The issue of "being responsible" and preventing pregnancy in unwed
women is more complicated than the typical simplistic reactions. Middle-class
parents commonly do, in fact, get teenagers to be responsible and not conceive. In poor communities, bigger problems exist and cycles of teenage pregnancies perpetuate poverty. (This issue is discussed more in Chapter 14.)

Fetal Research

The Edelin case also raised issues about fetal research, issues which went beyond those of abortion, because such research involves experimentation on
beings at the borderlines of personhood—fetuses, primates, and comatose patients. Fetal research can occur in utero or on aborted, live-born fetuses.

In 1973 and 1974, both kinds of research occurred. One study then of an
artificial placenta used eight fetuses—obtained by hysterotomy—weighing between 300 and 1000 grams.[22] If the artificial placenta had worked, it could have
kept alive premature babies with undeveloped lungs. Could an artificial placenta deliver oxygenated blood to fetuses whose lungs had not developed?
Warm saline solution mimicking the amniotic sac and tubes were placed in
veins and arteries of aborted, live-born fetuses.

The artificial oxygenation system was not successful and the fetuses died
after a few hours. The largest fetus made frantic "gasping" efforts and limb-
stretching movements as it died. Critics say such fetuses experienced pain;

physiologists and anatomists deny this. As with Karen Quinlan, no proof of lack of pain was possible. Harvard ethicist Sissela Bok said that because such nonviable fetuses could not experience pain and were dying, they could not be harmed.[23] Critics said this reasoning was too quick and specious.

Another experiment on fetuses studied whether the brain of a fetus could survive if the mother went into diabetic shock and failed to provide glucose to the fetal brain. To study this, heads were removed from twelve, nonviable fetuses whose heartbeats had stopped and before lack of oxygen damaged brain tissue. The heads were maintained artificially and it was thereby discovered that glucose could be replaced in an emergency with a synthetic liver fat.

These experiments incensed antiabortionists. As writer Maggie Scarf said, "Some types of scientific research, particularly those that may serve to harden or brutalize the investigator (and the society he or she serves as well), may simply not to be worth the moral price they exact."[24] Medical researchers reply that laypeople have no idea how brutalizing medicine already is, that these experiments aren't any worse, and that physicians aren't thereby turned into Dr. Frankensteins.

In 1974, HHS put a moratorium on both embryonic and fetal research, a moratorium which was to be lifted by Congress upon a favorable report from the newly created National Commission for the Protection of Human Subjects in Biomedical and Behavioral Research (the predecessor of the President's Commission). The commission's first job was to report on the ethics of embryo/fetal research (as reported in the last chapter). Although allowing research on early embryos, it suggested prohibiting research on live-born fetuses. Such research today remains under federal moratorium for institutions receiving federal funds.

Scientists say the moratorium stunted research on premature babies, and, in 1988, mounted a campaign to overturn the ban. Scientists argued that embryos and very small fetuses lack normal criteria of personhood such as consciousness, rationality, language, and autonomy, and are much like animals, the normal subjects of experiments (see Chapter 8). Indeed, adult chimpanzees and pigs have much more awareness and sensitivity than human neonates. So why not use an aborted, brain-dead fetus in experiments to benefit future, wanted children? However, this campaign was unsuccessful in ending the ban.

Opponents of fetal research see fetal experimentation as criminal negligence or worse. Paul Ramsey emphasized that the mother's decision to abort puts her in a conflict of interest with a live-born fetus. For Ramsey, experimentation on any such fetus is unconsented-to research and immoral exploitation of "a tragical case of a dying baby."[25]

A different issue concerned transplanting cells of aborted fetuses. Such transplants have been promising in research treating Alzheimer's and Parkinson's diseases, and juvenile diabetes. Preliminary work with rats, part of whose brains were destroyed, showed some restoration of memory after fetal-rat cell injections. Opponents of abortion fear such research would encourage abortions for the wrong reasons and would dehumanize researchers. Supporters emphasize the tragedy of neurological disease.

Abortion's Alternatives

Opponents argue that it is paradoxical for one unit to be terminating fetuses, as Edelin did, while down the hall, an NICU struggles to save a premature baby of the same age and weight. In the trial, Edelin was asked how two such babies differed and replied that they involved a difference in "intent" of the women: in one case, a woman did not want the fetus growing inside her, but in the other case, she did. Opponents replied that "being wanted" is too flimsy a standard for the value of life. Others retort: that's the way it is.

Opponents stress that there are not enough healthy babies to go around for adoption. If there were more, infertile couples would be less frantic to use in vitro fertilization. Supporters of Edelin say adoption isn't a viable alternative because babies of color are not easily adoptable, and this case involved a black, male baby. Second, a premature black baby is likely to have health problems or be retarded from lack of oxygen. Unhealthy, nonwhite babies rarely find adoptive parents.

Live-Born Fetuses and Abortion

Supporters of abortion often ridicule antiabortionists' reluctance to "draw the line" somewhere and say that embryos are not persons. The same argument can cut both ways. Is there *no* point where abortion is wrong? The issue raised in the Edelin case, of what to do with a viable or live-born fetus, differs from the issues where an abortion is performed on a nonviable fetus.

In 1977, physician Ronald Cornelson testified in California criminal court that, after a saline abortion resulted in a live-born baby, his colleague William Waddill choked a 2.5-lb live-born baby and suggested injections with potassium chloride to kill it. (This was the weight of the famous horse jockey, Willie Shoemaker, when he was born in Texas as a premature baby and put in a shoebox in a oven to keep warm.) Waddill was twice tried for murder, but the juries twice deadlocked.[26] In 1979, another 2.5-pound baby was live-born after saline abortion at the University of Nebraska Medical Center, and the physician doing the abortion told nurses to leave it alone and let it die, which it did after a few hours.

These cases perhaps explain why the Supreme Court granted legal protection to fetuses in the third trimester. The underlying view appears to be that the fetus becomes more of a person as it approaches birth, such that a 30-week old fetus might be called (somewhat awkwardly) "two-thirds of a person."

Because of such cases, physicians performing abortions today rarely do so after 24 weeks. By the late 1980s, the above problems were finessed by no longer using prostaglandins, which were safer than traditional methods but which increased the rate of live-born fetuses by 30 times. Physicians now use traditional, crude methods, which combine injection of hostile liquids (saline or urea) with D and E (dilation and evacuation). D and E isn't the more minor procedure of dilation and curettage (D and C). D and E surgically removes the fetus in parts and never results in live-born cases. To prevent infection in the mother from a remaining fetal part, the dismembered fetus must be reassembled to insure that all parts have been removed.

SUBSEQUENT ABORTION DECISIONS AND ISSUES

U.S. Supreme Court Decisions

A subsequent Supreme Court decision invalidated state laws requiring either consent of the biological or matrimonial father for women's abortions or consent of parents for abortions. The 1976 Danforth Court said consent of others over a pregnant woman amounted to a veto, and that the woman "is the more directly and immediately affected by the pregnancy."

In 1977, the Court said poor women can have abortions but government (Medicaid) needn't pay for them. In 1981, the Court said that a law requiring parental notification could be legal if it had an escape clause allowing a minor a chance to show a judge she was mature enough to make the decision herself. Several states then passed such statutes. In 1983, the court struck down Akron, Ohio's "informed consent" requirement, saying it was designed not to inform but to dissuade. After testimony from the American College of Obstetricians and Gynecologists that second-trimester D and C was no longer dangerous in clinics, the court overturned its previous second trimester hospital-admission requirement in *Roe vs. Wade.*

It was exactly such changes in medical technology that Justice Sandra Day O'Connor worried about in 1983.[27] She said *Roe vs. Wade* invited continued reinterpretation about viability, maternal health, and trimesters, and that the trimester framework "was clearly on a collision course with itself." She preferred getting the U.S. Supreme Court altogether out of the business of regulating abortion, and would let states handle such regulation.

The 1989 Webster Decision

In July 1989, the U.S. Supreme Court announced a widely awaited decision. During the preceding decade, President Reagan had appointed several justices to the court who were reported to be antiabortion. By some counts, the new court was 5 to 4 against abortion.

The 5-to-4 *Webster* decision held that it was legal for states to prohibit abortions in state-financed, public hospitals (consistent with its previous decision that Congress was not obligated to pay for abortions for poor women). Similarly, states could ban publicly paid employees from performing abortions. On the one hand, this merely continued the idea that a person may have the liberty to do something, but government has no obligation to provide her money so she can do it. On the other hand, some wondered why only this standard medical service was allowed to be prohibited.

The court also held, given the importance of viability, that states could require physicians to test for viability after 20 weeks, e.g., by ultrasound. (The 20-week point was chosen because of possible errors of 3 to 4 weeks in judging fetal age and because few fetuses are viable before 23–24 weeks because of lack of lung capacity.) As even Justice Blackmun noted in his dissent, nothing in these three decisions contradicted *Row vs. Wade.* In its actual effect, the decision was narrow, allowing almost all abortions in abortion clinics to continue as before.

However, the various opinions of the justices hinted at more to come. By scheduling three more cases about abortion for the next term, the court guaranteed continued controversy. Surprisingly, many of the justices seemed most concerned to get the whole issue of abortion out of their court. Justices O'Connor (in her previous opinion) and Scalia explicitly wanted such "political" decisions returned to the democratic process of the state legislatures. Justices Rehnquist and O'Connor seemed most concerned that the trimester system and viability necessitated the court's continual review of medical technology, and both seemed willing to go to some other system.

Even if subsequent decisions reject the trimester system and viability as a cutoff point, it is likely that legal abortions will be available in some places in America. As mentioned above, several states—including New York—had already legalized abortion before *Roe vs. Wade.*

Nevertheless, given the cost of traveling to states where abortions are legal, as well as the court's new position that states need not pay for abortions for poor women, combined with previous bans on federal funding for abortions for poor women, it appears that the country may be moving to a two-tiered system of access to abortion.

Antiabortion Activity

For over a decade, opponents of abortion have fought at state and federal levels for a constitutional amendment to ban abortions. They had some momentum but were never ultimately successful. Because polls consistently show 50 to 70 percent of Americans favoring abortions under some circumstances, an amendment to ban all abortions is unlikely.

In 1982, three abortion clinics were attacked. Two Texas men who attacked Florida abortion clinics were sentenced to 30 years in prison. One of them had previously kidnapped Illinois physician Hector Zevallos and his wife because Zevallos performed abortions. In 1983, two abortion clinics were bombed or burned. Peter Burkin firebombed a New York abortion clinic and went to prison. In 1984, 24 attacks occurred. The last, in 1983, came in Pensacola, Florida, on Christmas morning—"a birthday present to Jesus," said the girlfriend and co-conspirator of one of the convicted bombers.[28] Mathew Goldsby and James Simmons pleaded insanity but got 10 years. In December of 1984, a bomb destroyed an abortion clinic in a Maryland suburb of Washington, D.C., and just missed killing a security guard. As a result of these attacks, insurance premiums soared for abortion clinics and some had to close. Most stayed open but had to charge more for abortions.

The bombings of abortion clinics resulted in a backlash from most Americans, who began to perceive all antiabortionists as fanatics. As a result, antiabortion tactics drastically changed in 1988, when Operation Rescue began at abortion clinics across the country. It involved sit-ins modeled on the civil disobedience of the civil rights movement in the 1960s, and most important, it was nonviolent.

However, hours before the above announcement of the *Webster* decision, a fire broke out at a Concord, N.H., abortion clinic. A Fire Department captain said an arsonist had set the fire.

Involuntary Treatment in Utero

In 1973, the New Jersey Supreme Court forced a Jehovah's Witness to undergo surgery and blood transfusions to save her fetus. If delivered vaginally, the baby would have died, but if delivered by caesarean, the baby would have lived. The mother's religious beliefs forbade surgery: "God will decide what happens." The court said otherwise, saying that freedom of religion allowed her to refuse for herself, but not for her child, who as an adult might not accept her beliefs. Since then, many similar cases have been handled in the same way.

In 1985, Pamela Rae Stewart, who abused drugs, was charged with neglecting her third-trimester fetus.[29] Because Stewart suffered from *placenta abruptio*, a placenta likely to separate from the uterine wall, physicians urged her to return if hemorrhaging began. When she did not and the baby died, someone in the hospital notified child protective services, who notified police, who notified the deputy district attorney in El Cajon, Cal. Under a 1925 statute forbidding withholding of medical care, she was charged with "fetal neglect." The district attorney argued that there was no difference between withholding treatment from a 35-week, unborn baby and doing so from a newborn. Ultimately, a judge threw the case out, saying the old law wasn't intended to cover a case such as hers.

A 1986 case in Georgia raised slightly different questions, when 25-year-old Donna Piazzi lay brain dead in an ICU with a 23-week-old fetus growing inside her.[30] She was found in a drug overdose in an Augusta mall. Her husband wanted medical care stopped, but another man claimed to be the father of the child and wanted it. He asked physicians to treat Donna, so that the baby should live. The husband opposed this, saying Donna had a right to die, even if it meant the fetus' death. The husband did not prevail. Donna was maintained at Medicaid expense, and a month later, a fetus with multiple defects, which did not survive, was delivered.

In the late 1980s, conflict intensified between fetal treatment and maternal rights. Remarkable advances in fetal medicine allowed *in utero* treatment of congestive heart failure with digitalis or by surgical correction of cleft palates (the baby, at birth, has absolutely no scars). Such treatments could only normally occur with maternal consent. But what if a mother refused? At the same time, ob/gyn physicians saw more and more pregnant mothers who were addicted to drugs and who would bring such babies into the world similarly addicted (and sometimes, with the AIDS virus). As fetal medicine allowed physicians to do much more for fetuses, and as premature fetuses therefore became viable at earlier points, physicians increasingly felt torn between duties to *two* patients.

This conflict surfaced in 1987, in Washington, D.C., with "Angela C.," a 27-year-old woman who was rapidly dying of cancer, and who refused a cesarean to save her 26-week-old fetus.[31] Angela's hospital obtained a court order in 6 hours for the cesarean to save the baby. The operation took place against the explicit wishes of Angela, her family, and her physicians. The fetus did not live and Angela died two days later, with her caesarean listed as a contributing factor in her death.

The conflict about "two patients" also appeared in a different way in the 1989 case of the pregnant but comatose Nancy Klein.[32] Her husband, Martin, wanted to allow physicians to perform an abortion on Nancy on the chance that it might help her revive. Antiabortionists opposed his request in court to be appointed Nancy's guardian, but were denied. Amidst much controversy, Martin Klein allowed the abortion.

UPDATE

RU 486 is a new pill which dislodges an embryo implanted in the uterus. If it became widely available in America, as it is expected to be in China, England, and France, it could change the way abortions are done. For most women, abortion could be done completely in private and at very little cost. For this reason, antiabortionists waged vigorous campaigns to ban the drug in America. A similar campaign succeeded in France for 1 day and was then overturned.

In 1988, Newman Flanagan was still district attorney for Boston and was involved in another medical ethics case. This one involved prosecuting a Christian Scientist couple for manslaughter for not seeking medical treatment for their sick child. Kenneth Edelin today practices medicine in Boston.[33]

FURTHER READING

Larry Churchill and José Siman, "Abortion and the Rhetoric of Individual Rights," *Hastings Center Report*, 12(1):9–12 (February 1982).

John C. Fletcher et al., "Fetal Research: The State of the Question," *Hastings Center Report*, 15(2):12–16 (April 1985).

William Nolen, *The Baby in the Bottle*, Coward, McCann & Geoghegan, New York, 1978.

William Ruddick and William Wilcox, "Operating on the Fetus," *Hastings Center Report*, 12(5):10–13 (October 1982).

CHAPTER 7

The Baby Jane Doe Case

"Baby Doe cases" occur when parents and physicians face decisions about whether to decline or withdraw treatment to hasten death for defective neonates. This chapter focuses on the 1983 Baby Jane Doe case at Stony Brook, N.Y.

HISTORICAL BACKGROUND

In ancient Sparta, a Cyclops baby would be left to die in a country field. Both the *Republic* of Plato and the *Politics* of Aristotle advocated killing defective newborns. Romans thought it proper to discard babies who looked grotesque. For most of two millennia, Bedouin tribes of Arabia, the Chinese, and much of India practiced female infanticide. Males stayed with the family and were considered assets, whereas females left the family and were considered liabilities.[1]

The Christian church, as it began to be organized during the first three centuries A.D., condemned late-term abortion and infanticide. Around 300 A.D., Roman Emperor Constantine converted to Christianity and was persuaded to ban parental infanticide. His edict resulted in circumventions by parents who didn't want defective babies. While it was illegal to kill children, it was not illegal to abandon them in rural fields to die of exposure. The exposure of defective babies was a very common practice during the first four centuries A.D. and such "letting die" was not considered infanticide (or active killing).

Christianity strongly condemned both abandonment and infanticide, but had neither funds nor people to care for abandoned babies; it did not establish a foundling hospital until the 8th century in Milan. In his *History of European Morals*, William Lecky concludes ambivalently about Christianity's influence: it was the first to value "the castaways of society," but its role in protecting infant life "often has been exaggerated."[2]

During the Middle Ages, wet nurses aided parents wishing for others to raise their children or wishing to rid themselves of children. In the 18th century, Europe was overrun by exploding populations, resulting in exposure and infanticide functioning as birth control. Overpopulation revived institutionalized abandonment in France, Germany, and England. Well into the 19th century, parents continued to turn unwanted babies over to *balie* (wet nurses) or simply had them "put out" (abandoned) to rural baby farms where they were often fed gin to die painlessly. So many babies were abandoned during Napoleon's era that he established Foundling Hospitals, where parents could anonymously deposit a baby on a turntable, spin the wheel, and leave. In France in 1833, over a hundred thousand babies were abandoned.[3]

A hundred years ago, Thomas Wakley, founder of the *Lancet* medical journal, campaigned against such practices. The Infant Life Protection Society was founded in 1870 to oppose farms and "burial clubs" where parents collected from payouts on multiple life insurance policies on dead babies.

The 1960s witnessed the development of neonatal intensive care units (NICUs), which kept alive the kind of premature baby who had previously died. The 1970s saw development of small respirators and feeding tubes, which saved many babies, but which also salvaged some babies who were born dying. While often impossible to know from external observation, premature babies often suffered neurological hemorrhages or lung damage from respirators. Such care in NICUs, which is also very expensive, raises ethical questions about which babies should be treated and who should make such decisions.

BACKGROUND TO THE BABY JANE DOE CASE

The Baby Jane Doe case in 1983 took place against a background of several previous cases which had prompted the Baby Doe Rules, which were in effect during the case. These cases and rules are described below.

The 1971 Johns Hopkins Cases

Down syndrome, or trisomy 21, is a chromosomal abnormality discovered by Langdon Down in 1866, in which infants have 47 rather than 46 chromosomes in each cell, the extra chromosome being attached to chromosome 21. Down syndrome is a genetic condition always causing retardation and characteristic facial appearance; it is often accompanied by cardiac problems.

In 1971, in a NICU at Johns Hopkins Hospital in Baltimore, some Down syndrome babies were born with defects incompatible with life. During this time, few NICUs existed and few defective infants were treated aggressively. The same baby born today in an NICU would be treated very differently.

One mother in this case was a nurse who had worked previously with Down syndrome children; her 35-year-old husband was a lawyer. Her baby had duodenal atresia—a blockage between the higher duodenum and the lower stomach—which prevented passage of food and water. She was told that her baby had Down syndrome and that it would die if she did not consent to surgery to open the atresia. She immediately refused to sign, and the husband agreed. Pediatric surgeons and administrators honored the parents' refusal and did not go to court.

The film *Who Should Survive?* by the Joseph P. Kennedy Jr. Foundation describes a composite case created from the real cases at Hopkins where the above case supplied most of the details. The film portrays this case, but never gives viewers these parents' reasons for their decision.[4] Sociologist Renée Fox says the couple appeared to be "of modest means," suggesting they had middle-class income at best.[5]

One mother was told at the time by a physician that the degree of mental retardation and IQ score could not be predicted at birth, but that Down syndrome people range in IQ "in the 50–80 range, and some times a little higher."[6] She was also told that some rare Down syndrome adults score above IQ 65, but that the normal IQ range is between 25 and 60, with some severely defective individuals below 25. The same physician told the parents that children with Down syndrome were "almost always trainable. They can hold simple jobs. And they're famous for being happy children." (Whether this information is correct will be discussed later.)

In one case, the parents had two other children, in another case, five. One mother's reason for her decision was that "it would be unfair to the other children of the household to raise them with a mongoloid."[7] Commentator and theologian, James Gustafson, says one mother's decision was "anguished" and that when she heard her baby had Down syndrome, she "immediately indicated she did not want the child."[8]

One baby took 11, and another 15, days to die. Such a death would normally take 4 days, but some staff members, in sympathy with the baby, surreptitiously hydrated the babies. The babies were allowed to die, and not just killed, because it was thought to be more morally acceptable, and less likely to incur legal prosecution, to do it that way.

Neonatologists Debate Ethics

Because of the growing number of cases of this kind in NICUs, several well-known pediatricians went public in the early 1970s. English pediatrician John Lorber was one, and in 1971, he implied that some defective babies were so horribly deformed that they were better off without treatment (so they would die quickly).[9]

Lorber specialized in spina bifida babies, one of the defects of Baby Jane Doe. Spina bifida literally means "divided spine." Spina bifida occurs in one in 1000 live births and is the most common serious neural tube defect. Spina bifida may be in the form of meningocele (a balloonlike sac filled with cerebrospinal fluid) or a meningonyelocele (a similar sac with the same fluid, plus tissue from the spinal nerve or cord).

A meningomyelocele may be an opening without a meningocele, and consequently may leak valuable cerebrospinal fluid. The opening makes infants vulnerable to infections such as meningitis, often lethal in neonates. The baby, almost always paralyzed below the level of the opening, has attendant bowel and bladder problems, so that quality of life partly varies according to the level of the meningomyelocele. Quality of life also varies with associated problems such as hydrocephalus (swelling of cranial tissue), which commonly accompanies spina bifida and which was present in Baby Jane Doe. The swelling of hydrocephalus often causes increased intracranial pressure and decreased blood flow to the brain, and thus, mental retardation. Aggressive surgical treatment, with tubes called "shunts," can decrease such pressure and lessen chances of retardation.

Lorber developed prognostic criteria which predicted which spina bifida babies would die if left untreated. The higher the meningomyelocele on the spine and the larger the area affected of the spine and its coverings, the more likely the attendant problems and the greater the likelihood of death for the baby.

Lorber's criteria addressed the problem that some untreated infants do not die when left untreated. For them, nontreatment makes them worse off. (One untreated spina bifida person, who had been abandoned and "warehoused" for many years, reportedly tested at a Stanford Binet IQ of 80). Lorber's criteria seemingly solved this problem because *all* infants in his lowest category died.

Two years later, pediatricians Duff and Campbell wrote a ground-breaking article, which discussed unfortunate results from aggressive treatment.[10] Complicated neonatal cases from across Connecticut were referred to their NICU at Yale–New Haven Medical Center, which had the unusual policy of allowing daily access to parents.

The visiting parents, especially professional ones, affected the neonatologists greatly, creating in the latter "increasing doubts about the wisdom of many of the decisions that seemed to parents to be predicated chiefly on technical considerations." In cases with poor prognosis, the pediatricians allowed parents to withhold care. Of the 299 deaths over 2 years in the Yale NICU, 43 (14 percent) were "associated with discontinuance or withdrawal of treatment." These included, first, a spinal bifida child with hydrocephalus and multiple-organ anomalies and, second, a Down syndrome baby with idiopathic respiratory-distress syndrome and cor pulmonale (right ventricular strain secondary to pulmonary hypertension).

Some of the babies in the Yale NICU were so defective that they likely had little chance for personhood. Some babies were institutionalized in places which were described by one author (quoted by Duff and Campbell) as "hardly more than dying bins." Duff and Campbell quoted respected physician, Louis Lasagna, "We may, as a society, scorn civilizations that slaughtered their infants, but our present treatment of the retarded is in some ways more cruel."

Follow-up revealed no correlation between decision and religion, and a year later, no parents appeared traumatized by their decision. Some even claimed that the dying of their child had been a "deeply moving experience which had provided meaning in life." Duff and Campbell reported various objections by residents and attendings to letting parents make such decisions:

little parental understanding of medical conditions and prognosis, loss of "teaching material," and a slippery slope to conditions in medicine like those during the Nazi reign. But the same physicians said that, as parents, they also would have withheld treatment.

The surprising aspect of this article, which undoubtedly accounted for its influence, was its frank admission that 43 infants had died early because of cessation of treatment. At the time, the two physicians feared that the Connecticut attorney general might prosecute them.

The two pediatricians said parents should make the ultimate decisions. "Since families primarily must live with and are most affected by the decisions, it therefore appears that society and health professionals should provide only general guidelines for decision making." Physicians should not directly make the decisions. Moreover, they added, with a little education, "Parents *are* able to understand the implications of such things as chronic dyspnea, oxygen dependency, incontinence." . . .

The two pediatricians anticipated the Baby Jane Doe case and the "Baby Doe Rules" in discussing whether judges or legislatures should make such decisions. To this they said, "But we also ask, if these parties [physicians and families] cannot make such decisions justly, who can?" Finally, they wondered about the point of abstract moral rules, e.g., the rule about the sanctity of life: "the rules of society or the policies most convenient of medical technologies may become cruel masters of human beings instead of their servants."

The Mueller and Infant Doe Cases

On May 5, 1981, Siamese twins joined at the trunk and sharing three legs were born in Danville, Ill., to physician Robert Mueller and his wife Pamela.[11] Robert was in the delivery room with family physician Petra Warren, who delivered the babies. When Jeff and Scott Mueller were born, the Muellers and Warren together decided not to aggressively treat the twins so that they could die. An anonymous caller alerted Protective Child Services, which obtained a court order giving it temporary custody of the children.

Danville physicians divided deeply over the ethics of the Muellers' decision. The Muellers were charged with neglect, but a later hearing dismissed these charges while denying custody to the Muellers. In September, they regained custody after pediatric surgeons testified that the prognosis was bleak for successful separating.

The Danville Siamese twins were a precursor to the Infant Doe case about a year later.[12] On April 9, 1982, a baby with Down syndrome was born in nearby Bloomington, Ind. with tracheosophageal fistula. The baby subsequently became nationally known as "Infant Doe."

Physicians again divided over nontreatment. Tracheosophageal fistula is more serious than duodenal atresia. Prognosis tends to vary with the severity of the fistula or gap. In this case, the gap was fairly small. Surgeons said surgery had a 80 to 90 percent chance of success; others, merely 50 percent. The parents chose not to operate, based on information about prognosis provided by their obstetrician and because the child had Down syndrome.

Hospital administrators and pediatricians disagreed with the decision, and convened an emergency session the next day by Special Circuit Judge John Baker, who ruled that the parents had the right to make the decision. The county district attorney intervened and appealed the decision to the County Circuit Court, and after losing, to the Indiana Supreme Court. Each appeal failed; each time the courts ruled for the parents. The prosecutors appealed to Supreme Court Justice Paul Stevens for an emergency stay, but Infant Doe died before they arrived in Washington, D.C. rendering the appeal for a stay moot.

THE BABY DOE RULES

The Infant Doe case was followed intensely in the media and prompted President Reagan to direct the Justice Department and Department of Health and Human Services (HHS) to mandate treatment in similar future cases. Reagan opposed abortion and had appointed C. Everett Koop as his surgeon general—a pediatrician who had condemned abortion and nontreatment of impaired newborns.

Citizens may be accused of violations of the criminal or civil code of a state. Operating without consent is a criminal battery, operating incompetently is the civil violation of malpractice. In general, penalties for criminal infractions are more severe than for civil infractions.

Because crimes such as homicide and gross negligence are defined by state law, the federal government could not say that nontreatment was illegal. Thus an indirect route was used: the so-called Baby Doe Rules were implemented, rules which required treatment of all defective newborns and which defined nontreatment as a violation of Section 504 of the Rehabilitation Act of 1973, which forbade discrimination solely on the basis of handicap. In a new conceptual synthesis, *imperiled newborns were said to be handicapped citizens who could suffer discrimination.*

These rules were widely misunderstood: they did not assert that handicapped infants had a right to life but rather that denying them treatment violated their civil rights. Violators of such rules faced civil, not criminal, charges. The real pressure of the rules was that institutions violating the Baby Doe Rules were threatened with loss of funds. Through such rules, the executive branch can make social policy by reinterpreting prior congressional legislation. (The first civil-rights activity in the 1960s began with such executive orders by President Johnson.)

About a year after Infant Doe had died, HHS sent to NICUs notice of an "Interim Final Rule" which angered many pediatricians. Large posters were to be displayed by March 22, 1983, outside NICUs saying:

DISCRIMINATORY FAILURE TO FEED AND CARE FOR HANDICAPPED INFANTS

IN THIS FACILITY IS PROHIBITED BY FEDERAL LAW.

A tollfree 800-number was posted to report abuses—the so-called Baby Doe Hotline—which pediatricians feared would be used by irate nurses, disgruntled parents, ambulance-chasing lawyers, and anonymous cranks. So-called Baby Doe squads, composed of lawyers, government administrators, and physicians, investigated complaints. In the last 9 months alone of 1983, the hotline had 1633 calls; of these, 49 incidents were actually investigated.

What happened as a result of such squads? *Newsday* studied 36 investigations and discovered:

> ...in some cases, intervention has saved a baby with a fair chance of living a useful life; in others, extraordinary surgical measures have given babies no more than a few extra days of life at enormous financial and emotional costs. In one case, the medical bills mounted to $400,000 for a baby who doctors say "has zero chance for a normal life expectancy." In a few instances, parents had to give up custody of their children to the state after they refused to permit surgery.

> Records of 49 cases investigated by the Health and Human Services Department's civil rights office during the last 19 months show that in only six cases has government intervention appeared to have made a difference, with children given operations or treatment they otherwise would not have had. In 14 of the cases, mostly originated by anonymous calls, investigation proved that allegations of insufficient treatment were false or that treatment was medically impossible.[13]

During the time of their reign, Baby Doe squads operated under a great sense of moral urgency. Existence of the squads seemed to imply that evil pediatricians all across the country were conspiring with parents to kill handicapped newborns. The squads were ready on a hour's notice to rush to airports, fly across the country, and suddenly arrive—as one squad did one day at Vanderbilt University—like a surprise bank audit by outside accountants. Records were seized, charts were taken from attending physicians, and all-night investigations took place. The attitude of the squads was that time was of the essence because an innocent baby's life might be at stake. Besides Vanderbilt, the University of Rochester suffered (to use the terms used privately by some pediatricians) "a *blitzkreig* by the Baby Doe Gestapo." During the time the rule was in force, and according to the above *Newsday* investigation, the squads discovered no violation of federal antidiscrimination laws.

The squads made enemies of most physicians, even those who shared their goals. Medical staffs complained of their witch-hunting approach. Also, most pediatricians didn't want Uncle Sam looking over their shoulder. The American Academy of Pediatrics (AAP) went to court to fight the squads.

There was another reason the pediatric academy did this. Many pediatricians just did not believe that aggressive treatment was in the best interest of all severely defective babies. Some babies, they said, really might be better off dead.

Almost every physician had an intense opinion, one way or the other. *New England Journal of Medicine* associate editor, Marcia Angell, complained that the idea of such squads treated parents "as though they were enemies kept at bay" and she disliked the Reagan administration's primitive approach.[14] Her editorial irritated other physicians who emphasized that "the handicapped child is the patient," not the parents, and that physicians must be such patients' advocates. One of them wrote that "Elder Does" would soon be dying if Infant Does were allowed to die, and that, "Baby Doe was denied this routine surgery because he had Down's syndrome and for no other reason."[15] This last point was certainly true. However, and for various reasons, nobody wanted to admit it publicly.

The President's Commission on medical ethics, which had previously studied brain death, released its Baby Doe recommendations just before the Interim Final Rule became effective in March 1983. The pluralistic commission, with many conservative members, partially endorsed choice by parents in Baby Doe cases, but added the important caveat, "unless their choice...is clearly against the infant's best interests." Also, "an otherwise healthy Down syndrome child, whose life is threatened by a surgically correctable complication, should receive the surgery because he or she would clearly benefit from it."[16]

The original rule had neither been posted and nor had solicited comments in advance, as required by regulations. Citing the lack of notice and posting, the Court in 1983 invalidated the rules. Suitably chastized and this time soliciting comments in advance, HHS proposed *new* Baby Doe rules a few months later. The new rules required smaller signs, which were to be placed *inside* NICUs, so that only staff could read them. The squads were called off. The tollfree number remained on the signs.

THE BABY JANE DOE CASE

In early 1983, the revised Baby Doe Rules were about to go into effect but were being challenged in court by the pediatric academy. While this court battle was ongoing, Baby "Jane Doe" was born on October 11, 1983, at the St. Charles Hospital of Long Island, N.Y. Because she had several major defects, she was transferred to an NICU at University Hospital of the SUNY campus of Stony Brook.

Parents Linda and Dan A. had voted for Ronald Reagan in 1980 and were lower-middle-class people, working hard to be upper-class. They appeared months later on *60 Minutes.* They had been married 4 months when the 23-year-old Mrs. A. became pregnant, and the 30-year-old Mr. A. had built two extra rooms onto (what has been described as) their "modest suburban home" in the "flatlands of eastern Long Island." In another anticipation of the birth, the couple took natural childbirth classes.

Their baby was said to have been born with spina bifida, hydrocephalus, a damaged kidney, and an alleged microcephaly (small head, implying lack of brains). Pediatric neurologist Arjen Keuskamp advocated immediate surgery to drain the hydrocephalus and to minimize retardation. The baby's name was Kerri-Lynn, but was called "Baby Jane Doe" by the media and courts to protect her privacy.

Kerri-Lynn's defect must have been traumatic for her parents, for the spine was open with the meningocele protruding prominently. When the 6-pound, 20-inch-long baby was transferred to Stony Brook for the care of neonatal specialists, she was examined by George Newman, another pediatric neurologist, who told Mr. A. that evening that Kerri-Lynn could either die soon without surgery, or have surgery with a life of paralysis, retardation, and continual infections of both the bladder and bowels.

Like other physicians, Drs. Keuskamp and Newman intensely disagreed about treatment in such cases. Whether their different moral views caused them to see the facts differently, or whether their view of factual prognosis caused them to have differing moral views, is impossible to know. In any case, they differed.

Keuskamp withdrew from the case, citing moral disagreement with the parents' decision. Shortly thereafter, a suit was filed in state court. Keuskamp did not testify in that suit, but Newman did. He testified that:

> the decision made by the parents is that it would be unkind to have surgery performed on this child...on the basis of the combination of malformations that are present in this child, she is not likely to ever achieve any meaningful interaction with her environment, nor ever achieve any interpersonal relationships, the very qualities which we consider human.[17]...

So this is what Dr. Newman told Mr. A. about midnight on October 11, 14 hours after Kerri-Lynn was born. After a good deal of consulting with medical professionals, the parents decided not to allow the operation to drain the hydrocephalus, assuming that Kerri-Lynn would soon die. Four days later when she had not died, a social worker wrote that Mr. A. was in "despair" because Kerri-Lynn had not yet died and that Mrs. A. was determined to give Kerri-Lynn "as much love as possible" while she was still alive. "We love her very much," Mrs. A. said, "and that's why we made the decision we did."[18]

Reporter Kathleen Kerr, who broke the story for *Newsday* and who had numerous "firsts" on the story, was also the first reporter (and one of the only reporters) to interview the parents. She describes the interview:

> Each time he began a sentence, Mr. A. let out a deep sigh, as though seeking strength to answer. Mrs. A. continually touched her husband's arm and rubbed it soothingly. Mr. A. shed his tears openly....

> Mr. A. said, "We feel the conservative method of treatment is going to do her as much good as if surgery were to be performed. It's not a case of our not caring. We very much want this baby."

"We're not being neglectful, and we're not relying on our [Catholic] religion to give us the answer to what we're doing here."[19]

The parents acted on the distinction between extraordinary and ordinary care, disallowing surgery but allowing the so-called merely palliative care of food, fluids, and antibiotics. Nevertheless, Kerri-Lynn didn't die. As occurs naturally in some cases, the open spinal wound closed.

About this time, Lawrence Washburn, a municipal bonds lawyer who resided in Vermont, and who was active in right-to-life organizations, filed suit in Kerri-Lynn's behalf in a state court to force treatment. Because Washburn did not have legal standing to sue, attorney William Weber was appointed guardian *ad litem* for the baby (like the one for Karen Quinlan), and was temporarily empowered to make medical decisions.

Weber had initially supported the parents, but at this point, an interesting development occurred. After talking to the pediatric neurologist, George Newman, Weber abruptly changed his mind when he read what Newman had written in Baby Jane's medical chart.[20] Newman had written, Weber said, that after surgery Kerri-Lynn would be able to walk with braces. Weber concluded that what Newman had told the parents and what he had said in court conflicted with what he had written in the chart. On another important fact, Newman testified that the baby had microcephaly and would never be able to recognize her parents. To which, Weber retorted, "A lie. The hospital records shows that the initial measurement of the skull was 31 centimeters, which is within normal limits."

Understanding the subsequent legal battle in this case is a primer of modern law. Weber authorized surgery, but a day later, an appellate New York court reversed the decision. The justices decided that the law left decisions up to parents when choice was available between two "medically reasonable" options. In this judgment, they contradicted precedents, which held that "medically reasonable" decisions were ones both supported by some evidence and, more important, in the interests of the child (see below).

Weber appealed but lost in New York's highest court, the Court of Appeals, which noted that if the crime of neglect had occurred, state child-protection agencies, and not unrelated individuals such as Washburn, were the proper ones to bring the parents to court. (The high court called Washburn's involvement "offensive.") The appeals court said that Weber should never have been empowered to make decisions for baby Kerri-Lynn over the wishes of her parents. In this decision, the appeals court—along with everyone else in the country following the immense publicity—had perhaps become too wrapped up in the case. It completely forgot about the traditional doctrine of *parens patria* in which the state protects the helpless against those who would otherwise hurt or neglect them.

At this point, the parents thought they had won, but the Justice Department filed suit against the hospital in federal court, charging possible discrimination against the handicapped. Attorney General Edwin Meese and Surgeon General Everett Koop personally sent Justice Department lawyers to the federal court. The first step was for the Justice Department to see the medical records, so it sued the hospital to get them. The parents were outraged by the federal action: "They're not doctors, they're not the parents, and they have no business in our lives right now."[21]

In late November, federal Judge Wexler ruled that the Justice Department couldn't have the medical records and that the parents had not decided against surgery for "discriminatory" reasons. The parents were pleased but exhausted. "I'm drained physically, mentally, and emotionally," Mr. A. said. "I believed that you couldn't look at what we were doing and say we were wrong."

The case finally reached the federal Court of Appeals for the Second Circuit, which ruled that Congress had never intended Section 504 of the Rehabilitation Act of 1973 to apply to imperiled newborns. This judgment came in February 1984, just 10 days after HHS announced its revised Baby Doe Rules. The Justice Department appealed to the U.S. Supreme Court.

In 1984, the AMA joined pediatricians and sought an injunction prohibiting HHS from implementing its final Baby Doe Rules. Such an injunction was granted by the same Federal Appellate Court for the Second Circuit in December 1984. The U.S. Supreme Court in *Bowen vs. American Hospital Association et al.* in 1986 found for the AMA and Stony Brook Hospital, holding that no records needed to be released. The highest American court ruled that, because parents are not "federally funded recipients," Section 504 did not apply.

During this process, Mrs. A. said,

> I just want [all this] to end. Just to have a baby like this and deal with it is so much to go through right now. Just let us be with our daughter and leave us alone.

> If there's hell, we've been through it.

ETHICAL ISSUES

Selfish Parents

Theologian James Gustafson criticized the parents in the Johns Hopkins cases. Living one's life for others is the primary ethical requirement of Judaism and Christianity, he said, and the parents didn't want to do that. In attacking this criticism, Jesuit John Paris put Gustafson's concern more succinctly:

> That concern, as the spate of press commentaries indicates, finds its roots in a fear that the "me" generation is reverting to the ancient practice of exposing defective infants to the elements, or worse, that a "consumer" society is demanding the elimination of its less-than-perfect products.[22]

Episcopal priest and medical ethicist John Fletcher disagreed and didn't see religious values as Gustafson did. Fletcher, once the chief consulting medical ethicist for NIH, said he could "stand by the parents" in the Johns Hopkins cases and "would not want to come down real hard on them" for letting their baby die.[23]

Others questioned whether everyone saw his purpose in life in living for others. For a couple where both work, raising a disadvantaged child usually means that one must give up a job, with loss of that income. Moreover, Down syndrome is a lifelong condition, with an average lifespan of 40 and maximal age of 70. Does, or should, every person think that he or she is "called" to spend an entire life caring for such a person?

Champions of the retarded argue that a disadvantaged child cannot be allowed to die merely because it doesn't fit into a couple's life plans. After all, they say, we are not talking about what people want to do, but about what it's right to do. They see parents who let their Down syndrome babies die as lacking a morality, not as accepting a different morality.

Kinds of Cases

Euthanasia cases are often run together. This is confusing and possibly dangerous. It's one thing to permit terminal patients to die, but it's quite another to let nonterminal Down syndrome babies die by starvation. Similarly, it's one kind of case to let an irreversibly unconscious Karen Quinlan die, but it's quite another to prevent a Down syndrome baby from developing into (what could be) an ordinary range of happiness. The cases really are different.

People often incorrectly lump these different kinds of cases together under "euthanasia." It is important to differentiate voluntary killing of terminal adults from either Baby Doe or Karen Quinlan cases. These latter cases involving incompetents should be kept separate because the strength of reasons needed to justify them is much greater. Similarly, cases involving babies—who might develop and have an entire life ahead of them— should be kept separate from cases about brain death in people whose lives are mostly over.

Some ethicists, such as Robert Weir, try to determine permissible from impermissible nontreatment by the kind of neonatal defect involved. The most controversial cases are midway in the spectrum.[24] The happy side contains harelips, atresias, and fistulas in otherwise healthy babies, hyaline membrane disease (respiratory distress syndrome), as well as correctable, congenital heart defects. The opposite end contains anencephaly, trisomy 18 (Edwards' syndrome), trisomy 13, cri du chat syndrome, Lesch-Nyhan syndrome, Tay-Sachs disease, and infantile polycystic kidney disease. Weir thinks the former kind of case should live and that it's permissible to let babies die in the latter. Cases in the middle, such as Down syndrome and spina bifida, are the most troublesome.

Links to Abortion

Many pregnant women today undergo amniocentesis (sampling of the amniotic sac by needle for fluid for genetic analysis) and, if the results indicate a serious defect, many couples abort and try again for a healthy baby. Even though the aborted fetus is large (late second trimester) and may be at the stage where some "preemies" are saved, such abortions routinely occur.

Therefore it is quite natural to reason as theologian John Fletcher argues in *Who Should Survive?* If spina bifida is a good reason for aborting a 20-week-old fetus, why is it also not a good reason for letting a baby die? Birth triggers great emotions and symbolizes that a certain success has occurred, but it doesn't change the underlying condition.

This logic is neutral. If X justifies abortion, it should also justify letting die. If Y is a good reason against abortion, it should count against letting die. Indeed, this point is made both by the parent-supporting Fletcher and the parent-condemning theologian, Paul Ramsey.[25]

Such logic raises the question whether couples should be asked to justify their decisions in such cases or simply be left alone. When women have abortions, no reason is asked, perhaps because people would use disputes about good reasons to mask their real positions on abortion. Some abortions may be for silly reasons, others for profound ones. More important, almost all aborted fetuses have greater potential for quality of life, relationships, and contribution to society than defective neonates. Yet no one asks women considering abortion to give their reasons. One explanation for this asymmetry is that we value a baby more than a second-trimester fetus. However, that value may diminish when a baby is born malformed.

Nonpersonhood of Neonate

Only persons can be murdered. Faced with these problems, some people champion a radical view of personhood. They argue that newborns are not persons until some time after birth. For philosopher Peter Singer, neonates should not be regarded as persons until "a few months" after birth; for physician-philosopher H. T. Engelhardt, neonates are not persons until they have self-concepts around the age of 2; and for philosopher Michael Tooley, they are not persons until they can use language.[26] All these criteria face the formidable meta-ethical problem of explaining why one particular empirical aspect of human development—e.g., language, a human face, or birth—and not others, instills a human with the rights of personhood. All such criteria face the perils of crossing the fact/value gap.

Critics say these radical views of late personhood must be rejected for sake of a consistent public policy. It is one thing to allow parents to allow an imperiled newborn to die at birth. It is quite another to say that a baby is not a person until it's 2 years old. Not all couples are humane, and there are problems about infantile child abuse, especially with maternal postpartum depression.

Active vs. Passive Euthanasia

An important moral issue here is whether it would not be more compassionate to simply mercy kill imperiled newborns than to just let them die slowly. (This issue was discussed in Chapter 3.) Legally, mercy killing is—at worst—homicide, whereas "letting die" is—at worst—criminal neglect. Legal experts agree that there is much less danger of prosecution from letting die than killing. Ethical experts disagree, however, about whether "letting die" is more humane.

Are infanticide and letting die really morally different? James Rachels argues that they are not.[27] If motives and results both aim at death of the baby, how can the two morally differ? The point is simple logic. Whatever makes one decision good (or bad) should also make the other case good (or bad). The kind of action itself, or its description as active or passive, should make no difference.

Some defenders of the distinction offer a fallibilist reply. People are not perfect, they say, and mistakes are made. Allowing a child to die opens the door for changes of heart and a better diagnosis. Killing the child is too final, too quick. Moreover, they say, we respect the value of life more by having parents and staff suffer through a slow death than by cheapening life with a quick end. A study by the Hastings Center, a medical ethics research institution, concluded that a public policy which allowed physicians to actively kill imperiled newborns was not in such newborns' best interests.[28]

Governmental Regulation or Private Decision?

An advocate for the American Life Lobby, Inc., criticized the parents of Baby Jane Doe: "Private individuals and private groups of individuals don't have the right to make life-or-death decisions in private in an unaccountable manner."[29] The New York ACLU said the opposite, arguing that government and right-to-lifers were unjustifiably interfering with family autonomy. Columnist Ellen Goodman said the Baby Doe squads were "clumsy intruders" into painful family matters.[30] Ironically, the Reagan team had won office by a campaign promising to get Big Government out of personal lives, but then it turned around and directed the Justice Department to intervene in just such matters. John Paris, a Jesuit medical ethicist at Tufts University, called the attempted federal intervention an "outrage."[31]

Mill's harm principle called for government not to interfere with personal decisions which put no person at risk of harm. But Mill's principle would not help in this case, because what was at issue was whether the baby was harmed by nontreatment and whether it was a person.

Another way to think about this issue is to ask about which kind of decision Kerri-Lynn's parents faced. Sometimes the way a decision is classified affects the kind of answers which are discussed. Was this a private "family decision" or was it a case of neglect? More fundamentally, what's the primary ethical concern in the case: euthanasia or procreation? Are Baby Doe cases in the same category as decisions about abortion or decisions about Karen Quinlan?

It is likely that some such cases on the margins of personhood will always be indeterminate. Morality and ethics cannot provide clear, tight answers for all cases. To believe so is to fall prey to the game of medieval scholastics known as casuistry, where "right" answers were attempted in advance for all possible cases. Second, to legislate that marginal persons *are* persons legislates against a family's range of choice. Part of the widest range of choice is the ability to decide which beings at the margins of personhood count as persons in one's own family.

But how far does that range go? In July of 1983, the state government of Tennessee intervened so that 12-year-old Pamela Hamilton had to get chemotherapy over the religious objections of her father and herself. In 1988, Boston District Attorney Newman Flanagan charged a Christian Scientist couple with manslaughter because they called a Christian Scientist practitioner, not physicians, when their young child became sick (the child abruptly died on the fifth day after seeming to get better). What's the principle here? Let parents decide to let defective babies die because of expected low quality of life, but oppose other parents whose minority faiths conflict with standard medical treatment? In cases involving children of Jehovah's Witnesses, courts have mandated treatment by reasoning that, first, religious freedom does not extend to imposing parental beliefs on one's children at cost of life, and second, that such children might have different religious beliefs later as adults. The difficulty is to explain why the same reasoning doesn't apply to all Baby Doe cases.

Difference over Prognosis and the Fact/Value Gap

Differences in ethics affect judgments about prognosis in defective babies. A very vocal critic of Lorber's predictive criteria is Lorber's colleague at Sheffield, R. B. Zachary, a pediatric surgeon. Zachary argues that the only real options for spina bifida babies are either killing them or doing everything possible for each infant. Zachary is basically saying that no middle category exists where spina bifida infants can be "let die." Pediatricians such as Lorber, who claim a high mortality rate for some spina bifida prognoses, not only omit treatment but "push the infant towards death" by giving

> eight times the sedative dose of chloral hydrate recommended in the most recent volume of *Nelson's Pediatrics* and four times the hypnotic dose, and it is being administered four times every day. No wonder these babies are sleepy and demand no feeding, and with this regimen most of them will die within a few weeks, many within the first week.[32]

Another critic of the Lorber-Duff-Campbell camp was C. Everett Koop, who wrote that allowing brain-damaged infants to die would create a slippery slope of killing other defective infants, ending with killing "all people with neurological deficit after an automobile accident."[33] In "The Slide to Auschwitz," he implied that physicians should veto parental decisions: "Why not let the family find that deeper meaning of life by providing the love and the attention necessary to take care of an infant that has been given to them?"[34] For Koop, "each newborn infant, perfect or deformed, is a human being with unique preciousness because he or she was created in the image of God."

Catholic theologian Richard McCormick says a child can only have a good of its own, i.e., an interest in whether it lives or dies, if the child can *potentially form human relationships*.[35] Anencephalic babies, born without higher brains, thus have no interests of their own. Unfortunately, this standard rules out few cases. Pediatric neurologist Newman believed that Kerri-Lynn's small head made her similar to an anencephalic baby, such that she would never recognize her parents. Neurologist Keuskamp seems to have disagreed. Associations of parents of spina bifida babies retort that someone's potential can never be known until the life is lived.

Good of the Child

Spina bifida and Down syndrome are agonizing cases exactly because many of those afflicted can attain lives worth living. However, it is only by maximally treating everyone, e.g., by immediately draining hydrocephalus before greater brain injury occurs, that each can obtain maximal potential. The same is true in maximizing a child's intelligence: early intervention can help maximize IQ in Down people, whereas "custodial care" will limit it.

The above problem, of evaluative views biasing judgments about prognosis, heavily affects judgments about intelligence in impaired people. Down syndrome is a good example, especially because of this condition's external characteristics. The last 40 years have seen a revolution in thinking about IQ in Down people, against whom most previous studies were probably biased. Most past medical studies focused on institutionalized Down people, reflecting a sampling bias and not taking into account that IQ might have been much higher in a supportive home.

Although almost all Down babies will have IQs below 70, probably less than a third (some studies say only 10 percent) will have IQs less than 25 and be "profoundly retarded" and untrainable.[36] This implies that most Down people, especially with good early care, will have IQs above 25 and an indefinite number will be above 50. Unless such people are simply defined as unhappy, it is an error to think they must be so.

Academics and professional people tend to equate intelligence with happiness and to take IQ as a measure of intelligence. Problems exist with both assumptions, but space dictates only elaborating upon the first. As the above-noted studies indicate, most Down people in the past were probably underrated. With maximal stimulation and support, most Down people will probably score somewhere between IQ 30 and 70. Whether one imagines such an existence by thinking of a 6-year-old or a beloved pet, the fundamental conclusion must be that, given reasonable stimulation, love, and supervision, *most Down people will have a life which can go better or worse for them*, i.e., they will have a life with a narrative history. Most are not better off not existing. Because there is no way to tell in the nursery whether a baby will be at the low end or high end of the potential of Down people, the best interests of that baby is maximal treatment.

But isn't it irrational to want to live with such low IQ? Who would want to live that way? Won't such people be unhappy in a society such as ours, where intelligence is so valued? In rebuttal, Livermore, Malmquist, and Meehl were discussing mental patients when they wrote the following, but their comments make just as much sense when applied to the retarded:

> When faced with an obviously aberrant person, we know, or we think we know, that he would be "happier" if he were as we are. We believe that no one would want to be misfit in society. From the very best of motives, then, we wish to fix him. It is difficult to deal with this feeling since it rests on the unverifiable assumption that the aberrant person, if he saw himself as we see him, would choose to be different than he is. But since he cannot be as we, and we cannot be as he, there is simply no way to judge the predicate for the assertion.[37]

This conclusion enables a discovery of sorts. The ethical frameworks loosely described as "sanctity-of-life" ethics and "quality-of-life" ethics are commonly held to be incompatible. Yet these standards actually *agree* on treatment of most Down babies in the nursery.

A similar conclusion is possible for most spina bifida babies. One may say that a spina bifida neonate has a good chance of a life, if not blissfully happy, at least not destined by IQ or genetics to be unhappy. Since it often cannot be known at birth whether the spina bifida neonate will be in the high, normal, or low range, and since most such children will not be profoundly retarded, it follows that unless low (but not profoundly retarded) IQ precludes any happiness in life, such children should live according to the standard of "their own good." Having a "borderline," "trainable," or even "imbecile" IQ does not make life so bad that it would be better, for the person affected, not to exist at all.

This crucial point should not be confused with what decision is best for the family. Some parents see the family's good as requiring nontreatment of a defective baby. Such a baby's care would divert time and money from other children and the parents' own lives. But that is not the above point, which is that criteria of sanctity of life and good of the child agree on maximal treatment for most Down and spina bifida babies. Only if the quality-of-life standard ranges over the good of the entire family, and not just the baby itself, can it generate a conclusion that the impaired baby should not be treated. And to interpret it that way is so different from its application for voluntary adult patients (e.g., terminal patients) as to be a completely different standard. One is concerned with numbers and total good; the other is not, and only concerns the medical patient.

The only exception is where treatment saves a child from living a life of misery and pain. It this could be known, it would be immoral on the good-of-the-child criterion to save the neonate. It is exactly these cases which traumatize pediatric neurologists and families. Because most (but not all) of these children die, nontreatment is best. Those who do not, will be worse off than before.[38]

This conclusion about the good of the impaired child cuts against some sympathies. Those who want to let Down babies die, frequently say that the best interest of the child is to die, and that such dying is not just for the family's good. Yet it is self-serving for a parent to assert that his or her child would surely want to be dead than exist as a Down person. Decisions to let imperiled newborns die can be justified in some cases, but justification begins with being clear about what is going on.

Who Decides What Is Enough Expected Quality of Life?

Many Baby Doe cases come down to taking risks about predictions of quality of life. Certainly, it is rare that a baby will have no relationships or will only live in utter pain.

The question of factual prognosis must be separated from evaluative questions. In estimating chances of recovery from persistent vegetative states or chances that pregnancy will bring on symptoms of multiple sclerosis, medical specialists are proper authorities. On the other hand, judging what risks are *acceptable* is not a "medical judgment" but a personal, evaluative one.

In writing about the Baby Jane Doe case, philosopher Bonnie Steinbock observed that questions of factual prognosis became confused with the question of whether considerations of quality of life should *ever* count in a family's decision.[39] Representatives of organizations of parents and professionals who work with the disabled implied that in no case should predictions about quality of life count. Many other people would disagree, saying that each couple must decide what is acceptable.

This is one way of seeing the 1963 Johns Hopkins case. The mother had worked as a nurse with Down children and was familiar with the worst possibility. She may have found risk of that possibility to be unacceptable.

National columnist and ABC News commentator George Will, who has a teenage Down syndrome son, wrote about the 1982 Indiana Infant Doe case, saying treatment should not have been withheld merely "because parents decide, on the basis of doctor's guesses, that the child's life would be inconvenient, disappointing or without acceptable quality."[40]

But in that case, surgeons disagreed about whether Infant Doe's chances of survival of surgery were 80 to 90 percent or merely 50 percent. Will claims that one physician testified that Infant Doe would never achieve a "minimally acceptable" quality of life, that "some" Down syndrome persons were "mere blobs," that Down syndrome people could not be self-supporting or hold regular jobs, and "are quite incapable of telling us what they feel, what they sense...." Will says the "moral squalor" of this physician's statement "is [only] exceeded by its ignorance," and concludes, "Parents who conjugate French verbs for their superbabies are unnerved by what they think is the meaninglessness of a life that will not include reading *New York Times* editorials."

Will confuses several ideas here: whether quality of life counts at all, whether some specific standard of quality should be used for life-or-death judgments, whether specific kinds of defects meet such a standards, and last, whether parents should make decisions when experts disagree about future quality of life. Will first implies that whatever standard is used, Down syndrome people meet it, but then that some couples use a standard which is too high. But the other two questions remain. Many Down syndrome people may have been underestimated, but that does not change the fact that others were not, nor does it change the fact that other children experience far worse genetic diseases. Does quality of life *never* count, Mr. Will?

The Place of Religious Values in Ethics

Secular philosopher Peter Singer started a controversy in discussing Baby Doe cases by writing in *Pediatrics:*

> Once the religious mumbo jumbo surrounding the term "human" has been stripped away, we may continue to see normal members of our species as possessing greater capacities of rationality, self-consciousness, communication, and so on, than members of any other species; but we will not regard as sacrosanct the life of each and every member of our species, no matter how limited its capacity or intelligence or even conscious life may be.[41]

Singer emphasized the asymmetry between our dramatic undervaluing of animals (see his views, next chapter) and our occasional overvaluing of humans.

Singer's point was obscured when letters from physicians inundated *Pediatrics* in protest of the phrase "religious mumbo jumbo." The letter-writing pediatricians averred that religion was the heart of medicine. For them, medical ethics was a branch of religious ethics, and indeed, they could make no sense of ethics without religion.

Important parts of such debates often are unsaid. Some people think physicians can be best motivated to uphold certain ideals from a religious orientation instilled at an early age, which should be emphasized for admission to medical schools. They think that religious institutions are the best place to teach moral values to young children. These are important, perhaps correct, claims, but they should be put on the table and not left unsaid. Especially because they are partly empirical claims, they are subject to evidence and proof. It could also be that parents and their examples are far more important than religious beliefs in molding character.

In many ways, the typically acrimonious debate between religious and nonreligious physicians is a red herring. This can be seen by distinguishing claims about the importance of religious values in medicine from those about the truth of a religion. Regardless of whether the Islamic-Judaeo-Christian religious tradition has correct metaphysical beliefs, it is undeniable that values associated with it humanize modern medicine. These values are respect for human life, family integrity, unselfish giving, humility, equal moral worth, and compassion. The last of these, compassion, literally meaning "to suffer with," has always figured prominently in Judaism, Christianity, and Islam.

Of course, one does not have to be religious to value compassion or any other "religious" value. Some clergy imply that atheists are less compassionate, respectful of personhood, etc., than members of their flock. So long as a common definition of compassion is used, that is an empirical claim which can be tested by observation. There may be as many atheists as laypersons among physicians, and anyone who encounters such people can judge for himself or herself, e.g., whether any six randomly selected atheistic physicians are less compassionate, less respectful of persons, etc., than any six randomly selected physicians who are strongly religious. The proof is in the pudding.

For most of medicine, secular physicians endorse many of the same values, and fight many of the same enemies, as deeply religious physicians. As Peter Geach observes, people don't have to agree on abortion to do 99 percent of the activities in hospitals.[42] Because medical ethics studies controversies, this "forest" is sometimes lost in the "trees" of specific disputes.

One such tree which creates intense passions involves overruling choices of patients. It is one question to accept or reject religious values in private life. Whether such values make good physicians is another question, but it is one internal to medical education. However, medicine involves patients, and it is highly controversial in Baby Doe cases whether a physician should impose his or her values on patients. Notice that, even though the typically publicized case is one of a religious physician overruling less religious patients, this question involves any physician's desire to overrule patients' choices from any set of moral principles. If a Christian doctor can overrule a non-Christian patient, why can't a secular physician overrule a fundamentalist patient?

The problem here is a difficult one. Medicine needs to create physicians who deeply care about their values and who try to live by them. This goal is emotionally inconsistent with toleration of patients with different values and whom the physician must treat. Toleration is a relative virtue and only extends so far. One does not tolerate voodoo in a dermatology resident's treatment of patients and one does not tolerate psychiatrists who have sex with their patients. The burning issue concerns the scope of the intolerable. Some physicians can't tolerate a resident who urges his prayers on his patients.

Most religious people, in fact, tolerate many ethical beliefs in others. Moreover, most religious people in fact accept not aggressively treating an anencephalic baby. Most nonreligious people think parents who raise Down babies are very good people.

Some physicians would overrule nontreatment decisions in Baby Doe cases because they believe that families will grow through rearing their special child. Again, this is an empirical claim, and not a religious one. Unfortunately, neither people who dispute this claim nor those who accept it usually attempt to discover any real evidence for their claims, but (at best) base their belief on a few cases which they happen to know. That's too bad.

Secular pediatricians do differ from Koop in believing that patients must choose those values and not have them forced on them by pediatricians. They see their role as helping families make such decisions by giving relevant facts as completely and neutrally as possible, by protecting life where situations are uncertain (emergency room cases), by referring patients where a physician's ethics conflicts with a family's decision, and by recognizing not only that people differ greatly about ethical beliefs but also that physicians' ethical beliefs may be mistaken.

It is just such acceptance of patient choice in Baby Doe cases that some ministers and physicians find intolerable. Their intolerance of parents' choices and their consequent intervention is just what other physicians find intolerable. At this point, it is not clear how much this dispute is about religious values (which appear on both sides) and how much it is about differing conceptions by physicians of their relation to patients and society.

Good of the Family

There is some truth in seeing the conflict in Baby Doe cases as that between familial selfishness and altruism. Some believe that judgments by a family of a Baby Doe's "best interests" may camouflage intentions to benefit other children.

On the other hand, *Newsday* writer Fred Bruning defended leaving the parents alone:

> This is a dilemma that transcends politics, or ought to. Who but parents can begin to interpret the meaning of a child born with terrible handicaps? Here is a situation in which "feelings" alone are inadequate.... Nor is sweet reason sufficient either. For every argument, there is a counterargument; for every epiphany, a corresponding burst of doubt. Everything is right everything is wrong. Morality has deceptive moves.

> Travelers familiar with Beirut claim it is a city lost to hope because consensus is impossible. Perhaps it can be said that parents of severely damaged children inhabit a Beirut of the spirit, a place where innocence has no armor, where there is no distinction between suffering and survival. The rest of us are strangers, and we ought to let the parents consult the doctors, reach their decisions, tend to their babies, grapple with their lives. We ought to respect their heartache and their wishes. We ought to leave them in peace.[43]

Eloquent, indeed. But, surely, there are limits. Can't we leave parents alone within certain parameters? Isn't that what this case is really about? Establishing those parameters?

Criminal and Civil Suits

In criminal law, most district attorneys are reluctant to prosecute Baby Doe cases, preferring instead to chase real criminals. The *Wall Street Journal* editorialized that the courts are already clogged enough without local judges being forced by Uncle Sam to second-guess doctors in the nursery.[44] Nevertheless, criminal prosecution for neglect remains possible, as the Muellers experienced. Moreover, one need only recall the Edelin case to see the vacillations of the law. At birth, the "fetus" becomes a "baby," and presumably has rights under all state laws to inherit money, not to be abused, and to live. When neonatologists disconnect respirators to allow a defective baby to die, they appear to be breaking some laws.

In civil law, where parents themselves are the ones who decide to sue, the courts are seeing many cases. The 42,000 defective babies born annually of the 3.2 million American births breed many suits, as few parents today stoically accept defects as God's will.[45] As standards and expectations rise, parents often blame the obstetrician for birth defects: hence the high fees for malpractice insurance for obstetricians. In New York City, lawyers run ads in the *Daily News* soliciting neonatal suits.

Pediatricians worry about civil suits charging wrongful life. Wrongful life suits are filed on behalf of severely defective infants. They charge that defects occurred because of professional negligence, i.e., care substantially below the norm of care, and that the child's resulting life is so miserable as to be a legal *tort* or harm. In 1967, Mrs. Gleitman sued her obstetrician Robert Cosgrove, who failed to warn her that German measles could cause defects in her baby.[46] Jeffrey Gleitman was born nearly blind and deaf, and Mrs. Gleitman sued for expenses of his lifelong care. She lost, because the judge ruled that, had she known, she would have aborted. Jeffrey, the Court felt, "would almost surely choose life with defects as against no life at all." Any child born defective as a result of bad advice, but who could have been aborted had the advice been corrected, is by *Gleitman* unable to recover damages from incompetent obstetricians.

The Paradox of Existence is here again. How is nonexistence measured against life with miserable defects? How is life with defects of one child measured against life without defects for the next (but merely possible) child? Recalling the two concepts of harm from Chapter 4, Jeffrey was not harmed on the baseline standard of harm. But the "first born child of the Gleitman's" was certainly less than he could have been, and on the maximal potential standard of harm, Jeffrey was indeed harmed.

A more successful suit against pediatricians has been the idea of wrongful birth, such as occurred in 1980 in *Curlender*.[47] In wrongful *life* suits, someone—probably a parent—sues on behalf of the infant and argues that it would have been better off not exsiting. Since the infant does exist, it is argued that damages should be awarded both as compensatory, to ameliorate his or her condition, and as punitive, to prevent further errors. In contrast, in wrongful *birth* suits, the parents argue that the child itself was harmed and sue for compensation for costs of its care. They do not argue that the baby would have been better off not existing, but argue that the baby would not need extra care if not for the error.

In *Curlender,* a California court recognized a wrongful birth claim against a lab which mistakenly told two parents of a Tay-Sachs child that they were not at risk. Since 1982, courts in New Jersey, Washington, and North Carolina have agreed that, while life itself can never be an injury, parents may recover damages to pay for care which otherwise would not have been incurred.

UPDATE

The Danville Siamese twins defied their dismal prognosis and weighed 30 pounds after 1 year.[48] Shortly after that, a long operation separated the weaker twin, who died. Jeff, the stronger twin, lived and later entered regular school. Pamela and Robert Mueller divorced.

During the court battles over Kerri-Lynn, Linda and Dan A. changed their minds and permitted surgery to drain their infant's hydrocephalus—a decision which only became known months later.[49] The infant had already been given antibiotics after contracting pneumonia, and had she not received antibiotics, might have died. As it turned out, Kerri-Lynn lived and was taken home.

Her parents later lost motions in court to have their $78,000 in attorneys' fees paid by the Justice Department. Such fees can be paid if the government's suit was later deemed "frivolous, unreasonable, or without foundation." The Justice Department denied this characterization and also pointed out that it had never sued the parents, who had voluntarily joined the suit against Stony Brook Hospital for the medical records. Senator David Durenberger (R-Minn) later introduced two bills in Congress to have the parents' legal expenses paid.

Two years after Kerri-Lynn went home, a Baby Doe study came under attack at Oklahoma's Children Memorial Hospital.[50] The study had used Lorber-like criteria to not treat a group of spina bifida babies. In this study published in 1985, all 24 babies placed in the lowest category were kept pain-free, but not given surgery or antibiotics, and all died. All but one of those in the treatment group lived. This time, the ACLU intervened against the hospital, joining a group called the National Legal Center for the Medically Dependent and Disabled, and claiming that the hospital failed, over 5 years, to treat 30 children with spina bifida. This case had other overtones because spina bifida babies assigned to the nontreatment group were all claimed by the plaintiffs to come from poor, minority, or single-parent families. The case went to court in Oklahoma City in 1988.

Congress in 1984 amended its Child Abuse Prevention and Treatment Act (not the Rehabilitation Act) to count nontreatment in Baby Doe cases as child abuse. The change was intended to make states responsible for such cases, not the federal government, and to get Uncle Sam out of the neonatal nursery. Pediatricians disliked these rules, too, and one study found that 60 percent thought the amendments didn't allow decisions adequately considering the infant's suffering.

The only exception to the child abuse regulations was where a child was "chronically and irreversibly comatose." As Chapter 1 explained, this phrase is very misleading. As defined by some neurologists, a "comatose" person, whether infant or adult, is not in a "chronic" condition but an acute one, i.e., his or her life is limited to weeks or months. On the other hand, a person in persistent vegetative state (PVS) is not "comatose" in this same sense and may live for years. Congress probably meant to include PVS in the exceptions, but it might not have known the difference. This illustrates the harm created when legislators replace parents and physicians at the bedside and try to determine permissible categories of treatment and nontreatment in advance of the complex details of actual cases.

This problem was illustrated in Minnesota in early 1986 by Lance Steinhaus, a 5-week-old infant who was severely brain-damaged by the assaults of his abusive father.[51] A physician testified in court that Lance was in PVS. Two or three documented cases have occurred of recovery from PVS and the hearing judge determined that treatment could not be discontinued because PVS was not a chronic, irreversible coma (as defined above). This judgment was later reversed after testimony of a pediatric neurologist, who said Lance was irreversibly comatose (and who probably thought that Congress had meant to include PVS in its exceptions). Lance was then allowed to die. Nevertheless, and as written, the law requires PVS babies to be kept alive, possibly for a decade like Karen Quinlan.

Nearly 5 years after Kerri-Lynn was born, she was living at home with her parents. According to Kathleen Kerr, whose stories about the case won a Pulitzer Prize for local reporting, and who visited the family over 5 years, Kerri-Lynn is

> doing better than anyone expected—talking, attending school for the handicapped, and learning to mix with her peers. She still can't walk and gets around in a wheelchair but her progress has defied the dire predictions.[52]

In this case, champions on both sides now say they would wage the same battle again. American Life League's president Judie Brown says, "If another case arises, we'll fight again, just the way we did the Baby Jane Doe case." The lawyer who defended the hospital against the intervention, New York Assistant Attorney General David Smith, said in 1987, "Basically, it's absolutely wonderful that Kerri-Lynn had done as well as she has, but saying that the child's progress has defied the medical prognosis doesn't alter the fact that physicians and parents should be left alone."

The 1986 *Bowen* decision by the U.S. Supreme Court said that laws protecting the handicapped against discrimination didn't apply to Baby Doe cases because the parents had made the essential decision and they were not, as required to be covered by Section 504, "federally funded recipients." In 1988, the U.S. Civil Rights Commission concluded that such decisions were, in fact, not made by parents but by physicians (who *are* "federally funded recipients"). The Disability Institute, a disability rights lobby, hoped to use this conclusion to overturn *Bowen*. The physician who, in 1982, delivered Infant Doe commented: "I hope that...the commission members may have the privilege of living in blissful isolation from the hard decisions of real life."[53]

One of the big lessons of these Baby Doe cases is that cases in medical ethics do not have neat, predictable solutions. Frequently, real-life endings embarrass those who have confident moral answers. For example, veteran medical reporter and columnist B. D. Colen began to cover the case for *Newsday*, after local reporter Kathleen Kerr's story attracted national attention. In one of his "side-bar" stories published at the time, he described the grueling life and bitter complaints of a mother whose anencephalic or hydrocephalic baby (strangely named similarly, Cara-Lynn) had been saved and who had *not* died but had already lived 2½ years. What is interesting in retrospect is not that story, but Colen's use of it as a base of comparison for the Baby Jane Doe case:

> While Cara-Lynn looks far more grotesque than Baby Jane Doe, whose
> fate is being argued in the courts, the two mistakes of nature have an
> almost identical prospect for a life filled with pain and devoid of
> self-knowledge.[54]

Colen's prediction recalls that of pediatric neurologist Newman, who testified in 1983 that Kerri-Lynn would never "achieve any meaningful interaction with her environment, never achieve any interpersonal relationships...."

The outcome of this case and the Mueller case raises disturbing questions about the reporting of controversial cases in medical ethics by the print and visual media. All major print and visual media accepted Newman's view as accurate, and almost all dismissed Weber, the court-appointed attorney for Kerri-Lynn, as a fanatic. Only Newman's account was taken as fact by almost all physicians, journalists, and medical ethicists.

But why did only Newman's account prevail? That is an interesting question. A scathing article about the reporting of the Baby Jane Doe case in the *Columbia Journalism Review* argues that the "press failed egregiously to meet" the obligation to accurately report the case.[55] What is astounding is that serious questions arose about the accuracy of the reporting in a story which won the Pulitzer Prize (albeit for "local reporting"). Neither *The New York Times* nor the *Wall Street Journal* independently checked Kerr's story, although the *Washington Post* eventually started asking questions on its own.

Although the author of this critical article was a public relations man for a right-to-life organization, his point is beyond doubt that pediatricians radically disagreed about what treatment was best for Baby Jane Doe. The public was led to believe that this was simply a moral controversy, not a medical one.

The Appellate Division of New York said parents had the right to choose between medically reasonable options.[56] This alleged right was in contrast to the denial of parental rights to refuse normal medical treatment, which could be the crime of neglect. For example, declining chemotherapy is not allowed by courts as medically reasonable because it's a normal medical treatment in the best interests of the child. But then the question arises, why was declining normal treatment for Kerri-Lynn allowed? The point here is not to push a moral judgment. The point is that, at the time, emotions ran so high—on a topic where minds were already made up—that the medical controversy didn't get reported. At the time, the media so seemed determined to make Koop and Meese's Justice Department the villains for parent-bashing that no one really dug into the side of the story emphasizing what was best, medically, for the baby.

The public was not reliably informed by newspapers that hydrocephalus generally accompanies spina bifida and does not necessitate retardation if shunted quickly. The public was not informed that Kerri-Lynn might have had a normal head, or that having a very small head did not necessarily mean profound retardation. The public was not informed that Stony Brook Hospital might have a less high-minded motive for not wanting Surgeon General Koop to inspect the written records to see if Newman had contradicted himself. The momentum of media, medicine, and medical ethics rolled strongly for the parents, whose own decision had probably been strongly influenced by Newman and who had already—secretly—reversed themselves. As with abortion, people read facts in the Baby Doe cases with their minds already made up.

As Anthony Gallo, a pediatric neurologist, emphasized in explaining the medical background of this case, the consensus in his specialty swung like a pendulum between the 1960s, 1970s and 1980s—between treating most spina bifida cases and not treating most cases.[57] He says that Lorber's criteria influenced many centers toward nontreatment in the 1970s, but that right-to-life groups swung the pendulum the other way in the 1980s—the way it was in the 1960s. However, and most important, he also stressed that key breakthroughs occurred in urology, neonatology, neurosurgery, and CAT-scan diagnosis, which allowed much higher accuracy in prognosis and improved quality of life. This had led to the understanding that

> mild to moderate degrees of microcephaly are compatible with normal
> or even exceptional intellect. This is particularly true in cases of
> untreated meningomyelocele in which loss of cerebrospinal fluid
> through the unrepaired hole in the back may decrease the total mass of
> the head. . . .

> Essentially all children with severe meningomyelocele have
> hydrocephalus....Children with hydrocephalus who are treated
> reasonably early and who do not develop meningitis have a better than
> 50 percent chance of being intellectually normal.[58]

Such new views lend credence to the revisionist view among liberals of Surgeon General C. Everett Koop, whose later leadership on AIDS and cigarettes changed many opinions of him. On November 6, 1983, Koop was grilled on *Face the Nation* by reporter Lesley Stahl, whose tone implied he was the champion of a parent-bashing, intrusive, federal government. Koop replied that his position, and that of the Justice Department, was that because there were discrepancies about the medical condition, he merely wanted to see the records to learn what was best for the child.

At the very least, the unexpected outcomes in these two cases (which have been discussed here because of their fame but were otherwise randomly selected), as well as the likely bias in early cases where Down babies were allowed to die, make the Spina Bifida Association not seem so much like fanatics. They argued, in a friend-of-the-court brief in another case, that

> since we have found it virtually impossible to predict at birth which
> infants with meningomyelocele will become competitive, ambulatory,
> and intellectually able, we have not relied on arbitrary guidelines to
> determine which children should or should not be treated. On the
> contrary, we believe that all such children should be treated, and we
> feel that our data show this philosophy to be correct.[59]

By 1990, a consensus has emerged among pediatric specialists that, given the political climate and given more promising treatments, most infants should be treated. A Down baby with duodenal atresia would not be allowed to starve to death in NICUs today, and spina bifida babies are generally treated aggressively. Quality of life factors could count, but only for the most severely malformed and hopeless cases. For those slightly better prospects, treatment occurs and parents—for better or worse—often don't have much choice. The desperation of such parents was illustrated in 1989 when Rudy Linares killed his PVS (but not brain-dead) baby, holding police at bay with a gun as his child died.

That someone like Mr. Linares would act as he did was a predictable consequence of the impact of the Baby Doe Rules and subsequent congressional legislation. If the range of physician and parental choice is decreased for the best interests of impaired newborns—which has been the net effect of 20 years of activity—then some parents may be driven to desperate acts.[60]

FURTHER READING

Baruch Brody, "Commentary: Case Study on Faith Healing for Childhood Leukemia," *Hastings Center Report,* 11(1):10–11 (February 1981).

David Coulter, "Neurologic Uncertainty in Newborn Intensive Care," *New England Journal of Medicine*, 316(14):840–44 (April 2, 1987).

Norman Fost, "Counseling Families Who Have a Child with Severe Congenital Anomaly," *Pediatrics*, 67:231 (1981).

Hastings Center Project on Imperiled Newborns, ed. Arthur Caplan, *Hastings Center Report*, 17(6):5–37 (December 1987).

Loretta C. Kopelman et al., "Neonatologists Judge the 'Baby Doe' Regulations," *New England Journal of Medicine*, 318: 677–683 (March 17, 1988).

John Moskop and Rita Saldanha, "The Baby Doe Rule: Still a Threat," *Hastings Center Report*, 16(2):8–14 (April 1986).

John J. Paris, "Right to Life Doesn't Demand Heroic Sacrifice," *Wall Street Journal*, November 28, 1983, p. 30.

Carson Strong, "The Neonatologist's Duty to Patient and Parents," *Hastings Center Report*, 14(4):10–16 (August 1984).

PART 3

CLASSIC CASES
ABOUT
RESEARCH

CHAPTER 8

The Philadelphia Head-Injury Studies on Primates

For 15 years between 1969 and 1984, Thomas Gennarelli systematically injured monkeys and baboons to mimic brain injuries in humans. His research illustrates ethical issues involved in using animals in medical research. Such research is controversial in modern societies. In the last 20 years, Hollywood personalities such as Loretta Switt, Lindsay Wagner, Clint Eastwood, and Johnny Carson have defended animal rights, as have movies such as *Star Trek IV* and *Project X* which paint an unsympathetic portrait of animal experimentation. Former game show host Bob Barker fought the USC Medical School's primate research program. In the last 20 years, treatment of laboratory animals has moved from an issue for a few small groups to one of national concern.

HISTORICAL BACKGROUND

Animals have always been used by man, but the specific issue of animal experimentation did not fully arise until the beginning of modern science. René Descartes, in the 17th century, set the premises of the modern debate. A mathematician, philosopher, and physiologist, he investigated the circulation of blood and dissected live, unanesthetized animals (anesthesia was not invented until the early 1900s).

Descartes' views on animals stemmed from his more basic Cartesian worldview, which deeply influenced Western science and philosophy. The "Cogito, ergo sum" of his *Meditations* grounded his argument that *res cogitans* or "thinking stuff" distinguished humans from other animals. What is essentially human is this substantial mind or soul. For Descartes, such mental substance holds together the transient mental states—perceptions, feelings, thoughts, and dreams—and grounds free will, reason, and moral value. All other animals lack souls and are, therefore, ultimately only *res extensa*, or "extended, physical stuff." In this bifurcated world, animals for Descartes are merely fleshy machines whose eyes mirror no soul, whose "pain behavior" does not exhibit real pain.

167

Descartes accepted the Church's notion that humans had souls created by God and that animals did not. He assumed that soul and mind were identical, so that if animals lacked souls, they also lacked minds. He also assumed that if animals lacked minds, they could not feel pain. To be human, for Descartes, was partly to be able to feel pain, and in order to feel pain, a mind was needed. There was no middle ground.

The most infamous of Descartes' immediate followers were at the Jansenist seminary of Port Royal. The Port Royalists were early physiologists and vivisectionists (researchers operating on animals without anesthesia). Here is a description by the 18th-century writer Fontaine of the Port Royalists:

> They administered beatings to dogs with perfect indifference, and made fun of those who pitied the creatures as if they felt pain. They said the animals were clocks; that the cries they emitted when struck were only the noise of a little spring that had been touched, but that the whole body was without feeling. They nailed poor animals up on boards by their four paws to vivisect them and see the circulation of the blood which was a great subject of conversation.[1]

In modern times, some behavioral psychologists argued against assuming that animals were conscious (especially rats) and distinguished pain from "pain behavior." Cows exhibited "pain behavior," but whether they had mental states and the experience of pain was another matter.

Cartesianism attempted to solve the tension between science and religion by demarcating proper areas for each. Science studied matter, math, animals, and the human body; religion and the humanities studied mind, art, and ethics. Christians since this time have struggled with how mind and soul are related, how these relate to morality, and whether animals count in the grand scheme of things (ministers are often asked whether pets go to heaven).

C. S. Lewis, the 20th-century Christian writer, answered in *The Problem of Pain* by distinguishing the sentience of animals from the self-consciousness of humans.[2] He argued that animals feel pain, but not as humans do. A rat receiving three electric shocks feels the pain of each shock, i.e., it is sentient, but it cannot think, "I have had three shocks." The latter thought requires what Lewis calls "consciousness or soul" (he runs these together). Lewis agrees with philosopher David Hume, who argued that self-identity requires a permanent self or mental substance which unites all a person's thoughts as "his."[3] Primates have "a succession of perceptions," but not the human experience of pain as "my pain."

What Lewis was trying to find (in 1940) was what Descartes lacked, a middle ground. Unlike Descartes and some "black box" behaviorists, Lewis rejected the assumption that animals felt nothing and argued that animals were, in some sense, conscious. But what sense?

Critics attacked Lewis' identification of consciousness with either deep self or soul. People might have deep selves but lack souls; selves might simply perish at death, with no soul continuing afterwards. Also, if Lewis were correct that memory requires self-consciousness, animals would never remember anything. Experiments in psychology about learning would be senseless. Yet everyone knows that animals remember. Dogs that have been kicked remember when mailmen return.

Defenders of Lewis reply that much behavior and learning is non-conscious, e.g., in driving a car, there is no conscious thought, "I will stop at this red light." Past painful events may be remembered without being perceived as "my" painful history. Moreover, and as Hume taught, consciousness should not be confused with self-consciousness. Mere memory might be "hard-wired" into the brain from evolution.

These problems of how much pain animals feel, and how much such pain is like human pain, are not simple. Questions about animal pain raise some of the deepest problems in philosophy of mind and lie behind many controversies about animal research: At what point, on the ladder of evolution from shrimp to baboons, do organisms become sentient? When do organisms react to pain? Anticipate pain? How much "mental" pain can a fish, cat, dog, or pig experience? When do they remember pain as "my" pain? How would we know?

Is there a difference between being sentient (being able to feel pain) and being conscious (being aware of feeling pain)? How would we know? If we don't, why are there two different words? Is there a difference between being conscious and having a mind (being aware of being able to feel pain and being aware that a "self" seems to be the subject of awareness)?

Such questions in philosophy of mind blend into those in ethics. What capacities qualify one for membership in the moral community? What does one need to *count* in the moral calculus? Sentience? Consciousness? A soul? Moreover, how do we verify such capacities in a species, especially if important ethical positions hang on the answers? If we have, as a species, conflicts of interest against accepting certain answers?

Contemporary Animal Research

Estimates vary greatly about the number of animals used each year in biomedical research, because no federal law requires such figures to be kept. The Office of Technology Assessment (OTA) estimates 14 million, Andrew Rowan (an activist-scholar) estimates 71 million, and *Newsweek* estimates 17 million.[4] Rowan says basic and applied research use 40 percent, drug development 26 percent, safety testing 20 percent, science and medical courses 8 percent, and other scientific programs 6 percent.

The three uses of animals in research most hated by activists are LD-50 tests, Draize tests, and psychology experiments. "LD" stands for "lethal dosage," and *LD-50s* determine the amount of a substance necessary to kill 50 of 100 animals. These tests are done routinely across species, for substances from soap to chemotherapies. They have been criticized as crude, blunt measures (one wry critic says they tell mice how much of something to take for mass suicide). Largely in response to such criticisms from nonscientists, use of LD-50s has declined 96 percent since the early 1970s.[5]

The *Draize test* measures irritation to human eyes of products such as cosmetics by dripping concentrations into the sensitive eyes of rabbits. Activists seek alternative tests in cell cultures and computer models.

Psychology experiments such as Harlow's study of maternal instincts in baby monkeys or Seligman's "learned helplessness" research on monkeys provoke scorn by activists as extremely painful and as producing trivial results. Psychologists retort that both pieces of research were landmark studies.

THE PENNSYLVANIA HEAD-INJURY STUDIES ON PRIMATES

In Philadelphia, on Memorial Day of 1984, five members of the Animal Liberation Front (ALF) quietly entered a building of the University of Pennsylvania Medical School, descended to a subbasement, and broke into a laboratory. They there found 32 audiovisual tapes of years of experiments that were designed to produce brain damage in adult baboons and monkeys. At the time that the ALF took the tapes, the medical school was deserted for the holiday.

Disagreement exists about how much other damage, if any, they did. One university official claimed "two million dollars' worth," and the *American Medical News* gave this figure prominent emphasis, but no evidence for this figure was offered. Subsequent newspaper reports dropped the claim. It is not mentioned in the final report to the National Institutes of Health.

Everyone agrees that the ALF broke the law in stealing the tapes. The tapes had been made over 5 years by neurologist Thomas Gennarelli in attempts to find a reproducible model for head injuries to baboons. Gennarelli began to use baboons in 1980 after his previous studies with monkeys failed to simulate head injuries in humans. His lab studied this topic for over 15 years between 1970 and 1985.

The ALF heavily edited the 60 to 80 hours of tapes to a 25-minute segment showing only abuses. Distributed widely to television stations, the edited tape was difficult to watch and emotionally persuasive. As a reporter for *The New York Times* said:

> One sequence showed a monkey strapped to a table pulling against its bonds. The animal's head was encased in a steel cylinder to a pneumatic machine called an accelerator. Suddenly, a piston drove the cylinder upward, thrusting the animal's head sharply through an arc of about 60 degrees.

> In another sequence, as an animal lay in a coma, a researcher's recorded voice was heard saying, "You'd better have some axonal damage, monkey," and calling him "sucker."[6]

One damaging aspect of the edited videotape was that researchers made several derogatory comments about the primates of the kind heard by adolescent, machismo males. There was also lots of profanity, unsterile surgery, and horribly sloppy care of animals. Another damaging aspect was that the researchers claimed the baboons were sedated and felt no pain, but several segments showed the baboons twisting their bodies to be free just before the pneumatic hammer smashed their heads. Perhaps most repugnant to many nonscientists, several segments showed the researchers making fun of injured baboons, e.g., holding them up by broken arms or laughing about conscious but brain-injured baboons. Emotionally, the tapes the researchers took of themselves were worse than any ALF skit ever would have been.

A member of the ALF break-in team identified only as "Lauren" defended the break-in:

> We may seem like radicals to you. But we are like the Abolitionists,
> who were regarded as radicals, too. And we hope that 100 years from
> now, people will look back on the way animals are treated now with
> the same horror as we do when we look back on the slave trade.

Thomas Langfitt, the principal investigator of the overall head-injury program and chairman of the university hospital's neurosurgery department, claimed that even though animals moved before the tests, they had been anesthetized and felt no pain. His claim is hard to believe in watching the videotape showing baboons struggling to be free.

Langfitt also claimed to be "on the threshold of major improvements in treatment."[7] Critics retorted that this hoary old claim is made about *every* piece of research.

In April 1985, an organization called "People for the Ethical Treatment of Animals" (PETA) turned over the stolen videotapes to the National Institutes of Health (NIH) for review. This took place after a year of negotiation between PETA and NIH. PETA believed that NIH was biased because it was the primary funding institute for medical research and that NIH might suppress damaging information. NIH claimed it could be objective, but would investigate the charges only after it received copies of the tapes.

Previously, in 1983, key congresspersons had opposed a bill to strengthen regulation of animal experiments. In May 1985, PETA held two briefings on Capitol Hill where the edited videotape was seen by staffers of Senator Weicker and Congressman Natcher, respective chairmen of the Senate and House committees responsible for the NIH budget.[8] The two chairmen and sixteen other congressmen decided that the public would not like what it saw. They sent letters to NIH demanding suspension of Gennarelli's studies.

Columnist James Kilpatrick reacted indignantly to the videotapes.[9] (No liberal, Kilpatrick had once opposed President Kennedy's civil rights programs.) Excerpts were shown on NBC's *20/20* programs and broadcast on major television networks. A public outcry forced Health and Human Services Secretary Margaret Heckler to review the studies. Pennsylvania officials denied "gratuitous" abuse of animals in the laboratory. Later, and after the Office for Protection from Research Risks (OPRR) had spent almost a year trying to get the videotapes from PETA, it discovered that the University had a 2½ hour videotape which had been overlooked during the break-in because it had been in the camera. When asked by OPRR why such a potentially significant research record had not been made known and transmitted to NIH, a University of Pennsylvania official said it hadn't occurred to anyone that the videotape was important.

To review the experiment's merit, OPRR appointed a committee of a neurosurgeon, a veterinary anesthesiologist, and a veterinary pathologist—all of whom used animals in research. They found Gennarelli guilty of nine (of ten) charges but did *not* find fault with the scientific integrity of his experiments: "The research, as proposed, is likely to yield fruitful results for the good of society."[10] The Committee assumed there was nothing intrinsically wrong with injuring baboons to study human head injuries.

They criticized lack of anesthesia, inadequate supervision, poor training, inferior veterinary care, unnecessary multiple injuries to single animals, humor, smoking, "statements in poor taste" around animals, and improper clothing. "Taken collectively, these conclusions constitute material failure to comply with the Public Health Service Animal Welfare Policy." In short, the lab virtually ignored all rules to protect animals, and the university had no mechanism at all to insure that rules were followed.

Widespread public pressure continued, and a few months later, Secretary Heckler suspended the research. It was the first time a lab had been closed because of abuse of animals. To the ALF, the closing was a momentous victory. To Carolyn Compton, a physician, pediatric researcher, and spokesperson for scientists using animals, it was a "tragedy."[11]

Subsequent ALF Break-Ins

Six weeks after its first raid on the Pennsylvania veterinary school, the ALF struck again and "liberated" three cats, two dogs, and eight pigeons. The school's dean said the raids "would set back research efforts, including a study to determine the cause of sudden infant death syndrome."[12] Another dean said the stolen cats were being used in studies of breathing during sleep, that one missing dog had a steel plate inserted to study osteoarthritis, that another was being studied for ear canal infections, and that the pigeons were in a study of broken bones intended to benefit all birds.[13] He said the work would benefit other dogs, that it had to be done, and that additional animals would end up having to be used.

That December, in 1984, in Duarte, Calif., two rabbits injected with oral herpes and numerous dogs with cancer were taken, along with 100 other animals, from the City of Hope National Medical Center in California. ALF members painted a sign in the lab: "ALF IS WATCHING AND THERE'S NO PLACE TO HIDE!" Ingrid Newkirk of PETA called the City of Hope "a concentration camp" where animals were "being used for painful experiments."[14] The center's associate director said the theft of animals disrupted $500,000 worth of research on emphysema, cancer, and herpes. The ALF had targeted a study testing tobacco carcinogens in dogs. The associate director refused to comment on whether the abducted animals had been cruelly treated, but did say that 36 cancerous dogs, 12 cats, 12 rabbits, 28 mice and 18 rats were stolen and said that, "we're concerned that very important research work may not now be completed."[15]

In April 1985, in what was the largest animal raid to date, the ALF hit University of California, Riverside's biology and psychology laboratories. It stole 467 animals, including a stump-tailed macaque whose eyes had been sewn shut to study a device to help the blind navigate. PETA said the animals had been in painful, unnecessary experiments, some of which involved starvation. NIH investigated the charges, but found no evidence of abuse. The university claimed that $683,000 in damages occurred, as well as lost research. In April 1987, an arson fire gutted the $2.5 million veterinary research animal lab at University of California, Davis. The ALF claimed responsibility for both acts.

ETHICAL ISSUES

Animal Liberation/Animal Rights

Before 1975, animal welfare groups focused on treating research animals humanely. Until recently, scientists dismissed such "little old lady" concerns and portrayed them as antiprogress. Such dismissals pushed reformers toward more radical measures.

The Scientists Center for Animal Welfare advocates, not the banning of animals in research, but rather—and idea dating from at least 1959—the "three Rs" of *reducing* the number of animals used per experiment, *replacing* higher species with lower species where possible, and *refining* techniques to cause less pain. Testing a new drug on 10 rats is better than testing it on 100 chimpanzees.

In 1975, Australian philosopher Peter Singer published *Animal Liberation,* where he assumed that animals morally counted for something.[16] Saying that animals did not count because of their natures was like saying that slaves and women did not count, for similar reasons. Just as racism and sexism were evil, so was *speciesism.* Every non-question-begging argument supporting equal rights for minorities and women also supported concern for animals. If sensitivity to pain, family ties, and reasoning grounded moral concern for children, minorities, and women, why wouldn't the same also ground concern for animals? Such arguments immediately put "speciesists" on the defensive: how can the principle of equality support equality among people (of greatly varying abilities and intelligence) and not support equality among species of animals (of greatly differing abilities and intelligence)?

Singer also used utilitarian premises, i.e., the same kind of secular, results-oriented moral premises which scientists used to defend their own research. The *utilitarian ethical theory* holds that right acts produce the greatest good for the greatest number, e.g., research on today's sick patients may help greater numbers of future patients. Previously the "greatest number" referred only to humans, but this begged the key question. Once animals count for something, however little, radical conclusions follow, so that experiments which inflict horrible pain on millions of animals cannot be justified by saving a few human lives.

Singer argued that a medical experiment could be nonspeciesist only if humans would be willing to substitute an irreversibly comatose human in the same experiment. Most people accept using chimpanzees in medical research, but cringe at substituting an anencephalic baby (a baby born lacking almost all its brain). Yet if a chimpanzee is gregarious, sensitive, and deserves to live, and a severely retarded human is mute, comatose, and without hope, why should the chimp be the victim? Simply because one is a human, the other not?

Singer's position suffers all the theoretical problems of utilitarianism. Its consistent application requires people to relieve the suffering of animals, to aide victims of famine, and to help future generations at great personal sacrifice. It requires that people give to famine-relief rather than send a child to a good college. Because many lives could be saved by giving $20,000 a year to CARE, and because one does not need to go to college even to be happy, much less to live, the cost of college education cannot be justified by utilitarian parents. Consistently applied, utilitarianism requires saintly conduct. Philosophers such as Susan Wolf have argued that such a model of moral perfection "does not constitute a model of personal well-being toward which it would be particularly good or desirable for a rational human being to strive."[17]

Such arguments are not necessarily seen as *reductio ad absurdum* positions by animal rightists. Such arguments take a premise (animal rights) to a valid but unacceptable ("absurd") conclusion (a human life must be sacrificed to save a dog's life). Not everyone agrees on *reductios*. What counts as an "unacceptable" conclusion varies among people.

Moreover, that an ethical theory requires high standards of conduct is not to say it isn't a standard. Christianity defines right conduct in such a way that, if consistently followed, saintliness is required (turning one's cheek, a rich man cannot enter Heaven, etc.).

For others, utilitarianism of such scope does not satisfactorily answer the question, "What is morality *for?*" For them, morality must first consider obligations to the "inner circle" of family, colleagues and friends, even if doing so decreases "the greatest good for the greatest number" or does not result in the most saved souls. Moreover, as Wolf emphasizes, being saintly conflicts with development of other good but nonmoral traits, such as mastery of medicine, excellence in tennis, or knowing the great novels.

Part of what the debate concerns here is the importance one places on hypocrisy in ethics. For some people, it is entirely appropriate to profess caring about starving people, animals, or the poor—either on Sunday morning or in ethical theory—but, then, not act consistently on that belief in actual life. Others seek some compromise, say, by donating 10 percent of income to promoting such beliefs. This solution may be practical but it is theoretically awkward. It is like saying that animals or the starving are important 10 percent of the time but not the rest.

Regan's Position

Behind the Pennsylvania head-injury studies is the more basic issue of whether scientific research on animals is ever justified. American philosopher Tom Regan thinks not:

> I argue that the whole system of animal experimentation, the whole system of commercial and sport trapping and hunting, are morally bankrupt institutions. The only way you change these things fundamentally is by eliminating them. In much the same way as with slavery and child labor.[18]

Regan argues that humans have rights because they have lives which can go better or worse for them. This is true independently of whether others value such people. Why? Because persons have inherent, not instrumental, value. That is, *they have a life*. Where Singer applies utilitarianism to animals, Regan emphasizes the rights-based idea of treating each animal's life as an end in itself.

Regan claims that many species of animals also have lives which can go better or worse for them. Then he makes the crucial inference: "They too have a distinctive kind of value in their own right, if we do; therefore, they too have a right not to be treated in ways that fail to respect this value."[19]

Critics say that Regan here runs several unjustified inferences together. First, because any being (human or otherwise) has a life which can go better or worse, does that fact give it a distinctive value? More important, does such a fact about animals entail equal value with humans? Can't human lives go better or worse in more complex ways than lives of cows and rabbits? But maybe that is the point of the additional phrase "for them" in "go better or worse for them." Then, no comparisons can be made. If each aquarium fish has a life and if such lives can go better or worse for them, such lives are as important as the lives of human children.

Regan avoids the issue of different values of species by arguing that if humans have a certain quality and thus, rights, and that if animals have the same quality, then it is inconsistent not to give animals the same rights. Anyone who wishes to assert a superior right of (animal) humans must overcome this onus of proof.

"I Am a Speciesist"

Opponents of the animal rights movement refuse to expand the scope of morality to animals. This aspect of the animal question parallels the similar debate about abortion. Medical-school philosopher Carl Cohen defends using animals in biomedical research by arguing that animals cannot share in the human community:

> Notwithstanding all such complications, this much is clear about rights
> in general: they are in every case claims, or potential claims, within a
> community of moral agents. Rights arise, and can be intelligently
> defended, only among beings who actually do, or can, make moral
> claims against one another.[20]

Because animals cannot make claims, they have no rights.

Writing in the *New England Journal of Medicine*, Cohen rejects the analogy between racism, sexism, and speciesism. The former are bad, not the latter. "I am a speciesist," he declares. Moreover, "Speciesism is not merely plausible; it is essential for right conduct, because those who will not make the morally relevant distinctions among species are almost certain, in consequence, to misapprehend their true obligations."

Philosopher Raymond Frey argues that talk of "animal rights" uselessly confuses an already confused moral terrain. Regan says animals have rights simply by coming into existence and being the sort of creatures they are. But if this is so, Frey argues, then:

> In the case of intrinsic or fundamental, unacquired moral rights, this
> divergence reaches a radical degree, and what grip we had on rights
> has, I think been lost. Rather, we are at sea in a tide of theoretical
> claims and counter-claims with no fixed point by which to steer.[21]

The question of the proper boundaries of the moral community can be confusing. Because many pro-animal rights philosophers are pro-parental choice about abortion and Baby Doe cases, antiabortionists say they value animals more than they do humans. One student compared the views of one such philosopher on abortion and animal research, entitling her paper, "I'd Rather Be His Pet." Such critics emphasize the oddity of expanding the circle of moral concern with animals, but contracting it with humans. Singer would respond that whether the "circle" should expand or contract at a particular point depends on the characteristics of the beings in question (sensitivity to pain, awareness, sociability, etc.), not on species membership.

Ethical Touchstones

Singer says that an experiment is nonspeciesist if we would substitute an anencephalic baby for a primate. This is one approach to distinguishing justified from unjustified research. What if such substitution could save a hundred primates? A thousand? Is the life of a nonconscious anencephalic worth more than a hundred primates?

From the opposite direction, another approach is to ask whether it wouldn't be justified to sacrifice an animal to directly save a life of a normal human. If only one can stay, and there is a dog and a man in the lifeboat, should the moral man toss a coin to see who stays? Philosopher Regan says that because "animals aren't there to be used as our resources," it is morally wrong to kill an animal to save a human. Scientist Charles McArdle agrees, "I would seriously have to question whether I would allow an animal to die just to protect me." Pediatric researcher Carolyn Compton says, "I love animals, but there's no question in my mind that if I were able to sacrifice an animal life to save a human being, that I would do it."[22] Both this touchstone and the one above are useful in evaluating absolutist positions.

The Place of Ad Hominem Appeals in Ethics

Both Singer and Regan criticize factory farming, meat eating, sport hunting, wearing furs, and circuses. They urge avoidance of such practices to end animal suffering. Such a "philosophy" places animal experimentation in a larger context. Furthermore, when a philosopher not only argues for acting in a certain way but also actually acts that way, his arguments gain a new force.

However, within philosophy, it is unclear what force such personal testimonials are supposed to carry. Although such appeals do carry weight in popular culture, it is not clear what their role should be in rational argument. Indeed, a traditional informal fallacy of argument is an ad hominem appeal, which literally means "to the man" and which involves an inappropriate personal reference when arguing with an opponent. For example, in a presidential debate during 1988, George Bush made an ad hominem point against Michael Dukakis (who opposed capital punishment) when Bush advocated capital punishment for a man who had raped and killed his own wife. Dukakis tried to respond logically to a point based not on reason but on emotion (whereas the appropriate debate trick is to express outrage and say, "I'd kill the bastard with my own hands.")

But we are not debating here. The strength of a philosopher's reasons should determine our allegiance, not his or her answers to personal questions. And the balance of reasons should determine our position on a moral issue, not its emotional impact.

Moreover, once the door is opened to appeal to personal life, many things can walk through. At one such conference, English philosopher Stephen Clark chided his audience for feeding meals which contained meat to cats and dogs. Other activists there followed Albert Schweitzer and revered all life, killing nothing. Others emphasized ecological purity and opposed all kinds of hunting, as well as extinction of any species. Still others were not just vegetarians but "vegans" (eating no animal products, such as eggs from captive chickens). Still others refused to buy any animal products. Others regarded zoos and circuses as demeaning captivity and refused to take their children to such places. The most radical even condemned pet ownership, which PETA's Ingrid Newkirk said was an "absolutely abysmal situation brought about by human manipulation."[23]

Despite this danger of holier-than-thou attitudes, criticisms of appeals to personal action on this issue are somewhat odd. After all, the general subject is ethics, and one reason why people find the subject interesting is that people do act on ethical beliefs. The proper relation of action to belief in ethics is certainly awkward and complex.

Scientific Merit: Basic Research

The question of scientific merit of the Gennarelli studies needs to be put into perspective. Scientific research is like an iceberg, with research applicable to humans the visible tip above the water. Such research could not be supported without basic research, which goes on quietly in labs and is rarely discussed in national media.

In basic research, many animals are used—vastly greater numbers than most people guess. For every practical human success such as cyclosporin or knee replacements, perhaps a hundred others failed on animals and a dozen failed on humans. To validate each success, hundreds or thousands of animals are used as guinea pigs. The 128 American medical schools and the dozen pharmaceutical and research institutions utilize millions of animals each year—mostly rats and mice, but also dogs, pigs, cats, rabbits, and primates. And that is just in America. In Germany, France, Switzerland, Japan, Canada, and Australia, scientists use great numbers of animals. Charles River Breeding Laboratories, the General Motors of the American animal-breeding industry, alone produced 10 million animals in 1983.

Because most research is basic, drawing the line in animal experimentation is agonizing. Few people would stop research with direct clinical benefit to humans. Few people would stop research with even likely *indirect* clinical benefit to humans. Critics want to stop "trivial" or "repetitive" research, but they often cite cases where researchers staunchly defend the importance of the work (e.g., Harlow's and Seligman's work on monkeys). If all basic research stopped, real medical progress might stop. On the other hand, if no basic research stops, animal experimentation proceeds as always.

One suggestion is to fund only "worthwhile" research. Deciding what this means is the job of NIH experts who determine funding for grants. Such experts say that if they knew in advance which projects would be worthwhile, they would fund only those, but they don't know. Sometimes, a seemingly insignificant project yields important results.

At bottom, researchers have a kind of faith that the costs of their enormous enterprise—in dollars, careers, and animal suffering—will one day be outweighed by the discovered benefits. At bottom, animal activists are skeptics denying that the benefits to humans outweigh the costs to animals.

Scientific Merit of the Gennarelli Study

For animal activists, Gennarelli's lack of sensitive care toward his animals in itself proved the immorality of his project. Is this a mistake? Could a researcher have an excellent project but be insensitive to needs of animals? These are certainly two separate issues. Researchers say that the "insensitive" behavior on the tape is like the cynical humor heard among medical residents. Activists disagree, saying the researchers undoubtedly think they are sensitive, but are blinded to their insensitivity by their conflicts of interest.

Activist and veterinarian Nedim Buyukmichi said Gennarelli's studies were too inconsistent to give a reproducible model and too limited in scope to adequately mimic the injuries sustained by human accident victims: "After 15 years and $11 million to $13 million, essentially nothing has come out of this research that hasn't already been known from studies of human head trauma."[24]

A peer-review committee reviewing Gennarelli's grant said his research contributed to studying the drug mannitol's effect on reducing brain swelling after trauma and to the management of metabolic balance in coma patients. Critics called these justifications ad hoc and said they papered over a lack of real findings. Langfitt later claimed that Gennarelli's research provided the first evidence of the possibility of regeneration of damaged nerve cells (the one great hope of all paralyzed patients with spinal cord injuries). Critics compared this to the ubiquitous heralding of the "first evidence" of a cure for cancer.

In all the material written about Gennarelli's research, it may seem amazing that no one on either side specifically criticized, or specifically defended, the actual hypothesis of his research. That may be explained because it is unclear that Gennarelli actually had a hypothesis. Other than the goal of creating one exact injury in one baboon after another, there seems to have been no hypothesis.

Gennarelli was at the base of the pyramid of basic research on head injury. For him, it was obvious that the first step was reliably to produce one head-injury in a precise way so that it could be studied by others. The alternative was simply to give up.

Animal activists criticized Gennarelli for bashing primate heads for a decade and getting nowhere. Even if he succeeded in devising a machine to make a reproducible model of head injury, they said that such a model offered little help in actually treating such injuries. Scientists deny this. Knowing how to produce different kinds of burns in animals, they say, is the first step in studying the physiology of burns and the metabolism of healing.

Ends and Means

Animal experimentation abolitionists often debate tactics for stopping animal research. One question is whether, in a moral struggle, tactics should be employed which others regard as immoral, i.e., do noble ends justify unnoble means?

Ghandi in India, and the Southern Christian Leadership Conference in the South, used nonviolent, public civil disobedience to protest evil policies. Philosopher John Rawls says that justified civil disobedience differs from terrorism in being: (1) public, where protestors are clearly identified—versus hiding under white sheets at night; (2) nonviolent—versus killing innocent people (3) accepting of legal consequences—children went to jail in Birmingham during the Children's Crusade; and (4) the last step after exhausting legal means.[25] According to these criteria, some acts of animal activists—especially in England—are not justified civil protests but terrorism.

The Animal Rights Militia in England has placed bombs outside of the homes of four animal experimenters. No one was injured, because the activists phoned police who dismantled the bombs. The most radical English animal-rights group is Hunt Saboteur, which has bombed meat-packing factories and butchers, and set metal wires to cut hunters chasing foxes. Leader Marley Jones has said:

> In Britain, we [animal activists] tend to think that most types of actions [which prevent cruelty to animals], short of killing someone, are morally justified. Physical violence, in my opinion, is justified as a last resort, if all appeals to reason fail and there is no other way to save the animals.[26]

In the United States, in 1988, the ALF destroyed a brand-new building for animal research at the medical school in San Diego and burned down a veal-packing plant in Oakland, California. Masked ALF spokespersons took credit in televised interviews for these attacks and vowed to continue "until the killing of innocent animals stops." In late 1988, Fran Stephanie Trutt was arrested in Connecticut for attempted murder, for planting a bomb outside a company which makes surgical staples and uses animals to train surgeons how to use them.[27] A month later in England, four bombs exploded in English department stores, including Harrods, in protest of their sale of furs.

A columnist in London's *Times* criticized this attitude:

> Of all the Single Issue fanatics who increasingly infest our society, with their conviction that nothing matters beside their particular cause and that any action, however violent, dangerous, or criminal, is justified in the pursuit of it, the most monomaniacal are those who claim to defend "animal rights."[28]

Other unnoble but legal tactics are supposedly justified by higher ends. Just as Joseph Scheidler urges antiabortionists to spy on pro-abortion groups, so PETA's Alex Pacheco obtained a job in a primate lab in Silver Spring, Maryland, to spy on psychologist Edward Taub and to videotape animals used in his research. Similar tactics are recommended by Donald Barnes, the Air Force psychologist whose radiation experiments on primates were portrayed in the movie *Project X.*[29] Like ex-abortionist Bernard Nathanason, Barnes abruptly changed sides one day and became a spokesman for the other side.

Barnes recommends monopolizing all the time in debates, making scientists appear arrogant, working up passion before public appearances, refusing to talk to experimenters in private, and currying favor with reporters. He counsels potential debaters: "You don't have to answer their questions, you know. Simply say, 'That is an improper question, ' and proceed to say whatever you want." He recommends avoiding questions of whether an experiment is good science or whether the benefits of a particular project might justify the costs. "As much as possible, avoid getting caught up in 'scientific' arguments which you can't win. Beat a hasty retreat to philosophy and brandish your weapons: Tom Regan's *The Case for Animal Rights* and Peter Singer's *Animal Liberation.*" He also says, "Bear in mind that the only rationale for using nonhuman animals in research is that 'The end justifies the means.'"

Mailings on both sides inflame passions and distort simple truths. PETA's mailings claim most experimentation on animals is "totally unreliable." The Foundation for Biomedical Research, formed to lobby for medical schools, pharmaceutical companies, scientists, and animal suppliers, portrays all animal activists as sentimental, antimedical hypocrites. Periodicals of each paint opponents as unreasoning bigots.

Surprisingly, animal activists and research scientists are very similar in income, other beliefs, and backgrounds. The subscribers to *The Animals' Agenda*, the major magazine of animal activists, are largely college-educated (84 percent, with 25 percent holding M.A. and Ph.D. degrees), overwhelmingly white, earn $25,000 to $50,000 a year, hold managerial and professional positions (80 percent), and are mostly nonreligious (65 percent agnostic or atheist).[30] Similarly, most subscribers to *The Physiologist* hold Ph.D.s, are overwhelmingly white, earn $25,000 to $43,000 a year, and are not very religious.[31]

Trust in Scientists: The Media and Democracy

Scientists since Galileo and the Scopes trial have fought external pressures prohibiting certain kinds of research and have grown accustomed to occupying the high moral ground—at least among educated people. Recently, such scientists themselves have been accused of being irrational, of ignoring evidence, and of conflicts of interest from large salaries and huge grants. Critics challenged experiments which inflicted pain on animals for trivial reasons, which lacked controls, which lacked hypotheses, and which proved the obvious. Scientists reacted under a siege mentality and fought reform.

Television and print media present the public with conflicting stories involving animal experimentation. The public has a limitless appetite for "medical miracle" stories, yet animal abuse stories always garner quick sympathy.

In such stories, the public is often manipulated by mass media. Focusing on the distant "Mad" Scientist, who supposedly callously tortures animals, is an easy target. A much tougher target is the neighbor who acts on replacement-pet-ownership: when the pet "runs away," the neighbor simply replaces the lost dog with a cute puppy. Many others refuse to pay to have their pets neutered, having the cumulative effect of creating millions of unwanted dogs and cats.

The "pet objection" is serious. In 1987, only about 180,000 dogs and 50,000 cats were used in medical research. In contrast, 56 million dogs and 54 million cats lived in the United States. Of these, and in that year, about 22 million were abandoned or got lost—almost all of which died miserably.[32] Especially for utilitarians, the "greatest good for the greatest number" of animals lies first, not in further reforms of animal labs, but in the reform of how Americans think about pets. About 230,000 dogs and cats are used in medical research, mostly pound animals who otherwise would have been dead, a total which constitutes about 1 percent of the number of cats and dogs who die each year. Scientists wonder why only they are defamed as Dr. Frankensteins when most animal-abuse occurs down the block.

UPDATE

Overall, experiments exposed by the ALF have fared poorly upon NIH review under public pressure. In addition to the termination of the head-trauma studies on baboons at the University of Pennsylvania, the City of Hope Medical Center in Duarte, Cal., lost its Animal Care Assurance (a semilegal document assuring NIH that it can trust the university to abide by federal regulations). City of Hope lost $1 million in grants and was fined $12,000 by the Department of Agriculture (which oversees some animal research). University of California at Riverside's animal research facilities underwent an 8-month investigation, but NIH concluded that "no corrective action" was necessary. At Columbia University in New York, NIH suspended all grants involving vertebrates (other than rodents) following a rare, unannounced site visit motivated by secret ALF pictures of poor lab conditions. Investigators found poor veterinary care, unsterile surgery, lack of ventilation, and bad housing for quarantined dogs. Columbia said it had already taken steps to correct the conditions before the investigation.

On the legislative side, a major victory for ALF occurred in Congress in 1985. Starting in 1986, every university conducting animal research must have an Institutional Animal Care and Use Committee to review such experiments. In 1985, the Reagan administration opposed formation of such committees, but the videotapes of Gennarelli's head-injury studies persuaded Congress. The new rules were sponsored by Senator Robert Dole and Representative George Brown. In being the key event causing the creation of such committees, Gennarelli's head-trauma study was the "Tuskegee Syphilis Study" of animal research in leading to federally mandated review (see next chapter).

Activists claim the committees are mere window-dressing. In contrast to similar committees reviewing experiments on humans which have a majority of nonmedical members, animal committees are almost entirely composed of scientists themselves (with one token member, usually a sympathetic nonscientist). Such committees only read proposals and do not inspect labs to see if researchers follow their proposals. Most committees have never completely rejected a single experiment. The Department of Agriculture is charged with enforcing standards in labs, but lacks funds and the will to do much.

One controversy surrounds use of chimpanzees for research on AIDS—a use which animal rights groups are fighting. Some primates appear to model various aspects of HIV infection and AIDS. Animal advocates claim that primates are unlikely to help much for a condition which takes years to develop and which varies highly in humans. In general, primates are scarce because other countries are reluctant to sell them to America for medical research and because they are expensive to breed and raise.

Although Gennarelli's research was stopped, many other kinds of research on primates continue. As the population ages and as medicine cures many traditional diseases, more and more people will experience neurological diseases such as Alzheimer's and Huntington's. Precisely because they are most like us, some primates are often the best—or only—models for research on such diseases. The future will likely see the continuation of the tension between those who, on the one hand, would accept such diseases as part of natural aging and for whom the cost to animals of injurious research is too high, and, on the other hand, those caring for relatives of such diseases (or themselves at risk) who want research done, even at a very high price to those primates who, in research, must be our unwilling "silent partners."

FURTHER READING

Carl Cohen, "The Case for the Use of Animals in Biomedical Research," *New England Journal of Medicine* 315(14) (October 4, 1986).

R. G. Frey, *Rights, Killing, and Suffering,* Basil Blackwell, Oxford, England, 1983.

Eugene Linden, *Silent Partners: The Legacy of the Ape Language Experiments,* Times Books (division of Random House), New York, 1986.

Tom Regan, *The Case for Animal Rights,* University of California Press, Berkeley, Cal. 1983.

Bernard Rollins, *Animal Rights and Human Morality,* Prometheus, Buffalo, N.Y., 1981.

Andrew Rowan, *Of Mice, Models, and Men: A Critical Evaluation of Animal Research,* State University of New York Press, Albany, N.Y., 1984.

Peter Singer, *Animal Liberation,* New York Review of Books, New York, 1975.

Susan Sperling, *Animal Liberators,* University of California Press, Berkeley, Cal., 1988.

CHAPTER 9

The Tuskegee
Syphilis Study

The Tuskegee Study of untreated syphilis in hundreds of poor, uneducated black men in Alabama is one of the most condemned experiments of American medicine. Before discussing this study, it will be instructive to survey major abuses of medical experimentation in the 20th century. This will provide perspective on experimentation, not only for this chapter but also for the following three.

A SELECTIVE HISTORY OF ABUSES IN 20TH-CENTURY MEDICAL EXPERIMENTATION

For centuries, the craft of medicine used trial-and-error methods to perfect drugs and remedies, but it was not until the science of medicine began that experimentation became a major part of medicine. In the 19th century, some gentlemen physicians carried on experiments in their leisure time, e.g., as George Eliot describes Dr. Lydgate in *Middlemarch*. Some became famous, such as William Beaumont, who, in 1822, saved Alexis St. Martin from a bullet wound to the stomach, which then healed strangely and left a hole. Dr. Beaumont proved that stomach juices digested food by employing Alexis St. Martin as his subject and servant. But even this early relationship had its problems, for when St. Martin refused to be a subject and ran away, Dr. Beaumont had him sought by police.

The early 20th century saw other physicians experiment, following the inspiration of Koch and Pasteur. The germ theory of disease opened a new book in medicine and some physicians read avidly.

However, it was not until World War II that medical experimentation became institutionalized. During this war, both Allies and Axis powers wanted cures for dysentery, malaria, and venereal diseases. In America, Franklin Roosevelt established the Committee on Medical Research and this committee approached its project with a wartime mentality which carried over to researchers' attitudes after the war. Disease was the enemy, researchers were the soldiers, and victory could be had—given proper funding and will. During the war, considerations of ethics and informed consent carried little weight:

A wartime environment also undercut the protection of human subjects, because of the power of the example of the draft. Every day thousands of men were compelled to risk death, however limited their understanding of the aims of the war or the immediate campaign might be. By extension, researchers doing laboratory work were also engaged in a military activity, and they did not need to seek the permission of their subjects any more than the selective service or field commanders did of draftees. . . .

In a society mobilized for war, these arguments carried great weight. Some people were ordered to face bullets and storm a hill; others were told to take an injection and test a vaccine. In philosophical terms, wartime inevitably promoted utilitarian over absolutistic positions.[1]

After the war, it became apparent that some researchers had gone too far in pushing for cures, especially researchers on the losing side.

Research of Nazi Physicians

As mentioned in Chapter 3, physicians sympathetic to Nazi party ideals participated in early "euthanasia" programs in which the insane and comatose were involuntarily killed. Some of the most prestigious professors of German medicine supported extermination of racially "inferior" people.

In Ward 46 of the Buchenwald concentration camp from 1943 to 1945, vaccines against typhus were inflicted on homosexuals, convicted criminals, Russian officers, Polish dissidents, Jews, and Gypsies. In one experiment, a medical professor from the Robert Koch Institute injected infected blood into 40 involuntary subjects, who served as a treatment group. All in all, about 1000 prisoners were used, of whom 158 died from typhus. No thresholds of infection were established, and high morbidity occurred in unimmunized controls, almost all of whom died.[2]

Anopheles mosquitoes were flown in from swamps across the world to transmit malaria to subjects. Dr. Grawitz, the Reich Physician of the SS, infected women in their lower legs with staphylococci, gas, and tetanus bacilli. Particles of glass and stone were injected into wounds to test the efficacy of sulfa drugs.

For the German Air Force, Dr. Sigmund Rascher, "The Captain," studied abilities to live during rapid altitude changes. He built the "Sky Ride Wagon," an enclosed box on wheels with monitors inside, and discovered that, "the blood does not yet boil at an altitude of 70,000 feet."[3]

Rascher killed about 70 of 200 subjects coerced into studies of reviving nearly frozen bodies. Jewish and Russian inmates were stripped and chilled in icy waters or blizzards. As ward clerk Eugene Kogon wrote, "When their screams created too much of a disturbance, Rascher finally used anesthesia." Nude Jewish women were used to thaw frozen subjects, and the Captain reported "in detail how revived subjects practiced sexual intercourse at 86 to 90 degrees Fahrenheit." Because it is unlikely that nude women would be available to revive downed Luftwaffe pilots plucked from icy seas, Rascher's "experiments" were mainly degradations. In 1989, a conference at Minnesota debated whether such data should be cited in medical articles.

Other Buchenwald experimentors implanted hormones to cure homosexuality, shot captives to study gunshot wounds, starved inmates to study the physiology of nutrition, and surgically removed women's limbs to study regeneration.

At the Auschwitz concentration camp, physician Josef Mengele, the "Angel of Death," participated in the execution of 400,000 victims. Raised a conservative Catholic, Josef was the oldest of three sons of a successful manufacturer of farming equipment. Although above average in intelligence, Josef got his As more by hard work than by brilliance.

Like many pioneering physicians, the young Josef Mengele was ambitious and wanted fame. The Mengele business was too limiting, so Josef chose medicine. He studied in Munich between 1930 and 1936, with a special concentration in anthropological genetics, a fashionable topic of the 1930s which was part of the eugenics movement so powerful then in Germany and America. In 1931, Munich was the center of Hitler's National Socialist German Worker's party and its theme of racial purity. To advance himself with his politically conservative medical professors, i.e., professors who accepted whatever powers controlled political life, he became a Brownshirt. In another astute move in 1934, he married a professor's daughter. One witness says that, "they made a dashing young pair: Irene—tall, blonde, and good looking; Mengele—handsome in a Mediterranean way, dapper, and with a passion for fast cars."[4]

Mengele cultivated professors favored by the Nazis and oriented his research to their interests, publishing a doctoral thesis on racial jaw morphologies. Captivated by academic medicine, his research aimed at securing a rare, prestigious, full professorship.

Mengele's 20 months at Auschwitz began by clearing typhus from the camp. He "triaged" the sick and gassed about a thousand Gypsies. His superiors admired his methodical efficiency and his lack of sentimentality.

As time passed, Mengele began to greet incoming trains whose boxcars were filled with Jews. He examined them, looking for twins and other subjects for his experiments. Those he selected with a flick of his wrist lived by participating in his experiments. Most of the rest died. He supposedly humiliated some Jewish women by having them parade naked while he watched incoming passengers for twins.

Mengele's plan for his future professorship was keyed to finding a way to overcome the effects of genetics by modifying the environment, i.e., by influencing the genotype to obtain a desired trait. He sought identical twins, who served as natural controls of any environmental difference between them. He wanted to find ways to guarantee blue eyes, blonde hair, and healthy bodies with no genetic disease.

He experimented with six children to see if injecting dye could make eyes aturn blue. When finished, he cut out the twelve eyes and hung them on his lab wall, along with some human organs, some of which had been supposedly removed from bodies while still alive.

He made female twins have sex with male twins to see if twin children would be produced. He interchanged blood of identical twins to see the effects, and then interchanged blood between pairs of twins. In one set of nonidentical child twins, one was a hunchback, the other not, and Mengele surgically grafted the hunchback to the sibling's back, creating a "Siamese" effect, accentuated by sewing their wrists back to back. Witness Vera Alexander reported that when the children came back to the barracks: "There was a terrible smell of gangrene. The cuts were dirty and the children cried every night."[5]

Mengele ordered between 150 and 200 of the twins killed. In some cases, he killed them himself. As one physician present later said,

> After that, the first twin was brought in...a fourteen-year-old girl. Dr. Mengele ordered me to undress the girl and put her head on the dissecting table. Then he injected the Epival into her right arm intravenously. After the child had fallen asleep, he felt for the left ventricle of the heart and injected 10 cc of chloroform. After one little twitch the child was dead, whereupon Dr. Mengele had her taken to the corpse chamber. In this manner, all fourteen twins were killed during the night.[6]

At another time, when Mengele discovered a hunchback and his son, he had both of them killed, their bodies boiled, their flesh stripped, and the skeletons dipped in gasoline for preservation for his anthropological studies of body types. He kept seven dwarfs alive—from a Romanian circus family—in order to exhibit them to visiting German physicians.

In other experiments, he tested the limits of human endurance to electric shock on 75 male and female prisoners, of whom 25 immediately died. He subjected a group of Polish nuns to high dosages of radiation in sterility experiments, burning the nuns severely.

Although his temper occasionally flared when anyone subverted his plans, he was noted for being cool, impersonal, and detached. When 300 Jewish children by accident escaped death in the gas chambers and fled to a nearby field, Mengele ordered a gasoline fire set in a large pit and watched as the children were put in. Some children, on fire and screaming for their lives, clawed their way over dead bodies to the top, where Mengele and SS men kicked them back in.

As the Russian army approached in 1945, Mengele fled and successfully escaped. Even though he used his real name and was listed almost immediately as a major war criminal, he made his way to Latin America, where he lived for at least 40 years in Brazil and Paraguay. Although Simon Wiesenthal and other Israelis tried to capture him, he always escaped. He reportedly died in the summer of 1985 in Brazil.[7]

In his later years, Mengele met his grown son Rolf, who says his father never expressed any regret for his actions or ever thought he had done anything wrong. In his mind, it was not Josef Mengele's fault that Jews were to be killed at Auschwitz, and since they were to die anyway, why not use them first in experiments to advance medical knowledge, to advance Nazi programs, and coincidentally, to advance his chances for a professorship? After all, it wasn't *he* who had decided that these prisoners would die. Today, he lives in history as a symbol of medical evil because he harnessed great ambition to an amoral detachment while furthering massive suffering.

The Nuremberg Trial and Nuremberg Code

At the Nuremberg trials in 1946, German physicians said they had been merely following orders, that their experiments had been properly related to solving medical problems of war, and that what they had done was not substantially different from research done on captives by American physicians.

In this latter claim, there was an element of truth (although not a justification). In 1941, American researchers experimented on orphans at the Ohio Soldiers and Sailors Orphanage. They also experimented on retarded Americans at a New Jersey State Colony for the Feeble-Minded and at a Dixon, Ill., mental institution.[8] In attempting to produce a vaccine, researchers injected deadened forms of shigella bacteria into such subjects. No one died as a direct result, but many subjects got very sick. Finally, the Tuskegee Study was occurring in America during this time and was being run, as in Nazi Germany, by physicians working for the federal government.

One problem faced by the Nuremberg judges was the lack of a code covering ethical experimentation on captive populations. The judges mention 10 ethical principles of permissible medical experimentation which came to be cited as the "Nuremburg Code" after the war. Its most important principle held that captive subjects should freely consent to participation in experiments.

Abuses by Japanese Researchers

During the same war, Japanese physicians secretly killed over 3000 Chinese prisoners in medical research, especially at Unit 731 in Harbin. Prisoners were injected with dozens of diseases to study their natural course, diseases including anthrax, syphilis, plague, and cholera. In one study, 700 Chinese died in a plague study and in another, a man's body was filled with a horse's blood.[9]

These experiments are not generally known today because the U.S. government protected the Japanese researchers from punishment in exchange for learning results of their research. Indeed, it was not until late 1981 that these experiments became known, whereupon both the experiments and the U.S. protection were criticized for the precedent they set.

Henry Beecher's Criticisms

In the United States, the war against the Axis ended but the war against disease did not: "... the prospect of winning the war against contagious and degenerative illness gave researchers in the 1950s and 1960s a sense of both mission and urgency that kept the spirit of the wartime laboratories alive."[10]

By the 1960s, the sense of the times had changed. Rachel Carson's *Silent Spring* showed the ravages of pesticides and the Cuban missile crisis showed just how close nuclear destruction could be. "Miraculous" drugs were discovered to have terrible "side effects," such as DES children and thalidomide's monsters. Faith waned in the inevitability of scientific progress, and with it, faith waned in medical research.

In 1966, Harvard medical professor Henry Beecher, in the *New England Journal of Medicine,* criticized 22 experiments of fellow researchers.[11] All the studies had been published in medical journals, none had obtained informed consent, and several bordered on abuse. Moreover, Beecher claimed the 22 studies were not exceptions but the norm of medical experimentation. About the same time, Dr. Henry Pappworth similarly criticized 500 medical experiments.[12]

Both critics suggested that the dangers of medical research were unjustly inflicted mainly on "captive populations" such as prisoners, inmates of mental institutions, clients of nursing homes, and poor patients. Both suggested that if all people benefited from the results of such research, then all should participate as subjects.

The abuses cited here differed greatly from those of Nazi physicians. Although abuses, the problems stemmed not from a systematic contempt of some people (like the Nazi contempt for Jews and people of color), but more from a conflict of goals of physician-researchers. After World War II, the chief ethical problem of medical experimentation concerned balancing the interests of the individual subjects with the goals of both helping future patients and advancing careers.

THE TUSKEGEE SYPHILIS STUDY

Because the Tuskegee Study was investigated behind closed doors, its ethical issues never became widely known. Hence the historical background of medical and racial issues are especially important in this case.

Social History of Venereal Disease

Until the availability of penicillin in 1948, the common fate of kings and peasants was to suffer the sequelae of venereal disease once the first symptoms appeared. So suffered Cleopatra, Judea's King Herod, Charlemagne, Henry VIII of England, Napoleon Bonaparte, Frederick the Great, Pope Sixtus IV, Pope Alexander VI, Pope Julius II, Catherine the Great, Columbus, Paul Gauguin, Franz Schubert, Albrecht Dürer, Goethe, Friedrich Nietzsche, John Keats, and James Joyce.[13]

For hundreds of years, venereal disease was blamed on sin. Between the 12th and 16th centuries, syphilis was first separated from other diseases with similar symptoms and was then associated with prostitutes. Efforts to eradicate it by punishing prostitutes failed because customers were never treated similarly.

In the 18th century, standing professional armies arose and, with them, acceptance of high rates of venereal disease began. In one study around 1900, one-fifth of the British army had syphilis or gonorrhea.

Between 1900 and 1948, and especially during the two World Wars, American reformers mounted a great antisyphilis campaign, which was called the Social Hygiene Movement or Purity Crusade. The campaign emphasized "syphilophobia," which led people to believe that visiting prostitutes would uniformly infect customers with syphilis, which was supposedly always fatal. The campaign emphasized clean, active sports as an alternative to just-say-no attitudes.

According to historian Alan Brandt, reformers split twice, once over giving out condoms during World War I and once again over giving out penicillin during World War II.[14] The split came because some reformers fought the physical harm of syphilis, while others fought illicit behavior. In each case, generals fighting wars overruled moralists and ordered release of the controversial item. When the troops came home, the practices continued.

The Racial Background

Like American society, American medicine of the 1930s was racist. Most physicians condescended to black patients and sometimes used them as subjects of nontherapeutic experiments. Historian Todd Savitt described how J. Marion Sims, the father of American gynecology, practiced techniques for closing vesical-vaginal fistulas on slave women.[15] John Brown, who wrote a book about his former life as a slave, described how a Georgia physician kept him in an open-pit oven to produce sun burns and to try out different remedies.

The best-known account of the racial background of the Tuskegee Study is James Jones' *Bad Blood.*[16] In the late 19th century, Social Darwinism swept America (see Chapter 14), and some whites predicted that by 1900, the black race would be extinct in the competition for "survival of the fittest." As Jones describes them, white physicians were obsessed by aspects of black anatomy. Defects in whites went unreported, but medical journals described defects in blacks in great detail, ostensibly confirming the biological demise of blacks through evolution. Genital and brain development were said to vary inversely.

Pre-existing stereotypes of blacks led physicians to see their racist attitudes as "facts." When some physicians in 1914 were advocating the germ theory of disease, others were writing, in the *Journal of the American Medical Association,* that:

> The negro springs from a southern race, and as such his sexual appetite is
> strong; all of his environments stimulate this appetite, and as a general
> rule his emotional type of religion certainly does not decrease it.[17]

Jones describes how blacks were seen as dirty, shiftless, promiscuous,
and with bad personal hygiene. For white physicians of the time, syphilis
was a natural consequence of the innately low character of blacks, who
were (as one such physician said) "a notoriously syphilis-soaked race."
Forty years before the Tuskegee Study started, a rural Georgia physician
wrote, "Virtue in the negro race is like 'angels' visits—few and far between.
In a practice of 16 years in the South, I have never examined a virgin over
14 years of age."[18] A Chicago medical professor wrote in 1919 that black
men were like bulls and elephants in *furor sexualis,* unable not to copulate
around females. It went without saying that blacks would not seek treatment for venereal disease.

Historian Brandt wrote, "There can be little doubt that the Tuskegee researchers regarded their subjects as less than human."[19] Brandt suggests that
it was a rare white Southern physician who was not a racist in the early 1900s,
and that this situation continued throughout the study.

Medical Background

The spirochete causing syphilis was discovered by Schaudinn in 1906. In 1909,
the German Paul Ehrlich and the Japanese S. Hata discovered, on the 606th
combination of arsenic, a "magic bullet" targeting spirochetes. Ehrlich modestly called it "salvarsan."[20] Seeing that it cured syphilis in rabbits, Ehrlich
gave it to syphilitic patients. None of them was asked, as it was common practice not to do.

At first, salvarsan seemed to work wonders and, in 1910, Ehrlich received
standing ovations at medical meetings. But later, disease recurred in some
patients, and they died. Moreover, salvarsan itself seemed to kill some patients. Ehrlich maintained the drug had not been given correctly and developed a less toxic form, neosalvarsan, but it still killed some patients. The two
magic bullets also didn't work on endstage patients with neurological lesions
and infectious chancres. Neosalvarsan was better because it could be given
more easily, but as a physician of the time said, the treatment was "erratic,
and generally without rhyme or reason, —an injection now and then, possibly
for a symptom, some skin lesion, or when the patient had a ten-dollar-bill."[21]
Moreover, few physicians then could start an intravenous line without causing infection or great pain. Finally, Ehrlich had patented neosalvarsan, and it
was expensive. Few blacks during these Depression years could afford a dollar
a week for months of the weekly treatments, much less to take off time from
work to get the treatments.

When the Tuskegee Study began in 1932, the only study of the natural
course of untreated syphilis was Boeck's study between 1891 and 1910, of 1978
Norwegians. In 1891, Boeck thought that no treatment at all might be an im-

provement over treatment with neosalvarsan because such "heavy metals" removed symptoms of syphilis while not curing the underlying disease. Worse, the metals suppressed what would now be called the immune system. Boeck first defined syphilis by symptoms; the Wasserman test, a simple blood test for syphilis, didn't come until 1906. Boeck's student and successor, Bruusgaard, selected 473 of Boeck's patients for evaluation in 1929.[22] The selection included the more severely affected, who were more likely to have hospital records. Bruusgaard was surprised that 65 percent were symptom-free, and was even more astounded that, of those with syphilis for more than 20 years, 73 percent were asymptomatic.

One reason these results were surprising was because they contradicted the Syphilophobia Campaign. Bruusgaard's results showed that although syphilis was a terrible disease, it was not uniformly fatal for everyone. Bruusgaard's results also supported the possibility of spontaneous cures.

THE CASE FROM 1929 TO 1972

The First Phase of the Study: 1932–1933

The Tuskegee Study partially arose when physicians appreciated that long-term syphilis might not be as bad—perhaps not even fatal—as the sin-denouncing, antisyphilis crusaders had claimed. In 1929, America had several counties where venereal disease was extraordinarily prevalent, and the Julius Rosenwald Foundation—a Philadelphia philanthropy—started a project to eradicate it. With help from the United States Public Health Service (USPHS), the Foundation planned to treat all syphilitics with neosalvarsan in six counties with rates of syphilis above 20 percent.

When the Depression occurred, money became tight and the Foundation decided in 1930 that only one site could be funded. Macon County, Alabama, the home of the town of Tuskegee, was chosen because it had the highest syphilis rate, 40 percent. The Rosenwald Foundation began to treat syphilitic blacks with neosalvarsan, but ran out of funds and gave up. However, many black men in Macon County who had syphilis had been identified.

A Study in Nature

USPHS officers decided that such identification presented an ideal opportunity for a *study in nature* of syphilis. In 1865, the famous experimenter and physiologist, Claude Bernard, distinguished between such a study and an experiment. A study in nature merely observed what would happen anyway in nature, whereas in an experiment, a factor was manipulated. The Tuskegee physicians saw themselves as ecological biologists, merely observing what regularly occurred in nature.

Physicians often quoted Sir William Osler, who said, "Know syphilis in all its manifestations and relations, and all other things clinical will be added unto you."[23] Before the study, medicine for a century had emphasized the crucial importance of discovering the natural history of each disease. Unless physicians knew the natural sequence of symptoms and final outcomes, they could not recognize key changes. The natural history of syphilis had not been documented in 1932.

In the Tuskegee Study, men with early, infectious syphilis were screened out. In 1932, the USPHS repeated the Rosenwald survey and tested 4400 black adults, finding 22 percent with syphilis. (USPHS's 22 percent was lower than the Rosenwald's 40 percent because children were excluded and congenital syphilis in Macon County ran at 62 percent.)

According to some people, when the study started in 1932, it was to last a year. This is inconsistent with the claim that it was intended to be a "study in nature" to observe the natural history of the disease. Most likely, the idea for a continuing study in nature came after someone else's idea for a 1-year continuation of efforts along the lines of the Rosenwald Foundation.

A crucial medical point is that the 400 black male subjects had *late* syphilis (which was generally noninfectious). Syphilis is classified into two broad stages with subcategories in each: early infectious (primary, secondary, and early latent) and late noninfectious (gummatous, cardiovascular, neurosyphilis, and late latent). Today, syphilis is known as the Great Pretender because of the difficulty of diagnosing its latent and late stages (causing speculation in the late 1980s that AIDS was a form of syphilis). After the chancre subsides, syphilis silently spreads until a later outbreak of secondary symptoms—fever, rash, swollen lymph glands—and then becomes latent for many years. It may reappear under a variety of symptoms in the nervous or circulatory systems.

Tuskegee subjects were in the *early latent stage* with *noninfectious syphilis* of 3, 6, and 9 years' duration. Penicillin, which is now used to treat syphilis, was not available until 1943, and then only to servicemen and patients in demonstration studies. Penicillin became available to the general population in the late 1940s. In the Tuskegee study, men with early infectious, syphilis were screened out.

In 1936, a paper in the *Journal of the American Medical Association* by the USPHS surgeon general described the study as "an unusual opportunity to study the untreated syphilitic patient from the beginning of the disease to the death of the infected person."[24] It mentioned that it consisted of "399 syphilitic Negro males who had never received treatment."

As mentioned, when the Rosenwald Foundation identified the 20 percent of citizens of Macon County with syphilis, it treated some with neoarsenamine and mercury, which it hoped the USPHS would continue, but USPHS did not. The 399 subjects with untreated syphilis were selected mainly from the other men who had received no heavy metals treatment. These men, the surgeon general himself suggested, should be merely observed and not treated.

The Study's Middle Phase, 1936–1943: Spinal Taps and Deception

The Tuskegee Study was not a model of scientific experimentation. Names of subjects in the study and control groups were often mixed up. Except for a black nurse assigned to Tuskegee, the study lacked continuity of medical personnel. There was no central supervision, no written protocols, and no person clearly in charge.

There were also big gaps. The "federal doctors," as Tuskegee's denizens called them, came back rarely after gaps of many years. Visits are documented in 1939 and then not again until 1948. Seven years passed between visits in 1963 and 1970.

Lack of money explained some of the gaps. The federal public health budget dropped from over a million dollars before the Depression to less than $60,000 in 1935.

When the physicians returned after such gaps, and because of poor records, they wanted to know first, that they had a subject in the study group, and second, how far a known subject's syphilis had progressed. To discover this, spinal punctures ("taps") were conducted in 271 of the 399 syphilitic subjects. In this procedure, a 10-inch needle is stuck between two vertebrae into the cerebrospinal fluid, whereupon a small amount of fluid is withdrawn. During the process, patients are counseled to stay *very* still, lest the needle swerve and puncture the fluid's sac, causing infection and other complications.

Subjects were understandably reluctant to leave their farms, especially when they had no pressing medical problem, to undergo such painful taps. For this reason, the physicians provided them free transportation. Physicians also felt it necessary to dramatize the effects of "bad blood" (left vague) and to call the taps a "treatment" for bad blood.

A letter, sent by USPHS physicians to induce subjects to meet the federal physicians, was written under the imposing heading of "Macon County Health Department," with subheadings of "Alabama State Board of Health and U.S. Public Health Service Cooperating with Tuskegee Institute" (all of whom were indirect participants in the study). It read:

> Dear Sir:
>
> Some time ago you were given a thorough examination and since that time we hope you have gotten a great deal of treatment for bad blood. You will now be given your last chance to get a second examination. This examination is a very special one and after it is finished you will be given a special treatment if it is believed you are in a condition to stand it.[25]

The "special treatment" was the spinal tap for neurosyphilis, a purely diagnostic test. The physician-author wrote that men wanting this should meet the public health nurse for transportation to "the Tuskegee Institute Hospital for this free treatment." The letter closed in capitals:

REMEMBER THIS IS YOUR LAST CHANCE FOR SPECIAL FREE TREATMENT. BE SURE TO MEET THE NURSE.

Subjects and controls also received free hot lunches, free physical examinations, and free burials. Free burials were important to poor subjects, who often died without money for even a pauper's burial. In return, physicians did autopsies to see what damage syphilis had or had not done.

Around 1943, penicillin was discovered. It began to be available a few years later. The Tuskegee subjects never received penicillin, even in the 1960s or 1970s. How much subjects with late noninfectious syphilis were harmed by not getting penicillin is unclear.

The Denouement: 1965 to 1972

In 1966, Peter Buxtun, a young venereal disease investigator in San Francisco, learned of the Tuskegee Study and criticized the USPHS officials running the study.[26] By this time, the physicians supervising the study and its data collection had been moved to the newly created Centers for Disease Control (CDC) in Atlanta. These officials avoided Buxtun's questions about the morality of the study and focused only on whether continuing the study would physically harm the subjects.

A small group of physicians were convened in 1969 by the federal government's Department of Health, Education, and Welfare (HEW) to decide whether the Tuskegee Study should be stopped. The committee was convened at CDC in Atlanta and consisted of William J. Brown (CDC's Director of Venereal Diseases), David Sencer (the Director of CDC), Ira Meyers (Alabama's state health officer from 1951 to 1986), David Olansky, an Emory Hospital physician knowledgeable about the study's early years, Lawton Smith, an opthalmologist from the University of Miami, and Gene Stollerman, chairman of Medicine at the University of Tennessee. The minutes of this meeting record Meyers saying, "I haven't seen this group, but I don't think they would submit to treatment."[27] Ophthalmologist Smith pressed the hardest for continuing the study. Only Stollerman repeatedly attacked continuation, on both moral and therapeutic grounds. At the end, the committee overrode Stollerman and voted to continue the study.

Also involved in the decision to continue the study in 1969 were most of the physicians in the Macon County Medical Society, which had changed from an all-white membership in the early 1930s to nearly all-black in the 1960s. The black physicians were told about the study by Ira Meyers in 1969 and did not object. Indeed, they were given a list of all individuals in the study and agreed not to give antibiotics for any condition (at all) to subjects who saw them in their offices. This was the second time during the study that researchers actively prevented subjects from getting medical treatment. During World War II, researchers contacted the local draft board and prevented any eligible subject from being drafted (and hence, being treated by the military with penicillin for syphilis).

A monograph on syphilis sponsored by the American Public Health Association, published in 1970, and presumably written in 1969, had the goal of giving useful information to public health officers and venereal disease (VD) control officers. This monograph stated that treatment for late benign syphilis should consist of "6.0 to 9.0 million units of benzathine penicillin G given 3.0 million units at sessions seven days apart."[28] The first name on this monograph is William J. Brown, head of CDC's Tuskegee section from 1957 to 1971, and the same physician on CDC's 1969 panel who argued for continuing the study in which subjects with late benign syphilis received no penicillin.

Peter Buxton pressed CDC for 2 years, at one point traveling to CDC to be harangued by Drs. Brown and Cutler. He had expected to be fired from his USPHS job, but was not. His inquiries and protests had already caused the 1969 meeting at CDC to reconsider the study. Finally, in July 1972, Buxton told a friend and an Associated Press reporter on the west coast about the study. Jean Heller, an Associated Press reporter on the east coast, got the assignment.

The Associated Press Breaks the Tuskegee Story

On the morning of July 26, 1972, Jean Heller's story ran on the front pages of some newspapers around the country.[29] It described a study run by the federal government in Tuskegee, Alabama, where poor, uneducated black men had been used as medical "guinea pigs." Had not a bigger story broken the same day—that Democratic vice-presidential candidate Eagleton had received electroshock therapy for depression—the story might have had more impact.

Some congressmen were shocked to hear of the study, and Senator William Proxmire called the Tuskegee Study "a moral and ethical nightmare." After describing the terrible effects of tertiary syphilis, the story said that a 1969 CDC study of 276 of the study's untreated syphilitics proved that at least seven had died "as a direct result of syphilis." As many as 154 men died of heart disease in the same group, but this rate was identical with the rate of cardiovascular deaths in the control group. CDC's Venereal Disease Chief, J. D. Millar claimed the study "was never clandestine," pointing to 15 medical-scientific reports and noting that the subjects were told that they could get treatment for syphilis at any time. "Patients were not denied drugs," he stressed. "Rather, they were not offered drugs."[30] He also emphasized that, "The study began when attitudes were much different on treatment and experimentation."

The public scorned Dr. Millar's explanations. One editorial cartoon showed a frail black man being studied under a huge microscope by a white man in a white coat with a sign in the background saying, "This is a NO-TREATMENT Study by your Public Health Service."[31] Another cartoon showed poor black men walking past tombstones with the caption, "Secret Tuskegee Study: free autopsy, free burial, plus $100 bonus." Still another showed a white physician with a sheet covering a dead black man in a hospital bed, while at the end of the bed, the chart says, "Ignore this syphilis patient (Experiment in Progress)," and in the background, a skeptical nurse holds a syringe of penicillin and says to the physician, "NOW can we give him penicillin?"

CDC and the USPHS had always feared a "public relations problem" upon revelation of the Tuskegee Study, and now they had one. The Macon County Medical Society had its own problems, too, when its president told *The Montgomery Advertiser* that its members had voted to identify remaining subjects and give them "appropriate therapy." When the USPHS in Atlanta contradicted this and said the local physicians had backed them (not saying at the time that they had even agreed to deny subjects antibiotics for other conditions), the Society's secretary acknowledged their agreement to continuing the study but claimed they didn't know about withholding treatment. A USPHS spokesperson promptly documented their complicity.

The two Alabama senators, both Democrats, authorized a federal bill to give subjects $25,000 in compensation. Black votes, once largely Republican, had been key factors in the elections of Democrats Kennedy and Johnson, as well as of many southern congressmen in the 1960s and 1970s, including these senators. When Senator Edward Kennedy's subcommittee held hearings, two black subjects of the study were brought forward to testify: Charles Pollard and Lester Scott. These two men revealed the story of the Tuskegee Study and one of them appeared to be blind from late-stage syphilis. Pollard said some subjects had been told they had "bad blood" but not that they had syphilis. Other thought "bad blood" meant having something like low energy. Still others were told nothing. Senator Kennedy condemned the revelations and proposed regulation of medical research on humans.

Subjects went to federal court for compensation. They were represented by Fred Gray, a former Alabama legislator and the first elected black Democrat since Reconstruction. Gray made the suit a white-and-black issue of race, omitting from the suit Tuskegee Institute, the black nurse, Tuskegee Hospitals, and the Macon County Medical Society. By December 1974, the Justice Department decided it wouldn't win in federal court. If the department had fought the suit, it would have been tried in nearby Montgomery in the court of Frank Johnson, the liberal Alabama judge who had desegregated southern schools and upgraded the country's mental institutions.

So the federal government settled out of court. "Living syphilitics" alive on July 23, 1973, received $37,500, and "heirs of deceased syphilitics" received $15,000 (since some children might have had congenital syphilis). "Heirs of living controls" received $16,000 and heirs of "deceased controls" received $5,000. The controls and their descendants received compensation because they had been prevented from getting medical treatment during the years of the study.

This settlement occurred a year after Jean Heller's story had appeared. By then, even *The New York Times* followed the story only in a short paragraph or two on its inside pages. A federal panel was appointed in 1972 to investigate the Tuskegee Study.[32] For some reason, this panel met in secret to evaluate the study. Such secrecy prevented reporters from hearing about the study and by the time the *Report* finally appeared a year later, the public had forgotten about the study. At this time, members of the panel were shocked to read a cover letter from its black chairman mysteriously disclaiming his approval of the formerly unanimous recommendations.[33]

James Jones, the author of *Bad Blood*, later found many documents filed by researchers in the study. His *Bad Blood* was published 7 years later in 1981, 9 years after Heller's first story in 1972, and nearly 50 years after the Tuskegee Study began.

ETHICAL ISSUES

Deception and Informed Consent

One ethical issue in the Tuskegee Study concerns deception. J. D. Williams, a black physician who was 73 in 1972 and who interned at Tuskegee Institute Hospital when the study began, said the subjects did not know they were part of a study, what syphilis was, or that they weren't getting drugs they could have gotten.[34]

If the subjects were deceived, was it justified? This has been a repeated criticism of the Tuskegee Study. A federal panel faulted researchers for deception and for failing to obtain informed consent, a legal notion first heard in state court decisions in California in 1957 and in Kansas in 1960.

One apologist for the Tuskegee Study is R. H. Kampmeier, an emeritus professor of medicine at Vanderbilt Medical School and a former syphiologist in the decades of the study. Kampmeier thinks the condemnation of the study because of lack of informed consent was unfair. He thought it judged 1936 research by modern standards and that the criticism was "tilting at windmills" because it suggested that the Pasteurs of the past (who never bothered with informed consent) were unethical. Kampmeier said USPHS' 1943 study of penicillin did not obtain informed consent, and during the time of the Tuskegee Study, physicians simply walked into a patients' room and announced that they were taking out gallbladders.

Patient rights' champions reply that this shows what created the need for laws about informed consent in the first place. Moreover, it is illegitimate to compare not getting informed consent for procedures which could possibly benefit patients to not getting consent for procedures which could possibly *harm* subjects. To use an oft-abused distinction, one is therapeutic, the other is experimental. Even if telling patients the truth wasn't legally required and even if truth-telling wasn't always a medical norm, is it really true that it was ethical in 1930 to lie to subjects?

Medical historian and physician Thomas Benedek dismisses the criticism about informed consent as "anachronistic," noting that USPHS did not adopt the informed consent requirement until 1966.[35] That requirement was prompted by federal court decisions in the late 1960s mandating such consent in medical experiments. Before then, informed consent was not a legal requirement of experimental medicine. But the presumption always was that physicians would neither harm patients nor allow harm to occur. Also, Benedek emphasizes the *legal* requirement, not the moral issue of lying.

Was the Tuskegee Study Racist?

Was it a coincidence that all the subjects were black males? In Alabama before the civil rights movement? Would white males have been treated the same way between 1932 and 1972?

In *Bad Blood*, Jones builds on the background of racism in American medicine to see the Tuskegee Study as a natural result. Kampmeier emphasizes the historical context of the study, but such emphasis does not minimize how bad those times were for blacks—when the black students of Tuskegee Institute in the 1930s feared rural white toughs just outside their campus grounds. The fact that America (and American medicine) was uniformly racist does not excuse the racism.

Moreover, to believe the Tuskegee Study was not racist, one must believe that some reason existed *only* to study blacks with untreated syphilis. Some physicians believed syphilis ran a different course in different races, but if so, why not include whites in both groups? Furthermore, it is hard to imagine a parallel study where white middle-class patients would be similarly deceived.

Study Design

Were the studies, as claimed, good science with a clear hypothesis and good design? Many of the "controls" later contracted syphilis, and had to be switched to the other group. Records were often lost or had long gaps. James Lucas, a CDC physician, said the study was "bad science" and that the study's value had been undermined because "effective and undocumented treatment had been given the vast majority of patients in the syphilitic group."[36]

The criticism here is that the study proved nothing, i.e., that if these subjects were inadvertently "sacrificed to Science," that nothing for science was gained. Because many of the 399 syphilitics got some neosalvarsan or penicillin during the later years of the study, researchers could not be sure what the true untreated consequences of syphilis were.

An important thing about the study is that the "controls" were healthy men who initially did *not* have syphilis. Nothing about the effectiveness of treatment versus nontreatment in syphilitics was ever learned or intended. Kampmeier's justification of the study rested on the claim that untreated syphilitics fared no worse than those treated, but it is important to stress that *the Tuskegee Study did not compare those two groups*. It was known before the study began that syphilitics had higher morbidity and mortality than healthy subjects. It was also known from Bruusgaard's work that not all people with late latent syphilis would die of syphilis or its complications.

Moreover, the control subjects were somewhat naively assumed to remain unaffected, even though Macon County had an extraordinarily high (40 percent) rate of syphilis. Researchers supposedly treated early, primary syphilis when it appeared, but they only came once a decade and couldn't have distinguished latent syphilis of 2 years' duration from that of 15 years' duration.

Media Coverage

In October of 1972, Kampmeier criticized both the "great hue and cry" in the news media a few months before and the claim that "treatment was purposefully withheld to evaluate the course of untreated disease."[37] He said about *Time* and *AMA News* (later called *American Medical News*): "In complete disregard of their abysmal ignorance, members of the fourth estate bang out anything on their typewriters which will make headlines."

But this hardly seems true. Indeed, and in contrast to today's coverage of such cases, the media in 1972 botched the Tuskegee story. It was a complicated story to cover and within days, smaller and smaller articles moved farther and farther back into the last pages of newspapers. Kampmeier mistakenly criticized the media for reporting that the study withheld treatment. Yet that is *precisely* what was intended. If anything, Jean Heller and the press were too restrained. They were too fearful that science might be hurt. Subsequent events buried the story, so that few Americans today know much about it. Heller and the print media should have pushed the story harder.

Over the previous decades, the Tuskegee Study was casually reported in medical journals in at least 17 articles between 1936 and 1972. In 1964, an article in the *Archives of Internal Medicine* was titled, "The Tuskegee Study of Untreated Syphilis: The 30th Year of Observation."[38] Although it was true that no attempt was made to conceal the study, neither did anyone write to newspapers about what was going on.

Today, Americans receive news of controversies in medical ethics before physicians read about them in journals. It has not always been that way.

Was Tuskegee a "Study in Nature"?

If USPHS had never gone to Macon County, Kampmeier claims that subjects with syphilis would have gotten no treatment and would have been no worse off. This is an instance of the problem in logic known as "counter factual conditionals," which takes the form of "if so-and-so had not happened, then such-and-such would not have happened." Claims about past "counter factuals" look deceptively simple but really are not. In this case, an infinite number of other things might have happened had not USPHS conducted this study in nature, the most important of which is that USPHS might have given everyone neosalvarsan. Also, had USPHS not gone in at all, some other agency, such as the Rosenwald Fund, might have provided neosalvarsan. John Steinbeck could have written a novel about Tuskegee, arousing national indignation, as he did in the *Grapes of Wrath*. Another way to put this is: given that many physicians and some federal funds were going into Tuskegee to study syphilis, was this the *best* thing to do?

Harm to Subjects

One of the most important ethical issues concerns whether subjects were harmed. The issue of harm appears first in judging spinal taps. Some physicians regard spinal taps as insignificant harms justified by the necessity of proving presence or absence of neurosyphilis; hence lying about such insignificant harms is no large concern. From the perspective of physicians who daily see terrible disease and disability, such taps are not tremendously significant. Physician experimenters see patients with life-threatening heart attacks, terminal cancer, kidney failure, and psychotic self-mutilation. Vehement protests about a few spinal taps only come from people with no such medical perspective.

On the other hand, critics emphasize that spinal taps are not like taking blood samples. A small minority of patients will experience bad side effects, such as being unable to stand without headaches, which may last 2 to 3 weeks. One patient in a million will become paralyzed. Moreover, being "tapped" today without consent is, legally, battery.

Physicians say unconsented-to spinal taps are not traumatic. Defenders of patient rights say that attitude is just the problem. Physicians become blinded to wants of people who are outside of medicine. Physician/experimenters have special conflicts of interest, torn between serving patients and serving science. That is why ethics must come from outside medicine, not inside.

Modern researchers needing spinal taps offer as much as $500 to recruit healthy volunteers. Even these people are unrepresentative of the general population, and some people will not undergo nontherapeutic taps for $10,000. Economists believe that compensation to workers inversely correlates with preferences, so that dangerous or distasteful tasks require higher pay. That some people will not voluntarily consent to nontherapeutic taps today tells us that some would not in 1936. Patient advocates emphasize that most researchers have never had a spinal tap and that their professions lead them to see spinal taps as insignificant. In December 1988, a malpractice suit for $2.7 million was settled out of court by the Medical Center Hospital of Vermont after 28-year-old Pauline Pichora went into a coma after a resident "tapped" her.[39]

The more crucial issue is harm from nontreatment of syphilis. Some physicians argue that no proof exists that blacks were ever harmed by being untreated in the Tuskegee Study. Perhaps this is true for neosalvarsan, since it is unlikely that subjects would have gotten this expensive, cumbersome treatment of controversial benefit. But penicillin is another matter.

Kampmeier argued publicly (for many physicians who argued privately) that latent syphilis is a "chronic granulamatomous self-limiting disease." However, retired internist Benjamin Friedman, who practiced syphilology during the same decades as Kampmeier, disagrees:

In the 1940s it was known that patients receiving as few as 20 injections of arsenicals rarely developed symptomatic aortic disease. Since we could not determine in advance which of the latent syphilitics would, after 20 or 30 years, develop symptomatic aortic disease, it was necessary to treat all of them. One cannot maintain that some small number of syphilitics deprived of treatment did not therefore suffer injury.[40]

Kampmeier says that "incontrovertible evidence" shows that the late manifestations of latent syphilis have occurred by 20 years after infection "in almost all instances." Subjects at the beginning in 1932 had latent syphilis of 3, 6, and 9 years' duration, so in 1948 (the year Kampmeier takes penicillin to have become a proven therapy and widely available), the subjects had latent syphilis of 19, 22, and 25 years' duration. But penicillin was discovered in 1943 and tested across the country in public health clinics during the next 5 years. Why wasn't it given then?

In answer, apologists look back to Ehrlich's experience: the previous "magic bullet" had been idiosyncratic, not hitting its target in some cases, in others, killing patients. Who could know in 1943 that penicillin might not do the same? It was not until as late as 1958, Kampmeier says, that definitive proof of penicillin's efficacy was published. And this proof was only for early, infectious syphilis, not late latent syphilis. About the latter, Kampmeier said dramatically in 1974, "Today 26 years later we know no more about the effectiveness or ineffectiveness of penicillin in late latent syphilis than in 1948."[41] (Except for the Tuskegee Study, which did *not* compare giving and not giving penicillin to syphilitics, all latent syphilitics have been given maximal dosages of penicillin since its introduction. So Kampmeier is correct, there is no proof, but to get such proof, an unethical study would need to be conducted). Physician/medical historian Thomas Benedek, after reviewing the medical evidence available in 1940, concluded that untreated syphilitics in 1937 had lived longer and better than those partially treated.[42]

Most physicians disagree. The claim that penicillin was not proven effective until 1948 is especially weak. Friedman retorts, "penicillin replaced all the above [heavy metal treatments] and was available in adequate doses after 1946." Moreover, he says, "after Mohoney's studies in 1943 it became apparent that penicillin in adequate dosages was effective" (for early syphilis). Finally, prophylactic effect of penicillin in latent syphilis was expected and has been achieved: "the progressive decline in syphilitic heart disease since 1930 from the fourth highest cause of heart disease to almost total disappearance is strong indirect evidence that penicillin has a preventive effect."

Yes, the study's defenders say, hindsight is 20/20, but at the time, the picture was less clear. Benedek emphasizes that physicians in the 1940s knew neither optimal dosages nor a quick way to determine if penicillin had any effect on long-term syphilis. As for Friedman's claim about aortic disease (which is more frequent in black syphilitics than white), Benedek retorts that it only occurs in 10 percent of untreated syphilitics and then begins 15 to 20 years later, after which time it has done its permanent damage. Of the 70 syphilitic subjects examined in 1948, all had syphilis for at least 18 years. So giving them penicillin in 1948 would most likely have been too late to be effective.

Kampmeier insists that seroreversal in latent syphilis has never been proved to be associated with decreased morbidity or mortality. (This may be like AIDS, where having a positive antibody test doesn't necessarily mean one has the HIV virus.) Penicillin achieves seroreversal in early latent syphilis, and modern textbooks recommend this, but a 1984 textbook notes: "The clinical significance of dose-related seroreversal is controversial."[43] Other texts recommend penicillin in latent syphilis of long duration, but with a noticeable lack of footnotes to studies proving the benefit. The accuracy of the Venereal Disease Research Laboratories test (VDRL test) and of central spinal fluid tests for diagnosing or excluding neurosyphilis is especially controversial. Some people with tertiary syphilis have negative VDRLs.[44]

Medical historian Benedek concludes that giving penicillin to latent syphilitics in the 1940s "might have exerted a definitely beneficial effect on the prognosis of only 12.5 percent of the subjects." He notes that of those syphilitics who managed to live until 1973, virtually all outlived their nonsyphilitic peers. His 1978 review article concludes,

> The Tuskegee Study had been in progress for 12 years when the possibility of dramatic improvement of treatment appeared, for 16 years when new insights into the ethical implications of research began to be advocated, and was 39 years old when it abruptly became the subject of severe criticism for ethical deficiencies.... The righteousness of the ethical critics fails to take into account that in the context of the 1930s thoughtful physicians could detect no ethical dilemma in an investigation such as the Tuskegee Study, and also refuses to accept the evidence that very little would have been accomplished therapeutically by initiating penicillin treatment in the 1950s.

An especially troubling fact to critics was that no effort was made to survey syphilis in wives and children of subjects. Benedek read correspondence in the National Library of Medicine and discovered that "virtually all subjects were or had been married" and that subjects had an average of 5.2 children. Wouldn't husbands want to know they had syphilis? That they might become re-infectious and infect wives, maybe even giving their children congenital syphilis? Did researchers believe the racist myth that black men couldn't refrain from sex, and so did not tell?

Researchers know *now* that late syphilis is almost never re-infectious. Different researchers over 50 years ago did not know. They took a chance with subjects' wives and children (which is why, in settling the suit, the federal government also compensated the heirs).

More generally, the study can't be excused, as CDC tried to do, by saying that it didn't really harm anyone. It's lucky for researchers that it didn't cause more harm than it did. The crucial point about harm is that, in the late 1940s when penicillin became available, *it should have been hypothesized that penicillin might help subjects in the latent stage of syphilis.* For all anyone knew at the time, penicillin would have prevented lethal aortic heart disease. At the very least, why couldn't untreated, latent syphilitics have been divided into two groups, one of which received penicillin? The answer seems to be that everybody else was getting penicillin and the Tuskegee subjects were unknowingly used to serve as "controls."

Deontological Criticisms

In these disputes, physicians at USPHS and CDC often seemed to be arguing that unless harm be proved from withholding treatment, it was permissible to so withhold. This is a strange argument, which would wreak havoc if applied to other areas of medicine, e.g., there is no proof that patients do better in ICUs than normal hospital rooms.

If one adopts a moral view emphasizing motives, such as Kantian ethics, then proving harm is not ultimate. For such a view, the important point is that people do not exist to serve medical science. Whether black or white, people have rights to control their lives without risking harm from others. By systematically deceiving subjects, researchers deprived these black subjects of standard American rights.

Such deontologists emphasize the rights of subjects, their intrinsic dignity, and their right not to be treated as "means" to the goal of scientific knowledge. On such a theory, to violate people's rights is wrong *regardless of whether medical harm to them occurs.*

UPDATE

It is helpful to remember that by the time of CDC's decision in 1969 to continue the study, Rosa Parks had led a bus boycott in Montgomery (1955), students had integrated a reluctant Rich's in Atlanta (1960), the Freedom Riders had ridden (1961), the University of Alabama in Tuscaloosa had been integrated despite Wallace's posturing in its "school house door" (1963), the bodies of Cheney, Schwerner, and Goodman had been found buried (1964) under an earthen dam (as portrayed in *Mississippi Burning*), President Johnson had signed the Voting Rights Act (1965), and Martin Luther King Jr. had been killed (1968). In 1967 and 1968, frustrated blacks had rioted in Watts, Cal., and in Washington, D.C. By 1966, USPHS had become concerned about publicity about abuses in experimentation and instituted new rules for research—unfortunately not applying its rules to itself. So when CDC decided in 1969 to continue the study, it was not as if nothing had changed.

In 1973, and after the study stopped, remaining syphilitic subjects received penicillin. No allergic reactions occurred. The story immediately faded and soon only vague impressions remained of what had happened.

In 1972, the federal government required all institutions receiving federal funds and conducting human experimentation to have "Institutional Review

Boards" (IRBs) to review proposals for experiments before they were judged
for funding. Later on, IRB review was expanded to include research on humans in the social sciences. Today, IRBs are the frontline of prevention against
abuse in medical research.

   As part of its out-of-court settlement, the U.S. Government agreed to
provide free lifetime medical care for Tuskegee subjects, their wives, and their
children. By September 1988, the government had paid $7.5 million for med-
ical care for such subjects. At this time, 21 of the original male, syphilitic subjects were still alive—each having had syphilis for at least 62 years.[45] CDC
estimated that 28 of the original syphilitic group died from syphilis during the
study. In addition, 41 wives and 19 children had evidence of syphilis and were
receiving free medical care. Before revelation of the Tuskegee Study and the
accusations of Beecher and Pappworth, support for outside (IRB) review and
peer review of medical research was lukewarm. After these problems surfaced,
medical research was forced to come under regulation in a multi-stage process. Similarly, animal research came under quasi-regulation after revelation
of Gennarelli's head-trauma studies. Many researchers today resent the pa-
perwork of such regulation, but it is important to understand why both came
about.

   In 1988, questions were raised about whether it was ethical to cite the
twin experiments of Mengele and the cold experiments of Rascher. One compromise was to cite them, but with an acknowledgment as to how they were
obtained. One author argued that the general failure to teach about Mengele
and Rascher, with the continuing citation of their research, amounted to "denying the concept of evil in medicine."[46]

   Similar concerns could be raised about the Tuskegee Study. Few people
know about the study and it is not generally discussed in medical education.
It is unclear how much it it is cited, but there are only rare acknowledgments
of how any results were obtained. Perhaps most damaging, lack of understanding of Tuskegee continues the happy myth that evil in experimentation
was a problem of the Nazis, not American medicine.[47]

FURTHER READING

Thomas Benedek, "The Tuskegee Study of Syphilis Analysis of Moral Aspects Versus
   Methodological Aspects," *Journal of Chronic Diseases*, 31 (1978).
Alan Brandt, "Racism and Research: The Case of the Tuskegee Syphilis Study," *Hastings
   Center Report* 8(6) (December, 1978).
James Jones, *Bad Blood*, Free Press, New York, 1981.
R. H. Kampmeier, "Final Report on the Tuskegee Syphilis Study," *Southern Medical
   Journal* 67(11) (1974).
———, "The Tuskegee Study of Untreated Syphilis," Editorial, *Southern Medical Journal*
   65(10) (October, 1972).
Tuskegee Syphilis Study Ad Hoc Panel to the Department of Health, Education and
   Welfare, *Final Report*, Superintendent of Documents, Washington, D.C., 1973.

CHAPTER 10

Christiaan Barnard's
First Heart
Transplant

Along with Karen Quinlan's case, Christiaan Barnard's first heart transplant, in December 1967, began the interdisciplinary field of medical ethics. Transplantation created new ethical questions about whether heart donors were really dead, about conflicts of interest among transplanting surgeons, about costs, and about burdens on families. The Quinlan case involved conflicts about criteria of brain death and these conflicts involved needs for organs for transplantation. In 1975, just 7 years after Barnard's transplant, the complexity of issues in medical ethics perplexed many people and a new field had been launched.

HISTORICAL BACKGROUND

Early attempts to transplant human organs involved the skin (technically an organ), which Indian doctors transplanted as early as 600 B.C.[1] In the 16th century, Tagliacozzi transplanted skin tissue and recognized that the immune system rejected tissue from other bodies. Noses and ears severed in duels were successfully sewn back on victims, but never worked on another body. Lamb blood was transfused into humans with miserable results.

In 1900, Austrian Karl Landsteiner discovered that human red blood cells had types. He used arbitrary letters of the alphabet to name blood groups A, B, AB, and O. B blood contains antibodies which attack the protein markers in A blood, and A blood contains antibodies which attack protein markers in B blood. However, AB blood accepts either A or B Blood (because it "recognizes" its own blood types). Curiously, these three types can all accept O blood, even though O blood only accepts O blood. People with O blood are universal donors. This explains why transfusions worked surprisingly well among Incas, because almost all South American Indians have O blood.

206

Landsteiner's monumental discovery went unappreciated for many years until he finally received the Nobel prize in 1930. His work explained why the first transplants failed, in that blood contains antibodies which spot foreign substances, including different types of blood. Previous attempts to transfuse blood caused death, and countries such as England banned transfusions.

Because the cornea receives no direct blood supply, it is insulated from immunological rejection. Thus, corneal transplants succeeded in the early 20th century, and became routine by the 1940s.

In the early 20th century, the American physiologist Guthrie and the Frenchman Carrel learned how to sew together tiny, slippery, blood vessels, which if not perfectly sewn would leak or form clots.[2] In the early 1950s, Lawler transplanted a kidney from a cadaver but the patient died. Autopsy showed that the transplanted kidney had shriveled to a dead shell.

In 1953, Peter Medawar discovered that protein markers or "antigens" occur on the surface of cells, and that white blood cells called T-lymphocytes first recognize foreign antigens and then signal antibodies to attack. (In AIDS, the virus burrows inside T-lymphocytes and takes them over, destroying the body's ability to recognize foreign substances.) Highly specific antibodies develop against highly specific antigens. Medawar's work stimulated research both on how the immune system works and on suppression of its rejection of transplanted organs.

This progress was difficult. Medawar's work was the base of a pyramid whose apex was routine organ transplantation. Perhaps the most difficult part of building this pyramid was, like progress toward in vitro fertilization, overturning received truths. It was learned that antibodies did not mediate the immune system, as they had been thought to do. Most important, rejection was proved not to be a progressive, unstoppable process.

The kidney was first successfully transplanted by Thomas Murray in 1954 at Peter Bent Brigham Hospital in Boston from one identical twin to another. Four patients received liver transplants in 1963, but none of the four lived a month. Lungs were transplanted at medical centers in Mississippi and Pittsburgh in the same year, but with dismal results.

Three modern pioneers in heart surgery were John Kirklin, Michael De Bakey, and Norman Shumway. After moving from the Mayo Clinic to Birmingham, Ala., John Kirklin perfected cardiac surgery for congenital defects. As a medical student, De Bakey had devised a booster pump, which became the essence of the heart-lung machine and which, in the 1960s, made possible open-heart surgery. Like Kirklin, Shumway built on the work of his teacher, Minnesota's Owen Wangensteen, who trained many famous transplant surgeons such as Christiaan Barnard. Shumway discovered that cardiac nerve connections (severed during transplantation and too numerous and fine to be reconnected) didn't matter because the heart had an independent electrical "ignition system" through adrenal hormones which triggered its beats and rate. He also discovered that it was better not to transplant the whole heart, but to leave intact the upper walls (atrium or auricles) and reduce operating time in half.

CHRISTIAAN BARNARD AND
THE FIRST HEART TRANSPLANT

On December 3, 1967, a somewhat brash surgeon catapulted to international fame. Two weeks later, his face appeared on *Time*'s cover. South African Christiaan Barnard was then 44 years old—an early age for international fame in surgery. Barnard had jumped the gun on the prestigious medical centers around the world by successfully transplanting a human heart from one person to another. He had done so from an obscure hospital in Cape Town, South Africa, called Groote Schuur, meaning in Afrikaans "big barn."

The operation tapped deep symbolism in mankind. Some newspapers characteristically worried about "harvesting the dead," while others predicted that a form of immortality was at hand.

Christiaan Barnard grew up in a rural sheep-farming area of South Africa, the favored son of simple parents. Two Dutch Reformed Churches stood side by side in his town, one for the whites, the other for "coloreds." Barnard's father was minister to the second and was paid a third of the salary of the first. As such, the Barnards were poor and of low social status. Young Chris reportedly played soccer barefoot when his teammates all had shoes.

Barnard was able to attend college and graduate from European-style medical training. He joined a general practice in Ceres, a beautiful winegrowing area, as the second junior partner of an old family physician. As Barnard tells it, patients began to favor the youthful Christiaan over the senior physician, who forced Barnard out.

The second heart transplant patient, Phillip Blaiberg, ambiguously described Barnard as having the "personality of a genius."[3] Barnard was also described as cold, driven, and moody. Blaiberg identified cardiologist Velva Schrire as the "brains behind the transplant team." Owen Wangansteen remembers Barnard as lean, nervous, hardworking, intense, and as a person who didn't want to keep smoking but who did, anyway, by smoking other people's cigarettes. In many ways, Barnard fit the surgeon's stereotype, because few colleagues liked him. He was brusque and driven, offending nurses and staff. His wife said he was a perfectionist at home, unable to watch meat cut sloppily at dinner.

His daughter possessed great talent as a water-skier, and Barnard expected nothing less of her than a world championship. As he relates in his autobiography, *One Life*, he drove her ruthlessly and spent all his free time with her.[4] After she had several accidents, it became clear she would never be world champion (she was South African champion). He then decided to stop living through her and to seek fame himself.

Angered at being forced out of the country practice in Ceres, Barnard went to Cape Town, deciding to advance in other ways. He started studying bowel obstructions and experimentally operated on 49 dogs before finding success with the 50th. He then applied for a prestigious scholarship but did not win. The winner privately gave Barnard some troubling advice: he hadn't had a real chance of winning because his children went to an English-speaking, rather than an Afrikaans-speaking, school. For him to win high honors in South African medicine, his children would have to speak Afrikaans and belong only to the nationalistic Dutch Reformed Church. Raising children in English, rather than in the archaic Afrikaans, gave them the option to one day leave South Africa.

Losing the scholarship left Barnard open to accept a lucky opportunity to study in Minnesota under surgical pioneer Owen Wangensteen. Ambitious and dedicated, Barnard jumped at the chance, even though it meant opposing his family's wishes.

When Barnard's plane arrived in New York's Kennedy Airport, he was surprised when the black workers did not "Sir" him as had Cape blacks. Unlike South African blacks, Barnard observed that American blacks "were more Bantu,...tough, proud, and filled with an untouchable substance of self."[5]

In Minnesota, Barnard lived in poverty for 2 years in Minneapolis-St. Paul. South African physicians were not paid anything like the pay of American physicians, and Barnard shocked other physicians by working as a night nurse and doing menial jobs in the neighborhood to earn money to bring his family over. Other physicians felt he shouldn't have demeaned himself this way.

His wife disliked America. Both Barnards hated the cold winters of Minnesota. Sensitive to being viewed as racists, Barnard's wife felt Americans were hypocrites because they wouldn't send their children to school with blacks and avoided integrated neighborhoods. Americans preferred to symbolically fight racism by criticizing South Africa, not by looking around them. She felt the South Africans were more honest. Raised on the typical television images abroad of America, she perceived potential violence everywhere. She soon fled home with her children.

At Minnesota, Barnard completed a 5-year course of study in 2 years, earning a doctorate in medicine. To do this, he had to assist Wangensteen during the day as an attending assistant physician and study pathology and German at night. Already a young surgeon at home, Barnard resented being treated as a medical student by Wangensteen but swallowed his pride.

On Saturdays, he and two other surgeons-in-training sometimes drove down to the Mayo Clinic in Rochester, where Barnard learned how to close a defect in a ventricle without causing heart block from John Kirklin, who later became famous for cardiac surgery in Birmingham. Barnard also spent a week with cardiac surgeons Michael De Bakey and Denton Cooley in Texas. Cooley impressed the young surgeon, only for different reasons. Where Kirklin and De Bakey were methodical, quantitative, and cognitive, Cooley was brash and intuitive. Where other surgeons sliced away piece-by-piece to open a femoral artery, Cooley made one decisive cut. Where others took 3 hours for a cardiac operation, Cooley took one.

The technological key to Barnard's future heart transplant was the heart-lung machine, developed between 1931 and 1953 by the physiologist John Gibbon, and further improved in the early 1960s. The heart-lung machine opened doors not only to heart surgery but also to actually replacing "the pump." Before this machine, what operations could be done had to be done in a minute while the heart was stopped and the brain was without oxygenated blood. Early heart-lung machines were marred by clots which formed on surfaces of synthetic Mylar. In the later machine, air bubbles supplied the blood with oxygen and were removed by a greasy foam. If the bubbles were not removed, or if the debubbling mixture returned to the blood (as sometimes happened), the patient died. The slightest mishap with the heart-lung machine—electrical failure, leaks, or contamination—made the machine a killer.

At Minnesota, Barnard pushed to learn how to operate the newest heart-lung machine. About this time, Barnard began to develop arthritis—a devastating occupational handicap for a surgeon. Where other physicians would have switched specialties, Barnard tenaciously held on.

According to his autobiography, Barnard's days at Minnesota were not without mishap. One day, while his father watched Barnard from above through a glass dome, he operated on his 7-year-old son to repair a heart defect and ordered an assistant to cut a bit of tissue protruding from the vena cava.[6] When it was cut, a hole ripped in the heart wall and blood gushed up. Barnard panicked and, rather than simply putting his finger in the hole to stem the loss of blood, attempted to clamp the hole shut. This enlarged the hole further and by then, it was too late as the boy's blood pressure rapidly dropped from 85 to 65...to 42, and then his heart stopped. Immediately they connected the heart-lung machine, repaired the damaged wall, and attempted to restart the heart, but it never restarted. Barnard had made a cognitive mistake, one of many small judgments made each minute during surgery, and because of it, a young boy had died.

After returning to South Africa, Barnard made six trips abroad, and whenever possible, came back to America to train more. He always said he had learned the most from American surgeons. By 1966, everyone realized that the difficulty in doing a heart transplant was not the surgery but getting the heart not to be rejected, so he spent 3 months training under surgeon David Hume at Richmond, Va. where Barnard learned the few things then known about immuno-suppressive agents.

"The" Operation

When Barnard returned to South Africa, a key decision occurred which later infuriated some American surgeons. Owen Wangansteen magnanimously called Washington to arrange a small grant of $6000 to send Barnard home with a new heart-lung machine. It is obvious that Wangansteen, the mentor of most American transplant surgeons, did not expect Barnard to perform the first heart transplant. As Barnard himself said, Wangansteen treated him as a student, not as a surgical colleague.

Barnard returned to Groote Schuur Hospital in Cape Town, South Africa, in early 1967. The hospital is set deep into the slope of a mountain above Cape

Town. It is visible from all over Cape Town below and is a landmark to tourists. It looks like a resort hotel with evenly spaced windows and double wings, while ancient, mountainous, forests surround it on both sides. From a highway below, ambulances bring the injured from the city below to two entrances, one for white Afrikaners, one for nonwhite.

After perfecting techniques on dogs, Barnard quietly began to assemble a team to perform the first human heart transplant. Barnard had previously helped develop synthetic heart valves, and claims to have developed many other techniques. Now he was ready to go further. Even so, facilities at Groote Schuur were much more primitive than at American transplant centers.

Barnard asked fellow cardiologists to refer him a possible candidate. Physicians at Groote Schuur kept quiet Barnard's plans, about which American hospitals were ignorant. No one expected anyone to do a transplant until the problem of immune rejection was solved.

A dying patient named Louis Washkansky was selected. He was a 55-year-old, white, groceries salesman with a fondness for gambling, drinking, eating, smoking, and living life fully. He had been a youthful weightlifter and athlete, and later served in the army during World War II. He was a big, intelligent man with a ferocious desire to live. He was exuberant, extroverted, and well-liked. A married man, he played the machismo role to the end, pretending to his wife that everything was fine, snitching cigarettes, never slowing down, and flirting with nurses.

Louis Washkansky had diabetes, coronary artery disease, and congestive heart failure. He was about as sick as a cardiac patient can be and still live. His heart was so swollen and flabby that it extended across the inside of his large chest from wall to wall. Originally referred because he could not breathe at night, he was kept breathing through drugs. He returned to selling groceries and one day felt an attack coming on. Getting to the hospital an hour later, he got out and climbed the stairs to the cardiac unit—where his heart collapsed.

In April 1966, cardiologists had given him a couple of months to live and were amazed to see him live 2 more years. But he was still dying. In so doing, he was a physician's nightmare, taking 15 pills a day. At one point in September, he had so much edema (swelling from fluids) in his legs that holes were drilled in them for drainage. He spent 5 days without sleep—just sitting in a chair with water running down his legs into basins. His skin was almost black.

When approached in December 1967 about the transplant, Washkansky had no hesitation. He knew he was dying and his previous 2 years had been hellish. Barnard said he told Washkansky, "We can put a normal heart into you, after taking out your heart that's no longer good, and there's a chance you can get back to normal life again." After which, Barnard said Washkansky replied, "So they told me. So I'm ready to go ahead."[7]

After Washkansky had consented, Barnard waited 3 weeks for a donor. Washkansky then developed fulminant pulmonary edema—a sign that death was imminent—and Barnard worried that his chance would pass. This had happened to other surgeons, such as Mississippi's James Hardy, who years before had two waiting recipients die before a donor materialized.

On December 3, 1967, 25-year-old Denise Ann Darvall left her home on a Saturday afternoon, driving a car with her brother, father, and mother. Unknown to her, death was just minutes away. After parking the car, Denise and her mother walked a few blocks to a bakery. The bakery was a half mile below Groote Schuur Hospital. By odd coincidence, Mrs. Washkansky was then on her way up the mountain to see her husband and, during her trip there, saw a crowd gathered around the scene of an automobile accident.

The accident occurred without warning when an illegally speeding car had smashed into Mrs. Darvall as she left the bakery, killing her instantly and throwing her against her daughter. Denise had sailed through the air and was rendered brain-dead on impact but, most importantly for Louis Washkansky, her heart was still healthy. Denise was rushed up to Groote Schuur Hospital where Louis Washkansky unknowingly waited.

Shortly after arrival, Barnard approached the shocked father, who had just lost a wife to an insane quirk of fate, and who was now told that he had also lost a daughter. At a moment like this, everything depended on the public's trust of the medical profession, because not only did Edward Darvall have to accept the deaths of his wife and daughter, but he also had to accept Barnard's right to ask a very delicate question. Few questions which are this sensitive must be asked at such bad times.

When Dr. Barnard approached Edward Darvall, he said, "...we have a man in the hospital here, and we can save his life if you give us permission to use your daughter's heart and her kidney." According to Barnard, Mr. Darvall replied simply, "If you can't save my daughter, try and save this man."[8]

The Operation and Its Results

Mr. Washkansky had been already informed about the possibility of a transplant. Within 2 minutes of being told that a donor was available, he reconsented. Blood typing was done: Denise was O-negative, a universal donor; Washkansky had A blood. Calls went out to the transplant team, some of whom allegedly arrived at the hospital in pajamas or breathless when their car had broken down and after running up the mountain to Groote Schuur.

As he was rolled into surgery, Washkansky was still awake. For the first time, he felt "kind of shaky." The former amateur boxer said he felt like a person "going into the ring when you don't know who you're up against." Washkansky told Barnard he was his manager, but now he wanted to know what his opponent looked like. Barnard says he told the cardplayer nothing, but had nevertheless thought to himself, "I knew what he [his opponent] looked like. He was the *Skoppensboer*—the wild Jack of Spades. He was death and against him I had only the King of Hearts."[9]

Denise Darvall was declared brain-dead after her heart actually stopped beating. A few feet away, Washkansky had gone under anesthesia 45 minutes before. After her heart had stopped beating for 3 minutes, Denise was put on a heart-lung machine. (Waiting longer would have damaged her heart more, which was slightly damaged already from the 3-minute wait.) Meanwhile, Washkansky went on the heart-lung machine in preparation for excision of his heart because the two upcoming operations had to be precisely coordinated.

At this point, everything almost failed. Washkansky's femoral artery, where a tube attached, was so narrow from cholesterol that the machine couldn't force blood into his heart. The pressure on the tube climbed to 290, just short of where the lines would blow, spilling gallons of blood over the room. Frantically, Barnard and other surgeons reattached the line directly to Washkansky's aorta. Gradually the pressure dropped, saving Washkansky and the first heart transplant.

Barnard then walked to the next room where surgeons had opened Denise's body, preparing it for Barnard to cut out her heart. Barnard did so, leaving part of the wall attached to the heart, like a jack-o-lantern's lid. Then he put Denise's heart in an ice-cold basin and walked thirty-one steps back to Washkansky's operating room, where he gave Denise's heart to a nurse to hold. Then he cut out Washkansky's flabby heart and peered down into the huge, empty chest cavity. As he looked at both old and new hearts, he said, "This really is the point of no return."[10]

Then he sewed Denise's heart-plus-heartwall into Washkansky, where it looked quite small. Although both operations took 5 hours, cardiac surgeons regarded cutting out the old heart and sewing in a new one as relatively simple. The interesting question was first, whether the transplanted heart would start in a foreign body, and second, whether the new heart would be rejected.

After the surgery, an expectant operating team watched as Barnard began to start the transplanted heart. Reports differ about this scene. The hope was that the heart would start spontaneously as the blood temperature rose to normal (as it did in fact with the second transplant patient). This didn't happen. According to an upbeat UPI story, the new heart took up a fast beat after Barnard shocked it slightly, whereupon Barnard gasped, "Christ, it's going to work!"[11] Groote Schuur's chief surgeon described the heart's starting after the shock as "like turning the ignition switch of a car."[12]

According to Barnard's own account, things were not so simple. Like dog hearts, human hearts do not always start right up when shocked. After the first attempt, Denise's heart started and continued, then stopped. Moreover, the new heart didn't take over from the heart-lung machine. After another attempt, the heart started and beat regularly, whereupon the heart-lung machine was turned off.[13]

After working all night, the operation concluded at 7 A.M. Washkansky was quickly weaned from the heart-lung machine, and an hour later, regained consciousness and tried to talk. Thirty-six hours later and hungry, Louis Washkansky ate a soft-boiled egg.

Aftermath

Michael DeBakey in Texas graciously said Barnard had broken through a medical barrier and achieved greatly. *Time* magazine, reacting more to symbolism than understanding, called Barnard's work the "Ultimate Operation."

Intensely worried about immunological rejection, Barnard's team flooded Washkansky with gamma ray radiation from a cobalt unit and administered both prednisone and Immuran (azathoprine). The strong, burly man did not tolerate the treatments well.

Washkansky was encouraged to eat to get protein into his system, but his progress was slow. He had 5 rough days after surgery, when his urine output, enzymes, and heart rate were problematic. By day five, he said the constant tests were "killing me. I can't sleep. I can't do anything. They're at me all the time with pins and needles....It's driving me crazy."[14] But on his sixth day, after receiving steroids to prevent rejection, he began five very good days of happiness when he laughed, visited with family, and felt like going home. At this time, Barnard told a press conference that if Washkansky's progress held, he would have Washkansky home in 3 weeks.[15]

But this was the eye of the hurricane. When rejection really began, Washkansky began to feel horrible and his personality changed. A vibrant, forceful man became sullen, irritable, and suffered from chronic shoulder pain. Dark circles formed under his eyes, and he said he felt "terrible." As his heart and breathing rates climbed, an unknown shadow was seen on his lung X-ray on the 13th day.

The two threats to Washkansky were infection and rejection, but most symptoms of post-transplant patients could unfortunately indicate either. Worse, treatment of one problem could exacerbate the other. Thus, it was crucial to wait for a definitive diagnosis, even if doing so meant risking death.

By the 14th day, Louis felt that he was dying. He couldn't force himself to eat. He lost bowel control. The pain in his chest increased so much that he preferred to lie in his own feces rather than move. Barnard said he was "constrained" to put a nasogastric tube down his nose and throat to feed him, but Washkansky didn't want it. It didn't look to Washkansky that he was ever going to be normal again. He had lost his dignity and, hence, his will to live.

By the 15th day, Washkansky was breathing with difficulty. Spotty, mottled patches on his legs indicated circulatory failure. The patches meanwhile grew ominously on his lung X-rays and Washkansky gasped desperately for each breath. Barnard decided Louis had to go back on a respirator.

But Washkansky felt he was near his end, which was to come 4 days later. When Barnard approached him, Washkansky felt he would never be home by Christmas, i.e., never have a chance at a minimally normal life. Barnard disagreed, saying (on December 18th) that there was "a chance" Washkansky could be home by Christmas. Washkansky replied, "No, not now."

Inside an oxygen tent, Washkansky grabbed the tent's sides to prevent Barnard from entering to reopen his tracheotomy hole. Having been on a respirator before, Louis knew reconnection of a respirator meant giving up speech.

Washkansky refused, saying, "No, Doc."

Barnard replied, "Yes, Louis."[16]

Dr. Barnard put Washkansky on the respirator anyway. Washkansky would never talk again.

Mrs. Washkansky then called, telling Barnard that reporters said Louis was dying. Barnard lied and said reporters were lying. Both the surgeon and his patient perceived Mrs. Washkansky as weak and unable to bear the truth. New X-rays had showed that bilateral pneumonia, klebsiella, and pseudomonas had infiltrated Washkansky's lungs. Previously, he was given penicillin which had killed one organism, but allowed others to grow. The anti-immune drugs given to prevent rejection had also allowed all these organisms to flourish.

Mrs. Washkansky was allowed to see Louis (but wasn't told it might be the last time). Barnard urged her to make her husband keep fighting. On a respirator, Louis couldn't speak, and Mrs. Washkansky didn't understand why. She was told not to touch him because of germs. All Louis could do this last time was, with enormous effort, open his eyes and move his arm a bit.

After she left, Louis received 40 percent oxygen, but as his breathing worsened, it had to go to 100 percent. Between midnight and 1 A.M. the physicians struggled, giving him drugs to help his breathing, but it was too late. Germs had overrun his lungs and Washkansky began to suffocate.

After 2 hours of Washkansky's dying gasps, Denise Darvall's heart went into wild fibrillation from lack of oxygen and stopped. Even then, Barnard was not ready to give up. He rushed a team together to put Washkansky on a heart-lung machine. At this point, another physician challenged his decision, arguing passionately that it was "madness" to continue and that Washkansky was "clinically lost." Reluctantly, Barnard agreed. On December 22, 1967, after 18 days on a transplanted heart, Louis Washkansky died.

The next morning, Barnard watched the postmortem, which showed that lobar pneumonia had destroyed the lungs. The heart-lung machine would have been useless. The heart and Barnard's surgery were perfect.

ETHICAL ISSUES

Criteria of Brain Death

Although Barnard did not discuss it with Edward Darvall, he had to worry about whether his standard of Denise's brain death would be accepted worldwide. Everyone would inspect Barnard's criteria, looking for any sign of conflict-of-interest or Frankensteinian overeagerness.

Most transplant surgeons at the time realized that moral caution coincided with their professional interests. Such surgery depended entirely on altruistic, voluntary donations. Anything placing such donations under suspicion would sabotage them. Even as late as 1985, a Gallup poll showed that 44 percent of Americans hadn't signed organ-donor cards because they feared premature declarations of death to facilitate organ donation. (Criteria of brain death were discussed in Chapter 1.)

Some conservative critics of the time claimed that a heart should only be transplanted when it actually stopped beating. To them, taking a beating heart from a body, even a brain-dead body, was ghoulish. Pioneering cardiac surgeon Werner Forrssmann publicly criticized Barnard.[17] Forrssmann had developed cardiac catheterization and had experimentally put tubes nine times into his own heart. In 1956, he won the Nobel Prize for medicine. In 1968, he criticized the "macabre scene" where two teams of surgeons worked in adjoining rooms, one waiting with knives in hands for a young person to die, the other placing a patient on a heart-lung machine. Partly because of such worries, Japanese surgeons today do not transplant hearts.

Washkansky needed a heart in the best possible condition, and if Barnard had waited too long, he might have lost Denise's heart. Christiaan Barnard's brother, Marius, also a surgeon on the transplant team, described a disagreement between himself and his brother over when Denise's heart should be removed.[18] Marius wanted to take it out before it stopped beating to maximally help Washkansky. Instead, Barnard waited until the heart stopped beating, and then waited another 3 minutes to be certain it wouldn't spontaneously restart. The ethical question here concerned who was the patient, Washkansky or Denise Darvall? Didn't Marius Barnard have a conflict-of-interest? Whose interests came first?

Today it is law in all states that the physicians declaring patients brain-dead for possible organ donation can not be the transplant surgeons. It was also no coincidence that during the next year, 1968, the conservative "Harvard Criteria" of brain death appeared (which do not require a heart to stop beating before removal).

The philosophical problem of brain death is that there is no natural or metaphysical marker of the end of life. The abortion debate is full of fruitless searches for such a definition. Regardless of which end of life is under scrutiny, people desire to discover some factual event which would allow them to prove that a certain being is not a person. In both cases, the fact/value problem occurs. In both cases, whether a certain fact or event turns a being without, into a being with, moral value is not a discovery so much as a (usually slow, hard-fought) societal decision.

In defining death, what is familiar is cessation of breathing and heart-beat, but such crude criteria are not definitive. Denise Darvall's heart could easily have been restarted with a small electric shock, and with supportive treatment, could have continued in Denise's brain-dead body. Countless patients have been resuscitated and shocked back into life. Louis Washkansky could have been put on a heart-lung machine and could have been reawakened. He would have been paralyzed (from drugs given to prevent spontaneous breathing) and dependent on the heart-lung machine. Eventually, his heart-lung machine would have been contaminated, sprung a leak, or broken down, whereupon he would have "died" again.

These facts tremendously agitate some people, who perhaps would rather not understand the clinical details. Certainly many families would rather just hear that their relative had died and not be asked how much pain and money they would accept in choosing such-and-such criteria of death. On the other hand, perhaps Veatch is right that patients should be able to choose their own standard of death.[19] Barnard clearly would have violated Washkansky's wishes by putting him on a heart-lung machine, as he did before by putting him on a respirator.

Ethical Issues in First-Time Surgery

After the transplant, Barnard's feat was hailed at home as a South African achievement. American surgeons privately carped that Barnard's training in transplants, as well as his training on the machine, had occurred through the generosity of American medicine. Some complained that it was a mistake to have given Barnard such a machine when other surgeons had worked longer and harder to be the first to do a transplant.

More important, other surgeons had been more cautious about waiting until better immuno-suppressive drugs were available before going ahead. Wasn't there too much pressure to be the first? It would seem that the fame society gives those who are first is both good and bad for patients, driving physicians to new heights but also making them compromise what is best for their patients.

There is also something inherently arbitrary in remembering only the person who first did something. Less known is Adrian Kantrowitz, who at the time had been desperately trying to find one of the thousands of anencephalic babies born each year as he watched a baby turn blue in Brooklyn.[20] Kantrowitz eventually found a baby, obtained consent from the parents, and performed the grueling 24-hour operation 2 days after Barnard did the first such operation. Kantrowitz's baby suddenly died 6 hours after his transplant. In contrast, Barnard's patient had lived. Had it been the other way around, everyone would know the name "Kantrowitz."

By all rights, the first surgeon to implant a heart in America should have been California's Norman Shumway, who in fact transplanted the first adult human heart in America shortly after Barnard's transplant. Shumway had been gearing up for the operation since 1961, and could easily have done what Barnard did. He announced he was ready to do a human heart transplant in November 1967, the same time as Barnard began seeking a transplant recipient. In that year, perhaps a dozen surgical teams around the world could have done a heart transplant, *if* they hadn't worried about how long the patient would have lived.

The media, and the public's thirst for news about breakthroughs, helped create such problems. It was reported that, shortly after this time, Kantrowitz prematurely implanted a mechanical heart in a patient who died almost immediately. Another Brazilian patient first learned of the possibility of a heart transplant when he woke up with another heart inside him.[21]

Barnard both wanted the media attention and did not know how to handle it. He allowed the first real conversation between Washkansky and his son to be filmed live by a television crew. Also, allowing the germ-carrying media into Washkansky's room, even in sterile gowns, did not seem best for Washkansky, especially when he hadn't allowed Mrs. Washkansky to touch Louis because of the dangers of infection.

It is unclear, too, why the realities of Washkansky's gruesome death were underreported. Perhaps fellow transplant surgeons didn't talk to reporters; perhaps they were inured to such deaths. Certainly most reporters were undertrained in medicine to understand what was occurring. More important, the public was certainly more interested in the miraculous event than in clinical details of the demise.

Barnard seemed to relish publicity—much more so than William DeVries (see next chapter). Barnard held daily, candid briefings until doing so became overwhelming and the government information office took over. Critics were especially amazed that he favored American journalists and took monies from them in return for access to himself and Washkansky.[22] Barnard justified taking the money to benefit both his program and his future patients.

Quality of Life

Perhaps the most important ethical issue raised by the first heart transplant concerned quality of life, and this issue continued later with Barney Clark and Baby Fae. One criticism was that transplant surgeons equivocated about what counted as a success. When asked this question, Barnard replied that he couldn't really say when we would be certain of success. The first operations had the obvious criterion of simply making a transplanted organ work for a few days. But patients, physicians, and society wanted the richer criterion of a return to normal life.

Washkansky's case vividly portrays how dramatic surgery can turn a patient's last weeks into living hell. Did Washkansky know, at the beginning, how bad it could be? Did he give real informed consent? Was Barnard correct to say Washkansky had a chance to return to normal life, in getting his consent to operate, when it was unlikely that he did?

Because there was no real chance that Washkansky would live without better immuno-suppressive drugs, transplanting a heart in 1967 was like transplanting a head—a spectacular symbol, but with no therapeutic value to the patient. The 1954 Nobel prize winner of Columbia University, André Courman who worked on cardiac circulation, lashed out at Barnard for jumping the gun. "Merely demonstrating that it is technically feasible" to do a human heart transplant, Courman said, was unethical. Physiologist Norman Staub said Barnard's operation was merely "grandstanding" and that prevention of disease, not organ transplantation, should concern physicians.[23]

The public erroneously assumed that Barnard's skill as a surgeon allowed him to do the first heart transplant, but many surgeons had already emphasized that the surgery was relatively simple, despite its highly emotional symbolism. As Norman Shumway said, "It's not *who* does the operation, but *how*."[24] Shumway emphasized that post-operative, medical care was critical, not surgical cutting. Because no surgeon knew any new way to keep transplant patients alive in this post-operative period, none, except Barnard, had done a transplant.

In the early years of transplants, enthusiasm for the new operation obscured the fact that most recipients didn't do that well and only rarely returned to normal life. In 1968, the "Year of the Transplant," as many as 25 percent of transplant recipients became temporarily psychotic. Few reporters got this story because most practiced press release journalism and because the public disliked bad news. The truth was that the massive doses of immunosuppressive drugs produced initial euphoria (e.g., Washkansky's 5 days), followed by severe symptoms such as catatonia, depression, hysterical crying, and even temporary psychosis. These were listed as "side effects"—a slight misnomer.

Nevertheless, one spectacular success was all that was needed to unleash waiting cardiac surgeons around the world. That success came in early 1968 with Barnard's second patient, Phillip Blaiberg, a Jewish dentist who lived for 20 months.

Interracial Transplantation

Another ethical issue for Barnard concerned interracial transplantation. Barnard was told by Groote Schuur physicians that the first recipient absolutely had to be white. Otherwise, world opinion would charge them with exploiting nonwhite patients, who in South Africa were often illiterate. Earlier a kidney had been transplanted in South Africa from a black donor to a white recipient and the world press reported it as racial-physiological integration.

Such fears were accurate. The first question from reporters who called long-distance was whether Washkansky was white. When they found out he was Jewish, some asked him how he felt with a "Gentile heart" inside.

Barnard feared that apartheid might ruin his heart transplant. The heart of white, Protestant, Denise Darvall had gone to Washkansky, a middle-aged Jewish man, but her kidneys went to a black child. If Mr. Darvall had known where the kidneys were going, would he have consented? (He later said he would have.) The average South Afrikaner? What about in India, with its rigid caste system? Would a Brahman take a heart from a lower-caste person?

No fuss was raised about the interracial aspect, but the real criterion would come later when payment was determined. How many transplants to "coloreds" would be paid for by the government?

Perhaps like many South African physicians and professors in their dealings with their international professional communities, Barnard wished to isolate his achievement from the larger context of apartheid. Perhaps that is possible, perhaps not.

Philip Blaiberg got a heart from the 25-year-old "colored" Clive Haupt who suffered a cerebral hemorrhage one day. Later, Blaiberg's wife attended Haupt's funeral and both Blaibergs thanked Haupt's wife.

South Africa itself saw the racial issue in confused terms. Marius Barnard said that the first recipient could have been a nonwhite, but the realities of South African politics—and the world's view of South Africa—dictated otherwise. When Christian Barnard received a call informing him about a possible donor (Denise Darvall), he had to immediately ask, "Is she colored?" For if she had been, the operation would not have gone ahead. Earlier, a nonwhite had gotten a kidney from a white, and that was progress. But records of race of blood donors were still kept and, where a choice was possible (the usual case), recipients were allowed to choose the race of the donor.

South African physicians, like other physicians, said that medicine could not solve larger social problems. At best, medicine could make small progress in its own areas and not make larger problems worse.

Courage

Just as it is common for reporters to hail the "courage" of professional football players, so reporters hailed the bravery of the first two transplant patients. Neither of them agreed. Both said that this was their only chance to live, that they wanted to live, and that it took no courage to grasp at the held-out straw.

Socrates argued in the Platonic dialogue *Laches* that if no fears exist, courage is not possible, and that courage differs from being rash or daring in that it requires *worthy* goals.[25] Fools face fears, but for silly goals; thieves face fears and are daring, but do so for immoral goals. For Socrates, real courage requires facing fears for the right goals.

Under the definition, courage could not be exhibited in going ahead with the operation to avoid dying. What was feared was death, not continued life. Nevertheless, there are ways in which patients such as Washkansky could be courageous. One would be to decline the operation and accept a feared death. Another would be if patients such as Washkansky were really informed before they consented. If they understood the worst outcomes, including their likely powerlessness in those outcomes, and feared such possibilities, and if they then went ahead with the operations, then—at least according to Socrates' definition—they would be truly brave.

Good of the Family

In the first year of heart transplants, attention always focused on the recipient of the transplant, and the effects on the recipient's family often went unnoticed. Such families could not realistically object to transplants for their relatives. Their role was to support the recipient. Any previous problems between family members and the recipient had to be suppressed.

In both Washkansky's and Blaiberg's cases, the wives rode a roller coaster of emotions. Blaiberg had suffered a major heart attack 12 years before his transplant and was not told then that he could die any day. Only his wife and cardiologist knew the truth. (In retrospect, Phillip agreed with this paternalistic decision.) In the first transplant, Washkansky's wife, like Louis, expected him to return home, which he never did. Her life was a constant vigil by the phone.

Blaiberg did much better than Washkansky, but every time he suffered a setback, everyone feared it was his end. His first sore throat was major agony for his wife and his physicians. For his extra months of life, all care and attention focused on him. His daughter Jill, living on a kibbutz in Israel, became famous against her will and was unhappy at her loss of privacy.

A related issue was that of identifying the donor. Although such a policy encourages others to be donors (the Darvall family became famous), one South African journalist claims Mrs. Washkansky wanted the donor to remain anonymous. It seems that she felt it impossible to repay the debt but felt great obligation to do so, once Mr. Darvall was known. After 18 days, her husband was gone but her obligation to the Darvalls was not. (Note: Ethical issues about costs of heart replacements are discussed in the following two chapters.)

UPDATE

In January 1968, Barnard predicted that in 20 years, animal hearts would be successfully transplanted into humans. He predicted that if large pigs could be grown on special farms, their hearts could be easily transplanted into humans.[26] He thought primate hearts would be the next best candidates.

After Washkansky's death, Barnard flew to America to appear on CBS's *Face the Nation* and NBC's *Today Show*. While in America, he was quite busy, recording an episode for a show called "The 21st Century," meeting President Lyndon Johnson at the LBJ ranch, filming a full-hour show for NBC, and, when he came to San Francisco, received as much fanfare as the Beatles. He liked the publicity. He became the first surgeon to make a record album which, not surprisingly, didn't sell well. On the album, he was moderator of a discussion about transplant recipients, and one wit suggested the album might have sold better with a soundtrack by the Grateful Dead.

Magazines called 1968 the "Year of the Transplant." During those 12 months, 105 hearts were transplanted. After 1 year and 100 transplanted hearts, 19 patients had died on the operating table, 24 lived for 3 months, 2 lived 6 to

12 months, and 1 lived for almost a year. Of 55 liver transplants in the 15 months after Barnard's operation, 50 patients failed to live 6 months. Clearly, most of these early attempts were failures. The immune system was simply too powerful.[27]

In early 1968, Jean Dausset identified the first human leukocytes and proposed that white blood cells might be grouped as Landsteiner had previously grouped red blood cells. Building on Medawar's work, researchers matched white blood cells of donor and recipient. This matching is called "tissue typing."[28]

This discovery created a new ethical issue. In pondering the use of a donated organ, a surgeon could have a conflict between using the organ for one of his own patients in a risky operation or donating it for a safe operation at another center for benefit of a stranger. This anticipated the later problem of "designated giving," where a donor gives an organ only for a particular recipient, e.g., a particular baby needing a heart. If successful transplants needed good tissue matches, it would be impossible for one surgeon alone to match donor and recipient. Instead, such surgeons would need to cooperate in some system where donors would be matched with recipients. Such a system, with procurers and transporters of organs, would require—in surgeons— cooperative social skills rather than individual competition. The tension in such a system, between individual surgeons pushing for maximal organs for patients in their programs and pulling against the interests of unknown patients attended by rival surgeons in distant programs, persists in organ-procurement programs today.

Three famous cardiologists then suggested a 3-month moratorium on heart transplants until further evaluation could be done. Minnesota's Walter Mondale suggested a presidential commission to evaluate the research. Other surgeons disliked the idea of commissions and said surgeons should do the evaluating. Surgeon Walton Lillhei lashed out at "self-appointed critics" who "are better versed in the art of criticism than in the field under study...[and who are] frustrated by their own inability to create."[29]

These problems emerged in the "summit meeting" on heart transplantation in July 1968 between Barnard, Kantrowitz, and Denton Cooley. Cooley was reluctant to use tissue-typing, arguing that if he had a relationship with a dying patient, how could he give the donor-heart in hand to some distant stranger who had a better tissue match? Even if his dying patient might live only 6 months, could Cooley deny the patient that? Cooley indicated he wouldn't want his immunologists to stay his hand, simply because he didn't have a good tissue match. As subsequent events with the artificial heart showed (see next chapter), it was indeed difficult for anyone—even colleague Michael DeBakey—to "stay" Denton Cooley's hand. Cooley's desire to do the big operation for his patient conflicted with evidence about how transplants best worked.

After Dausset's proposal, liver-transplant surgeon Thomas Starzl and other surgeons declared a moratorium in 1968 on transplants until more was learned. Soon it was verified that leukocytes govern antigen rejections and that leukocytes could be grouped. Analysis of past operations indicated that matching tissues would increase successful transplantation.

Many cardiac surgeons criticized heart transplants. In the next decade, subsequent results were disappointing. The typical rate of 50 percent survival after 1 year was often quoted for recipients, but rarely was the figure for 3 years—17 percent. As the 1970s closed, the moratorium on transplants looked permanent. Massachusetts General Hospital, associated with Harvard Medical School, rejected a heart transplant program because of worries about costs and poor outcomes. In animals or humans, transplants of any organs between individuals rarely lasted a month, much less years. For knowledgeable observers, the death rates in early heart transplants were appalling. Rather than the Decade of the Transplant, it had been the Decade of the High-Tech-Last-Gasp.

Throughout the next decade, Shumway argued that very carefully selected patients could benefit from such transplants, and he did not follow the moratorium. Most surgeons agreed with the moratorium, and most transplant programs withered.

Such dismal news was broken in the early 1980s by cyclosporin, a drug which blocks the immune system's rejection of foreign tissue. Years before, and according to company policy, Sandoz workers vacationing in Norway had brought home soil samples. One of the samples contained an extraordinary fungus, which became the basis for cyclosporin. Cyclosporin suppressed the small part of the immune system responsible for organ rejection while allowing the rest of the system to fight normal infections. This miraculous drug was proven efficacious by the FDA in selected transplant programs between 1979 and 1983. In 1978, just when the door on heart transplants had almost closed, cyclosporin came along and blew it wide open. The number of transplants then soared dramatically, from 23 in 1975 to 172 in 1983, from 710 in 1985 to 1427 in 1986.[30]

The new success raised the issue of costs. As San Francisco heart transplant surgeon Oscar Salvatierra said in 1985:

> Presently, many transplant surgeons throughout the United States are being forced to perform an economic means test before a transplant.... To restate this more bluntly, it is easier for many potential heart and liver recipients to be maintained in a costly critically ill state, until death, by reimbursable alternative cul-de-sac therapies, than to be restored to normal life by organ transplantation, which in many instances is not reimbursable.[31]

By the late 1980s, some (but by no means all) insurance programs began to reimburse surgeons for heart transplants (kidney transplants were already covered under Medicare—see next chapter).

Christiaan Barnard stayed in the news over the next decades, but in different ways. His arthritis worsened, and—after several years—he could no longer operate. His name became associated in the 1980s with a cosmetics firm making disputed claims about collagen facial creams. He became a jet-setter, traveling in international social circles, going through two marriages, and entering a third to a famous model in 1987. He became a critic of keeping hopeless patients alive and criticized Karen Quinlan's physicians. Although one of the most well-known physicians in the world, he was not well-respected within academic medicine, and his medical career went steadily downhill in the 1970s, as if helplessly sliding down the slope of Groote Schuur.[32]

FURTHER READING

Christiaan Barnard and Curtiss Bill Pepper, *One Life*, Macmillan, Toronto, 1969.
Phillip Blaiberg, *Looking at My Heart*, Stein & Day, New York, 1968.
Renée Fox and Judith Swazey, *The Courage to Fail: A Social View of Organ Transplants and Dialysis*, 2d ed., rev., University of Chicago Press, 1978.
Peter Hawthorne, *The Transplanted Heart*, Keartland Publishers, Johannesburg, 1968.
Richard Howard and John Najarian, "Organ Transplantation: Medical Perspective," *Encyclopedia of Bioethics* III, Free Press, New York, 1978.

CHAPTER 11

Barney Clark's Artificial Heart

Although devices meant to replace the function of the heart were implanted before, Barney Clark was the first patient in whom such an implant was meant to be permanent. The success of this implant in keeping Dr. Clark alive affected many people, but it affected them in different ways.

HISTORICAL BACKGROUND

Relevance of the End-Stage Renal Disease Program

The kidneys clean the blood of poisons, and a hemodialysis machine replaces this function. Willem Kolff developed the first workable hemodialysis machine in the early 1940s in Holland, using a converted fuel pump from an automobile to keep a woman alive (who happened to be a Nazi) until she regained her health. Kolff later came to America's Cleveland Clinic, and then to Utah, where he hired Robert Jarvik to work with him in developing the artificial heart.

Prior to continuous dialysis, each session of dialysis (blood-cleansing) required surgery to attach tubes to arteries and veins, but after a few weeks, all major veins and arteries were used up. In 1970, Seattle's Belding Scribner devised a semipermanent shunt (tube) which could be opened and closed without causing infection, thereby creating long-term dialysis by allowing patients to dialyze three times a week and return to normal life.

Scribner had few machines and thousands of Americans were in renal failure. Each machine cost $6000 in 1970 dollars. Lacking funds for more machines, Scribner faced the ethical problem of who shall live when not all can. He let a committee of laypeople attack it. In doing so, he may have been humble about his own moral expertise and wanted local support. It was also true that any selection criterion would be controversial and attract publicity for more funds to make more machines.

The committee chose criteria favoring those who had jobs, family responsibilities, youth, good health, and strong motivation. Shana Alexander in *Life* dubbed it the "God Committee." She criticized the standards as social worth criteria, because they seemed to imply that some were more deserving than others.[1]

Funds were needed to pay for treatment of kidneys. Medicare (for the elderly) and Medicaid (for the indigent) programs were added by Congress to Social Security in 1965, yet 2 years later, over a thousand patients existed precariously on dialysis while others died for lack of money to make new machines. At this time, Kolff used modified Maytag washing machines for dialysis, sending patients home with bills of $360 rather than $10,000. The Maytag Company, worried about liability and the effect of such usage on its image, subsequently refused to let its machines be used.

By 1971, many stories had dramatized the plight of patients in renal failure. The dialysis breakthrough had created both a miracle and a tragedy: people were alive who otherwise would have been dead, but many others were dying for lack of machines. An NBC documentary contrasted the gigantic costs of the space program and Vietnam War with the small costs of dialysis machines. Shep Glazer, the president of the American Association of Kidney Patients, dialyzed himself before a House Ways and Means Committee and supposedly (in what may be an exaggerated story) disconnected a tube, letting his blood flow on the floor, saying, "If you don't fund more machines, you'll have this blood on your hands."[2]

In 1972, Congress passed the End-Stage Renal Disease (ESRD) Act. ESRD funded dialysis machines for all Americans. Because ethical controversy existed about selection criteria, Congress swung to the opposite extreme. From the former criterion of social worth, the ethical pendulum swung to no criterion.

Senator Vance Hartke, in 1972, said ESRD would cost $100 million the first year, with lowered costs thereafter, as decreasing costs per unit lowered outlays. Kolff predicted that his machines could be mass produced and sold for $200. By 1984, ESRD had cost taxpayers not $100 million but $2 billion a year—twenty times Hartke's prediction. (Some estimate that artificial hearts for 50,000 Americans a year would cost $7 billion.) By the 1980s, every possible candidate, no matter how hopeless, was receiving dialysis. Hartke and Congress had given little thought to incentives. In the next decade, Medicare's cost-plus funding of medicine encouraged physicians to treat everyone, no matter what the cost (this was one reason Congress phased in funding by diagnostically related categories of "DRG's" in the 1980s).

Meanwhile, few funds dribbled down to pregnant poor women for prenatal care. Some nephrologists (kidney doctors) made $200,000 a year. Seeing unlimited profits, hundreds of dialysis clinics sprang up from hospitals and for-profit medical companies.

Congress passed the ESRD act in a 30-minute session because it faced an unbeatable coalition: the American Medical Association, the elderly, blacks (who have high rates of kidney disease), the National Kidney Foundation, and a powerful national media. Such a coalition produced a hastily passed program. Other conditions such as hemophilia were not funded. The success of creating a political lobby around diseases of a single organ soon attracted copy-cats for the heart and lung.

Subsequent congressional laws added costs of kidney transplantation to ESRD, as well as payments to agencies which procured kidneys. Cyclosporin allowed success in kidney transplants to jump from 3730 in 1975 to 9000 in 1986. Such success obviated the old ethical issue of selection but created new ones, such as whether dying patients should be dialyzed, whether the monies for kidney treatment might be better used elsewhere, and whether government could effectively regulate medicine.

Among fiscal conservatives, ESRD became a paradigm of how *not* to fund medical services. Kolff said that Congress' open-ended funding defeated cost-cutting innovations. Nephrologists running dialysis clinics had conflicts-of-interests, sometimes discouraging their patients from getting kidney transplants because they only made money by keeping patients on dialysis.

Development of the Artificial Heart

After World War II, the federal government aggressively supported medical research on the heart. This support was led by Senator Lister Hill, the son of a surgeon, and Congressman John Fogarty, a victim of heart disease. In 1963, Michael De Bakey, who for years had been developing an external LVAD (left ventricle assist device) for the heart, testified to Hill and Fogarty that a larger, more complete device—an artificial heart—could be created and successfully implanted in humans, if such work were funded.[3] Michael De Bakey was a professor at Baylor College of Medicine and one of the greatest experts in the world on heart surgery. A colleague of De Bakey's at Baylor was Denton Cooley, a competitor secretly working on his own version of the artificial heart.

In a change in 1965, the NIH (National Institutes of Health) committed $40 million over 4 years for a fully implantable artificial heart and hoped to test one by 1972. However, in the early 1970s, NIH became pessimistic about artificial hearts and switched much of its grants into LVADs (left ventricle assist devices). LVADs were what physician-essayist Lewis Thomas called "halfway technologies" for diseases, halfway between real cures and no therapy at all.[4] Such technologies kept people alive in semisick states, and were better than death, but were not a complete cure.

In 1970, a dying patient was flown to the Texas Heart Institute in Houston to have his healthy heart transplanted into Haskell Karp, who was dying of a failing heart.[5] Before Karp became Cooley's patient, Cooley had privately hired a biomedical engineer to develop his own artificial heart. De Bakey's NIH-funded work on artificial heart components was available to Cooley, who secretly hired some of De Bakey's grant-paid staff.

Before the transplant could be done, Karp's heart deteriorated and Cooley implanted an artificial heart. Like Christiaan Barnard, Cooley wanted to perform a "first," and, on April 4, 1969, he operated on Karp while De Bakey was in Washington, D.C. He did not get permission from his IRB (institutional review board), the committee required by law to review the ethics of medical experiments, which was chaired by Michael De Bakey. Cooley later claimed that because the operation was therapeutic, not experimental, for Karp, no review by the IRB was necessary. Also, Michael De Bakey chaired Baylor's IRB.

In Washington, a furious DeBakey read in the front page of *The Washington Post* how Cooley had developed a similar artificial heart without informing De Bakey. Cooley had used some of the same personnel funded by De Bakey's federal grant to develop a similar artificial heart. De Bakey realized that the operation was not done to solve Mr. Karp's problems, but for Cooley to be first. In a subsequent paper, Cooley revealed that all of his experimental calves with artificial hearts had rapidly died. This study was done before he operated on Karp.

For 3 days Mr. Karp lived comatose after the operation. After her husband died, Mrs. Karp learned that her husband's operation was considered experimental and sued Cooley in court. She testified that neither she nor her husband understood that the operation was the first attempt to see if the device was clinically feasible in a human. She had not understood that it had little realistic hope of returning her husband to normal life. Neither Mr. or Mrs. Karp understood, when both signed consent forms, that the possibility existed that Mr. Karp would die in pain, nausea, and mental stupor.

In the resulting trial, the lawyer for the Karps argued that Cooley's attempt was not intended as therapeutic for Karp but rather was experimental. The incorrect extension of the legal doctrine of *therapeutic privilege* from normal medicine to risky experiments plagued medicine during this time, especially in surgery. This notion allowed one to lie to the patient in extreme situations for his own clear, immediate good. (Critically injured accident victims are consoled by friends: "No, of course you're not dying" to bolster their will to live.) Cooley had invoked therapeutic privilege by not informing the Karps of anything which might disturb them.

In the subsequent trial, at the last moment, De Bakey did not testify after previously indicating that he would. The prosecution then could not meet the onus of proof against Cooley's presumption of innocence, and the case was dismissed. Cooley subsequently resigned from Baylor College of Medicine, where Michael De Bakey continued to teach.

Two years later, Cooley again implanted an artificial heart without permission from his IRB, claiming it was an emergency and a matter of life or death. This time the patient was a Dutchman named Meuffels, who died after 2 days. *Life* praised Cooley and overlooked how he had technically broken the law.[6] Meanwhile, another unknown surgeon in Utah worked on artificial hearts and followed regulations without media attention. His name was William DeVries.

Throughout 1982, NIH continued to support both LVAD and artificial hearts, pouring $200 million into both over 2 decades. In early 1982, the FDA permitted DeVries to implant an artificial heart from Kolff's lab into a patient.

BARNEY CLARK'S CASE

In December 1982, 61-year-old Barney Clark was clearly dying. Why he was dying is important to this case because it was not emphasized during media coverage at the time. Barney Clark started smoking cigarettes at age 24 and continued for years, smoking one to two packs a day. His lifelong smoking caused his early demise.

As a dentist, Dr. Clark knew about the harmful effects of smoking cigarettes. Like many smokers, he had tried to quit for years without success. Perhaps like many smokers too, he had planned to finally quite before any damage was done, but in his case, he waited too long.

Barney Clark had three of the worst effects of smoking: heart failure (idiopathic cardiomyopathy), chronic obstructive pulmonary disease, and emphysema. At age 49 (12 years before his operation), and after 25 years of regular smoking, he finally quit. He said that doing so was "the hardest thing I've ever done," and there is no reason to think he was exaggerating. By then, he had developed the chronic bronchitis, shortness of breath, and fatigue which indicated early emphysema. This led to his early retirement at age 55 and to his inability to enjoy life. He especially missed playing golf. He told his wife many times, "I wish I hadn't smoked."[7]

Because Barney Clark not only had heart disease but also chronic lung disease, he was not the ideal candidate for the artificial heart. Ideally, a person with a dying heart but strong lungs should have been chosen.

Barney Clark's father died in 1933 when the son was 12 years old. An only child, Barney supported his mother, who was still alive at 85 when Barney died. He grew up in Provo, Utah, and life in 1933 must have been hard for a widow and a 12-year-old boy, with a mortgage to pay. In November, Franklin Roosevelt had defeated Herbert Hoover. When Roosevelt was inaugurated in March, most banks had closed, paralyzing the nation's credit. Roosevelt set up a federal welfare program, which was soon replaced by the WPA (Works Progress Administration), which created jobs for out-of-work teachers, businessmen, artists, and salesmen.

Barney sold hot dogs and worked odd jobs to help his mother. Later, he worked his way through Brigham Young University and the University of Washington Dental School. He met his wife, Una Loy, in the seventh grade and married her in 1944 when he was 23 years old.

Clark set up business in Washington State, where he practiced until he retired in 1977. Barney and Una Loy had three children, one of whom, Stephen, became a surgeon. Barney Clark mainly socialized with a group of men his age who played at his country club. He was twice president of the club. The 6'2" Clark was a man who liked to arm wrestle, drink alcohol, and play cards in the men's locker room. He was a Mormon.

In 1970, Clark began to feel poorly and finally gave up cigarettes. Perhaps he understood how sick he was and hoped for a reprieve. By 1978, he could no longer keep up with friends playing golf and the slightest exertion left him breathless. Physicians diagnosed emphysema, an incurable, obstructive lung disease, accompanied by congestive heart failure and cardiomyopathy, an incurable disease of unknown origin where the heart's muscles degenerate to uselessness and are finally unable to pump blood to the lungs or arteries. In June 1980, Clark had been sent home from a local hospital with poor prospects and was then described by his cardiologist Terrence Block as "all huddled up in a ball and icy cold."[8]

Over the next 2 years, Block kept Clark alive by using several then-newly released, powerful drugs, such as captopril and hydrazaline, which dilated his blood vessels and made it easier for his heart to pump blood. By March 1982, Block knew Barney was terminally ill and considered a heart transplant for Clark by Norman Shumway at Stanford. Unfortunately, Stanford had an age cutoff at 50 years. Ideally, Clark would have received a heart-lung transplant.

Block referred Clark to the University of Utah to obtain an experimental drug, and there Clark first learned of the artificial heart program and met William DeVries. According to Block, Clark initially scoffed at being a candidate for the machine and said he couldn't think of anything worse than being tied to such a device, but by November, when he couldn't get enough oxygen and was bedridden with fatigue, he changed his mind—as dying people often do.

A screening committee had been set up to pick the first candidate for the new artificial heart, called the "Jarvik-7." They decided that the first recipient had to be someone so sick that death was imminent. It was thought unethical to pick someone who might live another year when the artificial heart itself might well kill him. Only for someone who had only days to live could such a procedure even possibly be therapeutic.

When it became clear that he might be the first, officially approved, artificial heart recipient, Clark visited the barn where sheep and calves with artificial hearts resided. One calf was named Lord Tennyson and had survived for 268 days with a Jarvik-7. Clark also saw that many of the calves and sheep had died.

Clark was given an 11-page consent form approved by the IRB, which he took home to read with his family and personal cardiologist. After thinking it over for 24 hours, Clark signed the form the next day in front of IRB members. The same day, to test his determination to see the operation through, a group of physicians tried to change his mind.

Surgeon William DeVries was unmistakable to anyone who saw him. A six-foot-five, lanky athlete with a boyish mop of blonde hair and a tanned face, the 38-year-old had excelled in high school basketball and high jumping. He had seven children. He claimed to sleep only 5 hours a day, spending 16 hours a day at the hospital. The remainder of his time, when not spent commuting or skiing, was spent with his wife and kids. A churchgoer raised in Utah, he also earned his undergraduate and medical degrees in that western state.

Almost as important as DeVries in the public perception of this operation was 36-year-old Robert Jarvik, the inventor of the modestly named

"Jarvik-7." Controversy surrounds the claim that Jarvik actually invented the device which was implanted in Barney Clark. In the reporting of this story, the picture painted by reporters of Jarvik bordered on adulation. Not involved in care of patients, Jarvik was available to reporters when others were not.

According to the official story, the young Jarvik invented automatic surgical staples while watching his surgeon-father operate. According to Jarvik, at the time he had no interest in medicine. When his father later died of an aortic aneurysm, the son dedicated his life to cardiac care. But instead of admitting "the inventor of surgical staples" with open arms to medical school, 15 American medical schools rejected him. So he went to Italy and entered the University of Bologna, an open-admissions medical school which, like most such European medical schools, separates future physicians from the mass of self-selected students by rigorous exams at the end of the second year. After 2 years, Jarvik returned to America, where he did not pursue a degree at any medical school, but instead earned a master's degree in occupational biomechanics at New York University.

In New York, Jarvik met Willem Kolff, who was then at the University of Utah Medical School, which had lured Kolff away from Cleveland by giving him a free hand to set up a lab to make artificial organs. Kolff helped Jarvik get admitted to Utah's medical school, and during the next 4 years, Jarvik worked for Kolff. Upon getting his degree, Jarvik immediately went to work in Kolff's lab and did no internship or residency.

Jarvik and Kolff led the crude-mechanics school of organ transplantation, which adopted a nuts-and-bolts approach to building artificial organs. Nothing of the elegance of cyclosporin for them. Various kinds of artificial hearts were constructed in Kolff's lab, which employed other people, such as the Australian surgeon, Clifford Kwan-Gett. Critics called it the "tinker toy" lab, but Kolff dismissed them, pointing out that similar nay-sayers had dismissed his dialysis machines.

The Jarvik-7 largely consisted of molded polyurethane with two plastic-and-aluminum chambers holding an inner *diaphragm* (a chamber separated by a thin inner wall). Because diaphragm substituted for the *ventricles* (the powerful, lower part of the heart which pumps blood), it needed a source of power. This was supplied by compressed air (the kind used by auto mechanics), which came up through 6-foot tubes inserted through Clark's stomach. The air inflated the diaphragm, the right ventricle of which pushed blood into the lungs for oxygenation and then back to the left ventricle, which pushed the oxygenated blood through the rest of the body.

The Jarvik-7 also contained synthetic valves commonly used in valve-replacement operations. The opening and closing of these valves against the Jarvik-7's walls produced a clicking sound which could be heard when an ear was pressed to Clark's chest. The air compressor was carried around on what Utah physicians called "the grocery cart." Such a cart was necessary because the air compressor weighed 375 pounds.

Implantation of the Jarvik-7

Almost 15 years to the day after Christiaan Barnard's transplant of Denise Darvall's heart into Louis Washkansky, William DeVries scheduled Clark for his operation the next morning. Outside, snow began to fall on the Utah mountains as television reported that an operation, about to begin, would make history. Back in Washington state, a thief ransacked the Clark home, stealing photographs of Barney, perhaps hoping to sell them to eager reporters. (After the operation, two Jarvik-7's were also stolen from DeVries' office.)

Clark already suffered from chronic atrial fibrillation and after dark, he began to experience the potentially fatal condition of ventricular tachycardia ("V-tach"). During that night of December 1, DeVries said Clark's heart had weakened and was threatening his life. DeVries claimed at a television news conference afterwards that, had he not implanted the Jarvik-7, Barney Clark "probably would have been dead by midnight."[9] As a result, the operation began that night at 11 P.M. On his way to the operating room, Clark joked, "There would be a lot of long faces around here if I backed out now."[10]

As the operation began and at DeVries' command, the sounds of Ravel's "Bolero" filled the room. Upon opening the chest, the surgeon found a flabby heart—twice the size of a normal heart—which merely quivered rather than contracted, and was described by one physician present as looking like "a soft, overripe zucchini squash."[11] After cutting away the two ventricles (lower parts) of the heart, DeVries stitched two Dacron cuffs to the intact atria (upper parts) of the heart. The two plastic ventricles connected to the Dacron cuffs with Velcro fasteners. Because of previous steroid use, the atrial walls were paper thin, and the pressure of snapping the Velcro fasteners ripped the stitches from them. The cuffs had to be restitched into a new section of heart wall and then gently snapped into place.

The cuffs held but when the Jarvik-7 was turned on, it didn't work. The device did not pump blood out of its left ventricle. DeVries felt frustrated and, for an hour, tried to get it to work correctly. Three times he opened the ventricle by hand and each time ran the risk of introducing air into the blood and causing a stroke. DeVries would not know if he had done so until Clark awakened. At this point, DeVries reportedly exclaimed, "Please, please, please, work this time.!"[12] Finally, he replaced the artificial ventricle altogether from parts from another Jarvik-7 and got the machine working, 2 hours after it was supposed to start right up.

Throughout this ordeal, Jarvik was very nervous. He scrubbed up and entered when the machine was implanted and helped DeVries get it to work. Clark's operation took all night and concluded around dawn. When the anesthesia wore off in a few hours, an anxious DeVries watched Clark as he opened his eyes. If he could hear their requests and move his extremities, he would have missed a bad stroke. He was asked, without explanation, to move his arms and toes on both sides. He did so, and everyone felt relieved.

People are often shocked when they visit an intensive care unit or see a postrecovery patient after major heart surgery. Una Loy Clark was, as most people were later when they saw Barney Clark on videotape.[13] Clark also had a hole in his throat (through which a breathing tube ran), a feeding tube into his stomach, a bladder catheter, and, of course, the two air hoses through his upper abdomen into his internal Jarvik-7, and—from the bedside—the 375-lb. air machine.

Later that day at the press conference, university physicians enthusiastically described the operation as a "dazzling technical achievement" and as something "as exciting and thrilling as has ever been accomplished in medicine."[14] The *New York Times'* Lawrence Altman, M.D., who writes "Doctor's World," called it "one of the most dramatic stories in medical history."[15]

After the Implant

While the world anticipated news, hundreds of reporters swarmed about the University of Utah Medical Center in Salt Lake City. As occurred with William Steptoe and Louise Brown, reporters were highly frustrated by DeVries' protective policy toward Clark. From the beginning, DeVries had feared a "media circus."[16] Throughout the subsequent months, physician administrator Chase Peterson, Utah's vice president for health affairs, ran interference with the media and functioned as a hospital public-relations professional. At one point, reporters exploded when he said there would be no further news. The Clark family signed an exclusive deal with one magazine, and other reporters felt left out. Although the hospital changed its no-talk policy, reporters became angrier and angrier as the weeks went on.

Inside the hospital, everyone worried that Clark's immune system would rebel against the Jarvik-7. Like Louis Washkansky, Clark felt horrible after the operation. Although he had not suffered any massive stroke, he suffered from what was called "intensive care psychosis" (or "acute brain syndrome") involving massive memory loss, confusion, delirium, and semiconsciousness.

A week after the operation, a somewhat better Clark asked how he was doing and DeVries replied, "Just fine." Seconds later, Clark began seizures, or involuntary shuddering from head to toe, perhaps caused by the drastic increase in blood flow from presurgery to after-surgery on the Jarvik-7. Injections were given of a muscle tranquilizer (Valium) and an anticonvulsant (Dilantin). Suffering a seizure, Clark's unconscious body quivered for the next several hours; gradually the quivering became confined to his left leg and arm. Throughout the next months, spells of mental confusion continued.

The next days were bad. DeVries later said that during this time, there were times when Clark wanted to die and, at one point, said directly, "Why don't you just let me die?"[17] His lack of energy, difficulty in breathing, and mental stupor depressed him. Several times, he told a psychiatrist, "My mind is shot."

On December 14, things got worse when a commercial welded valve broke inside the Jarvik-7. The Jarvik-7 mimicked the natural heart in having four values (mitral, tricuspid, etc.) and used the commercial valves routinely implanted by heart surgeons. When the $800 valve broke, Clark's blood pressure dropped dramatically, threatening his life, and DeVries had to reoperate to replace it.

Nineteen days later in January of 1983, Clark was doing much better and DeVries said his chances were good of eventually going home. But, instead, complication after complication occurred. Drugs to keep Clark's blood thinned to prevent lethal clots also caused severe bleeding (from normal sores and cuts, which didn't clot and heal). A persistent, severe nosebleed had to be surgically sealed.

More serious was Clark's underlying emphysema, which created pneumothorax (air that escaped from the lungs into the chest cavity), requiring another operation to relieve pressure on the weak, smoke-damaged lungs. During these last months from January to March, Clark complained of conditions caused by his emphysema and unrelated to the Jarvik-7. He constantly complained of never being able to get a good breath. This was because he was suffocating to death.

In early March, Clark made several videotaped interviews with DeVries, one of which was edited and released to the public. Two videotaped interviews where Clark had nothing positive to say were not released. Cardiologist Thomas Preston claimed that the final short segment "came from an extensive interview in which, encouraged by Dr. DeVries, Clark issued a semblance of a positive statement."[18]

In retrospect, this clip clearly was the best moment to be found, and all the world saw the results. Barney Clark was not a happy man, tethered to a huge machine, barely conscious and in some pain. On the other hand, Clark himself claimed to be glad to be alive and not sorry he had undergone the operation. It seemed that he might improve.

But the next day Clark developed severe nausea and vomiting, leading to aspiration of some vomit, in turn leading to pneumonia. Fever developed and his kidneys weakened. This was the beginning of his end.

On March 23, 1983, Barney Clark died of multiple-organ collapse. The large dosages of antibiotics had killed most of the useful, benign bacteria in his colon. Necrosis of the colon developed and produced toxins which entered his blood. This was accompanied by increasing expansion of his extremely fragile veins to the point where they could no longer transmit blood. Both degenerations led to death of his kidneys, brain, and lungs, as little of the (increasingly septic) blood reached these organs. The Jarvik-7 continued pumping long after all his vital organs had failed.

Una Loy was called and asked if she wanted to be present when the key was turned off to stop the Jarvik-7. She said Barney was already dead and left the room.[19] Someone (it was not revealed who) stopped the machine after a few hours.

Weeks later, hospital officials corrected what they termed an "oversight" in not telling reporters that 3 days after Clark's death, another valve had broken and killed another experimental patient. This time it had been Ted E. Bear, a 220-lb ram (who inspired the continuing story on *St. Elsewhere* of the ram "Flash" with his "Craig 2000" artificial heart).[20] At his death at 297 days "on the pump;" the ram had lived longer than any other mammal with an artificial heart. It should be noted however, that such rams were healthy at the time of the implants, unlike subsequent human recipients.

ETHICAL ISSUES

Criteria of Success and Quality of Life

Ethicist Eric Cassell, M.D., criticized DeVries as lacking criteria for success—what would DeVries count as a "good result?"[21] If Clark's sorry condition was good, almost any result would qualify. Michael DeBakey, in turn, said success had to be defined as restoring a patient to normal life. Christiaan Barnard cheered DeVries on, urging him not to "give up" and telling him to ignore his critics.[22]

DeVries countered in two ways. First, "from a research standpoint," the operation was successful.[23] Most observers agreed that it had been proved that an artificial heart could keep a man alive much longer than had been expected. Moreover, and despite its several problems, the Jarvik-7 had done better than critics had expected. Lawrence Altman agreed, asking what other such radical experiments in medicine had ever been more successful for the first patient.[24] After all, the machine had circulated the blood and initially did not seem to form lethal clots.

Second, DeVries said it was up to Barney Clark and his family to determine if the quality of life was high enough, not others. Clark said the operation was "worth it if the alternative is that...[you] either die or have it done."[25] Mrs. Clark later called the operation only a "partial" success because there was no full recovery.

Chase Peterson called it a "modified success," but warned that the public would only put up with a few more such partial successes without a real one.[26] What was needed, he said, was a case (such as Christiaan Barnard's second transplant) where the patient could go home to lead a reasonable quality of life and conduct interviews with reporters.

Public opinion agreed with Peterson. The whole point of the program should be to restore normal life. Like Karen Quinlan, Barney Clark became a symbol of how not to die. He symbolized how mechanical technology could cruelly reduce the fragile richness of life to painful gasps for the next breath. Clark's attention in his interview seemed so focused on breathing that he hardly appeared to notice the video cameras.

A *New York Times* editorial criticized surgeons' "passion for the spotlight," saying "the primitive belief that the heart is the seat of life endows heart surgery with mystical glamor; the artificial heart is seen as a defiance of death."[27] But the *Times* didn't think death had been defied. DeVries had not given Clark an extra 112 days of good life, but an *extra 112 days of dying.* The newspaper concluded that "medicine's real triumphs lie in improving the quality of life for everyone, not in death-defying heroics that benefit, or torment, the few."

Certainly, the mental quality of Clark's life deteriorated after the violent convulsions a week after his implant. Stephen Clark said that his father "was never the same mentally" after them. In such a state, could Barney Clark consent to continue the experiment? If not, was his family ever asked?

One of the issues was the way Clark *looked* to the outside world and his family. As DeVries pointed out, people had unrealistic expectations. They simply had not experienced the mental confusion and bloated faces of such patients. One of Clark's nurses said public expectations about miraculous recoveries to normal life were "too high." One prominent anesthesiologist said such hopes were "terribly naive."[28] Indeed, people often forget that most patients seen by most physicians are over 50 years old, very sick, and suffering from memory loss and incapacity. Being a physician or nurse is not like being around healthy college students. Physicians and nurses are accustomed to treating impaired people and settling for small successes in arresting the downward pull of age, but the average citizen is not.

Self-Determination and Barney Clark's "Key"

During the first few days after the operation, Willem Kolff and Robert Jarvik both said Barney Clark had a "key" which could be turned off if he decided to die.[29] His consent form said he could withdraw from the project, even if it meant his death. But as soon as Kolff and Jarvik commented, Chase Peterson softened the statement, saying the "key" was only a metaphor, not an actual physical instrument, dispelling the implication that Clark himself could shut off the Jarvik-7. DeVries undoubtedly told Peterson to downplay the "key," lest the media get the idea that Clark could really kill himself. As Clark's breathing became forced and his consciousness murky, nothing more was said about the key.

The truth about the key was that a physical key did exist. The air compressor was locked "on" to prevent someone from inadvertently turning it off. The key to this lock was never intended to be a physical embodiment of Clark's ability to choose not to continue living. This was Jarvik's and Kolff's erroneous interpretation.

Neither Jarvik nor Kolff appeared to appreciate usual postoperative mental problems. Perhaps this was due to Jarvik's lack of actual clinical experience. In any case, so common is temporary mental confusion after major, traumatic surgery that patients in ICUs are commonly (and loosely) said to have "intensive care psychosis."

Jarvik also seemed not to understand the clinical realities when he said a key wasn't really necessary. He said it was easy for a patient such as Clark to kill himself. "People can die in many ways," Jarvik said, "and they are amazingly creative about it."[30] In truth, by the time a patient like Clark gets to the point where he is so miserable that he really wants to die, he is too weak to do anything. He can often barely lift his arm. At this point, he is also likely to be mentally incompetent.

Thus, Barney Clark never really had the choice of dying, and never had a real key, because the ethical issue was more subtle than was presented in popular and academic reports. Any time that Clark deteriorated and felt like dying, it could have been a temporary phenomenon, as happened in his early days, and as happened to Louis Washkansky. On the other hand, when Clark really was dying, he went downhill fast, and then it was too late for him to have any real choice. The dilemma about voluntary choice in Clark's case is poignant and a dilemma that many patients face. As Clark's early incompetence shows, such incompetence may be reversible. It must have pained Peterson to have Jarvik talking about Clark's "key," making life more difficult for Peterson with reporters, and oversimplifying the real ethical issues.

Benefit to Barney Clark: Therapy or Research?

Hours after the operation, DeVries claimed—when he decided to operate at 11 P.M.—that, without the operation, Clark would have been dead "at midnight." Cardiologist Thomas Preston disagreed, saying that the "imminent death" claim was made only to justify trying the artificial heart. Preston also disputed that Clark benefited from the Jarvik-7.[31]

DeVries claimed that a potentially fatal arrhythmia caused him to begin the operation just before midnight. According to Preston, the arrhythmia was most likely caused by medications Clark was on. Moreover, Preston claims that, during the previous year and a half, Clark had had identical arrhythmias, which were reversed. The only patient who is truly at death's door is one who had stopped breathing and who is being resuscitated. Even then, thousands of patients are revived each year. To surgeon Preston, if Barney Clark then was not immediately dying, he was more an experimental subject than a patient receiving new therapy.

The crucial question, then, is how much of a chance this particular experiment had with his particular, lung-impaired patient. NIH, which had funded the artificial heart for 20 years, considered DeVries' operation experimental, not therapeutic, and opposed DeVries' plans to implant the artificial heart.[32] The FDA also did not see the implant as therapeutic but gave DeVries an *exemption* from proving therapeutic benefit.[33] Critics such as law professor George Annas criticized the FDA for violating its own rules and exceeding its own authority.[34] Physician Pierre Galetti carefully noted that Clark's case only demonstrated the "clinical feasibility" of the artificial heart, not the more important "clinical usefulness."[35]

Some researchers try to get around this dilemma by talking about "therapeutic research." This blurs a useful distinction. Some experiments neither intend nor achieve therapeutic benefit for the specific subject, but hope to benefit future patients. Barney Clark himself didn't think the procedure was likely to be therapeutic.

Selection

The issue of cost raises the question of who would receive artificial hearts, if they were successful. With in vitro fertilization, only those who pay get the service, but they would like insurance companies to fund it. Companies such as Blue Cross-Blue Shield were originally created by surgeons so that patients could pay their bills, and surgeons such as DeVries hoped such companies would eventually pay for artificial hearts.

This raises the larger question in public policy of how insurance companies decide which medical procedures to reimburse. Such decisions are little understood, yet sometimes they amount to selecting which patients live and which do not. Insurance companies themselves decide which procedures, if any, to reimburse for each new medical innovation. Which treatment physicians prescribe can be heavily influenced by which procedures are reimbursed by insurance. Gastroenterologists, faced with making a diagnosis by an hour interview, for which they receive $100, or a 10-minute endoscopy (examining the bowel by fiber optiscope), for which they receive $600 and which decreases their risk of malpractice claims, understandably elect to "scope" most patients. If all other gastroenterologists act similarly, that establishes the "customary and reasonable practice" of routine (but expensive) endoscopy.

Another issue about selection concerns the family. After Clark's death, the Utah team claimed that one of the things it learned was the value of strong family support and announced that such support would be a criterion of selection for future candidates.

In April 1983, a potential recipient had been rejected because of lack of such familial support.[36] This rejection was criticized as subjective (the family supported the team, therefore the Utah team liked having families around), and unscientific. Robert Jarvik testily objected, "I have never seen an adult bull visit one of our calves and yet the calves do very well."[37] In opposition, nurses, social workers, and physicians cited long experience with dialysis and coronary patients and claimed that "everyone knows" patients did better with family support.

Costs

Two separate issues about costs came up in this case. First, was the artificial heart cost-effective for an individual patient? Clark's total bill topped a quarter of a million dollars. Utah administrators had initially not expected it to be so costly. Chase Peterson said they expected Clark to either die in a few days or be discharged in a few weeks.[38] Afterwards, it was decided that a second implant would not be allowed until costs of it—and the operation to implant it—had advance funding. The Clarks had contracted to pay for the treatment, but were released as costs zoomed. George Lundberg, editor of the *Journal of the American Medical Association*, denied that the cost per patient—a quarter million dollars per patient—was worth it, and that such implants should continue for the hundreds of thousands of heart patients each year, into whom a Jarvik-7 might be implanted. "How much is one more day of longer life worth?" he asked. "Is every life worth the same amount and if not, why not?"[39]

A second issue was cost to society. NIH invested over $8 million in the Utah project and over $164 million between 1964 and 1982. Was this the best way to spend such funds? Should such expenditures be continued? The Office of Technology Assessment estimated that 60,000 Americans might use artificial hearts at a Medicare cost of $5.5 billion a year.[40] Artificial hearts could easily become another exorbitant end-stage renal disease program, and cost over $7 billion a year.

Moreover, there were more subtle issues involving cost. Economists discuss opportunity costs of funds for artificial hearts, i.e., medical programs which could have been funded had artificial hearts not been. Everyone sees that $7 billion spent on Jarvik-7's could have been spent on bone-marrow transplants for leukemia patients, but there are also expectations and momentum. If artificial hearts were to restore normal life even for a few months, cries would start to fund the program. People would say, "How can society let these patients die?" Once a few patients were funded, other programs would jump on the bandwagon. Surgeons would lobby insurance companies for funding. A medical breakthrough which is dramatic, lifesaving, and popular is nearly impossible to stop—once any success at all occurs. Early on, DeVries said, "I think the snowball's started and I don't think anybody can stop it now."[41] Criticizing this process, Preston says, "in our medical system... what physicians establish is what we get, with indifference to relative social or medical value."[42] (This issue of cost of heart replacements is also pursued in the next chapter.)

Prevention

Some people believe that money is better spent on research into prevention of terminal illness than on expensive treatments at the end stages of disease. In discussing this case, the leftist magazine *The Progressive* wailed that a "medical establishment grown fat on chemicals and technological wizardry is not willing to empower people so they can prevent illness."[43] It said that artificial hearts, which might benefit a small number of cardiac patients who could afford the cost, were "qualitatively different from the basic advances in immunology which have saved million of lives, even among populations not directly treated."

Many people have trouble getting passionate about preventing statistical deaths. People volunteer donations to save an identified person such as Barney Clark but grow indifferent at saving unknown lives. Jonathan Glover and Leon

Trachtman argue that this approach is irrational.[44] A saved life is a saved life. If $3 billion could save more lives if spent in antismoking programs than on artificial hearts, we ought to prevent smoking. On the other hand, saved statistical lives are always mere *claims*. It is difficult to be certain that such lives would not have been saved anyway—there are just too many variables.

Part of the issue here plays emotion against reason. President Reagan called subsequent artificial heart recipient William Schroeder to urge him to fight on. It is always easier to think you have helped by making personal contact, but the president could have really saved lives in 1987 by continuing the unpopular 55 m. p. h. speed limit. Since the national drinking age was raised to 21, automobile deaths related to alcohol have decreased.

Perhaps the abstractness of saving statistical lives can be overcome by a "what if" scenario about Barney Clark. What if the lure of tobacco had been overcome at the turn of this century? Suppose Barney Clark had never smoked. If so, he might have lived into his eighties. Probably many people would not need artificial hearts in their early sixties if they had never smoked, drunk alcohol, etc. Priorities seem akilter when a quarter of a million dollars is spent per patient for perhaps a few extra years of life, when such problems need never have occurred in the first place. Such comparisons show the human cost of tobacco and alcohol in lost years of life, often just when a person is ready to retire and enjoy life.

Relationships with Media

Like many medical centers, the University of Utah both needed and resisted reporters, who in turn both needed and doubted Utah's physicians. Chase Peterson claims that the medical center knew the story would be big and DeVries claimed to have feared media abuses, and so they took steps to control the press. They designated a media room and Peterson became the media point-man. They prepared for months about how to handle reporters. Later, Peterson claims that the university and the physicians were naive in not anticipating the number of reporters and their intense interest.

Reporters were in a difficult position for several reasons. Utah had invited them to come, but then wanted to dish out news in controlled dollops. Reporters feared being manipulated. DeVries and the University of Utah wanted attention. The artificial heart program had been encouraged by the university for decades, ever since it hired Kolff, and a successful program would put Salt Lake City on the map, along with the Texas Heart Institute and the Mayo Clinic. Physicians were upset with reporters when unsubstantiated rumors appeared on front pages, as when a leak surfaced that the IRB (institutional review board) had not considered Clark a good candidate. Reporters accused physicians of lying about how the videotape was set up and about how the IRB functioned, as well as omitting data about financial, conflicts-of-interests.

Moreover, something in the story was fishy. Cardiologists around the country were saying privately that the whole project was "erector-set medicine" because the physiological problem hadn't been solved—the problem of how to permit blood to contact artificial surfaces without forming clots. And the question hadn't been answered about whether it was a "success" to live tethered to a huge machine and gasping for breath. When reporters asked these questions, they felt they only got back happy talk.

In his essay, "The Physician, the Media, and the 'Spectacular Case'," DeVries commented on these problems:

> It is one of the ironies of being involved in a spectacular medical case that physician/researchers are simultaneously criticized by some members of the profession for cooperating with the press and by others for not publishing enough data "even though this data is incomplete information from ongoing studies." . . .
>
> The many media teams covering a spectacular case compete intensely for innovative ways of *reporting, telling,* and *selling* the story. At times, they highlight seemingly unimportant events for unknown reasons. The medical team experiencing the story as it unfolds remains bewildered, wondering if the reporters really want to get at the heart of the story or would rather tiptoe around the edges looking for a dramatic detail that nobody else has.[45]

Reporters distinguish themselves by getting something others do not. That system rewards initiative and intelligence, but the university thwarted those qualities by giving all reporters the same information. Reporters panicked when the Clarks signed exclusive deals with *Reader's Digest* and when they felt that the university held back information to help the Clarks maximize profits from such sales.

In retrospect, part of the hard feeling on both sides can be attributed to incompatible goals. When any person becomes famous, reporters want to know as much as possible about him. Frequently this means losing privacy as *paparazzi* photograph one's every move. Hospitals frequently complain about this, while continuing to seek out fame. Hospitals in such cases always want to manage the news, partially to protect patients and their families, partially to protect themselves. Reporters want total, immediate, truthful access to all information, from scientific to intimate.

When a patient becomes a celebrity, things are different. Both hospital and reporters are placed in uneasy positions where pursuing their goals may conflict with a patient's best interests. Because hospitals and physicians have a primary obligation to protect patients and their families, the university agonized about a videotape made of the operation. Mrs. Clark objected because it smacked of "sensationalism."[46] Even though $150,000 had been paid for its production by several television stations and even though the university wanted to release it, physicians were torn between their own goals for publicity and the Clarks' desires for privacy. Ultimately, the medical center nixed the tape.

Reporters were also to blame here, acting as if Barney Clark were a presidential candidate—rather than a private citizen—and wanting access to him. In truth, Dr. Clark was a dying man who was limping along. He was not tough enough to be directly interviewed by reporters, but every reporter nevertheless wanted to interview him.

Scientific Contribution and Publication of Results

According to surgeon Stephen Clark, "Dad never really thought the artificial heart would work for him. All he expected to do was make a contribution to medical research."[47] But did he do so? The results are in dispute. Barney undoubtedly saw himself as the first step along a long path leading to success, and afterwards, several surgeons put forth this view. Stephen Clark first said the operation contributed to science, but later was unsure, saying, "Ask me in 20 years."

It can be argued that no contribution to science occurred, because Clark was the wrong candidate. His lung disease was too severe, and he ultimately succumbed to it. DeVries claimed that before the operation, he didn't know Clark had such severe lung disease, implying that if he had, Clark wouldn't have been chosen (undermining the justification of "anything goes with a dying man"). It can be argued that only the later recipients showed the true limitations of the Jarvik-7.

At a subsequent conference on the case in October 1983, DeVries was criticized for not having published results in professional journals. He said he was waiting until he had good news. The *New York Times*' Lawrence Altman pointed out that, after his first transplant, Barnard had published within a month in a peer-refereed journal.[48]

Three years after Clark's implant, no scientific review of the operation or subsequent implants had appeared. In a 1986 editorial, *New England Journal of Medicine* editor Arnold Relman criticized the lack of intent to do randomized clinical trials. For success, he said, there had to be

> a multicenter trial with established protocols and full reporting of results. [Otherwise] in the absence of protocols and cooperation among institutions, we are likely to see a proliferation of competing and unplanned efforts that will not advance the field and may even set it back.[49]

Perhaps patients could have lived longer, with less cost, by another treatment. Without clinical trials and proof, all that was learned is that some patients can be maintained for a few months.

For many, DeVries waited too long to publish his results. In early 1988, the *Journal of the American Medical Association* carried three signed, review-editorials. Doing further implants, the reviewers concluded, would only document greater problems. The surgical critics implied that it would be unethical to do more, that to do so would assuage the ego of the surgeon but harm patients. The Jarvik-7 was specifically criticized as causing some of the fatal complications:

> At the time of device implantation or at autopsy, thrombi have frequently
> been identified on components of the mechanical heart. Prolonged,
> although temporary, use of prosthesis, similar to a permanent heart
> substitution, only provides time to increase the number of thromboembolic
> events and to allow further establishment of infection.[50]

After Barney Clark died, DeVries was allowed three more operations by the
FDA, and he continued to claim that the Jarvik-7 would be successful, but his
was a voice in the wilderness.

Informed Consent

Informed consent in medical experiments is emphasized by lawyers but often
dismissed by surgeons as bureaucratic red tape. Few surgeons get full pro-
fessorships at renowned medical schools for excellent consent forms. It can be
argued that Dr. Clark had maximal resources for understanding what was
asked of him: as a dentist he knew basic science, his son Stephen was a surgeon, and Barney Clark had relationships with well-known cardiologists. For
understanding what could happen, what better patient could there be, other
than a cardiac surgeon?

Another point of view reminds us of why informed consent came about.
Surgeons such as DeVries in famous medical centers exercise Olympian power
over dying patients terrified of death. Such power makes it easy for a few
physicians to rationalize risky procedures which exploit patients, as occurred
in the Tuskegee Study. Informed consent, both a moral and a legal concept,
exists as a moral check against this inequality and as a legal recourse when
power is abused.

Ethicist Alex Capron doubted whether Clark really understood that the
roller coaster path of his illness might make him want to die.[51] Did Clark understand that he might feel compelled to continue the experiment, feeling that
not to do so would let everyone down? Lawyer George Annas faults the consent process for not anticipating these outcomes and strongly criticizes everyone for not making it clear who would decide when Clark became
incompetent.[52] Clark was treated as if incompetent at various points, and Una
Loy was asked to consent. Since it was his body and his life, Annas says,
surgeons should have first asked Barney when he thought it would be appropriate to give up, and second, who he wanted to make decisions if he
became incompetent. (He probably would have designated his wife, but this
should have been made explicit.) Moreover, Annas thinks the consent form
was simplistic, as if it just said, "Go for it! This is your only real chance," while
omitting that Clark might end up semicomatose and without "self-determination and dignity as a human being."

It's hard to know if Clark really cared about such legalistic procedures
designed to guarantee maximal autonomy. He probably cared more about,
respectively, a chance to stay alive, and a chance to regain a somewhat normal
life. Barney Clark was not Elizabeth Bouvia.

Law professor Annas insists that DeVries ignored the consent form (just as Denton Cooley did), which stated that "additional chest surgeries may be required in the event the device needs to be replaced or repaired which will be explained to me and will be done with a new consent form signed by me for each procedure." Annas claims this was not done for the valve replacement or the surgery for nosebleeds. But this is unfair. Because of the emergency drop in blood pressure when the valve broke, Clark lost consciousness and could not have given consent. And the minor surgery to correct the nosebleed did not require a new consent form. Besides, Annas admits that Clark verbally consented.

Much of Annas' criticisms about informed consent illustrate a problem in medical ethics. It is pedantic to harp on the letter of the law and miss the spirit of the operation. There is something foolish about criticizing the consent form's lack of anticipation of Barney's Clark's subsequent "halfway" state. There is something really mean-spirited about criticizing lack of consent for emergency measures. All these problems also affected the first heart transplant patients who took cyclosporin and lived for years. Such problems also affected the first patients on kidney dialysis or undergoing kidney transplants. Isn't it unfair to omit the successes, and to focus on the failures?

Annas would be unfazed by this criticism. He reiterates that simply because a patient is dying does not justify *any* experiment. Law professor and psychiatrist Jay Katz agrees, emphasizing that "all kinds of senseless interventions are tried" because physicians resist death.[53]

Perhaps the most important question about informed consent was never answered: did Barney Clark and his family understand how bad his death could be? He certainly did not have what philosopher Margaret Battin called the "least worst death" (see Chapter 2). Did he understand, from the consent form or the physicians, that the implantation ran, for him, a great risk of dying the "worst death?" It would seem not.

Others see informed consent as largely symbolic. The important thing was trust between the Clarks and DeVries. No matter how good the consent form, Clark would not have let strangers operate on him. Conversely, no matter how horrible the consent form, Clark would have undoubtedly wanted DeVries to operate.

Role of the IRB

After the Tuskegee Study became known, the federal government required all medical experiments to be reviewed by a committee known as an IRB (Institutional Review Board). This committee is composed of lay people as well as physicians and administrators, and is mandated to protect subjects from abuses in experiments.

New York Times reporter Altman criticized the IRB for operating in secrecy, for not making it clear what its proper role was (in selecting patients, reviewing consent, and monitoring progress), for not protecting Clark's best interest, for being inefficient in reviewing ongoing details in the case, and for having a conflict of interest between protecting the medical center and protecting the patient.[54]

IRBs operate loosely and according to local interpretation, under broad federal guidelines. They are more powerful than hospital ethics committees, which are purely advisory. An IRBs most direct charge is to insure that patients give informed consent to participation in medical experiments and to insure that patients are not exploited. Because patients sometimes are dying and willing to try anything, it may be difficult to decide what counts as exploitation. IRBs concentrate on risks versus benefits and may send a protocol back to a principal investigator for amendment, more peer review, or clarification. If the IRB turns a proposal down, there is no appeal.

Two different possible functions of IRBs should be distinguished: *prior review* and *monitoring* (enforcement). IRBs are not enforcement agencies. Like the FDA, they are yes-or-no committees, and once a "yes" is given, both institutions rely on the integrity of researchers to follow agreements. Because of the ability of local IRBs to interpret their own policies, and because of the importance of the Barney Clark case, the Utah IRB decided to go beyond normal procedures and to monitor the experiment. Ross Wooley, a professor of biomedical engineering and chair of the subcommittee overseeing the Clark case, saw Barney Clark up to 4 hours each day during the 112 days. He became deeply involved in the case, becoming a confidant of Clark and adviser to DeVries. He read the patient's chart, interviewed other members of the Utah team, and took on what sociologist Renée Fox called a "physician *cum* ethicist role" as the "moral watchdog" of the team.[55]

This was a new and rare role for an IRB. Monitoring or enforcement has been discussed as a function for IRBs, but not implemented for several reasons. First, members volunteer, and such public service already takes considerable time. In medical centers such as Utah, a hundred experiments a month may be reviewed, with each one containing between 10 and 200 pages of documentation. Second, most lay members are not medically educated and must turn to medical experts for assessments of risks. Third, members turn over frequently due to the heavy demands of this unpaid work (which goes unappreciated by the public at large). There is often a lack of continuity, because a member may miss several meetings and not understand new developments.

Within this structure, disagreements frequently occur about the primary purpose of an IRB: Is it to protect vulnerable patients against unscrupulous researchers and for-profit companies? Or is it to protect the institution and researchers against litigious patients? Or both? Disagreement about the role occurred among the Utah IRB members, as it does on most IRBs. Peterson claimed that no conflict exists if an IRB does both (like "therapeutic research"). This is a common view of researchers, but it is not what NIH had in mind in creating IRBs.

The problem with Wooley's deep involvement in the case is that it is easy to become identified with the operating team and lose perspective, especially if one must go back to the committee and make decisions. As the one with the most information, Wooley had a different role on the IRB than did other members. Gradually, other members began to realize this difference.

After Clark died, DeVries and Peterson had second thoughts about this role of "home grown ethicist," as DeVries described Wooley.[56] Wooley had no special medical or ethical training in this area, just strong feelings and interest. Could such a role be generalized across the country for any similar IRB member?

The IRB eventually decided that Wooley was too deeply involved and asked him to give up his IRB vote on matters about the artificial heart, which he did, evidently without resentment. The IRB then backed off on any monitoring role. It also turned down DeVries' request to implant more artificial hearts until he published his results in peer-refereed medical journals.

Different Standards for the First Time?

Texas surgeon Denton Cooley at first criticized DeVries for implanting the artificial heart in Barney Clark, saying the device was not ready at the time. On reflection, he dropped his criticisms.

If no one took any risks, not much would improve in life. In medicine, the one constant is that people die. In taking risks, physicians try new things which may help later patients. If previous physicians had not done so, the average expected life span for adults would still be 45, 55, or 65 years, instead of 75. From a utilitarian point of view, even if some patients are harmed, the benefit to the great future number of patients is justified.

DeVries makes a similar point:

> If many other experiments in the recent history of medicine had been subjected to the kind of scrutiny the artificial heart has received, we might today be without the following: dialysis, which did not succeed until the 17th patient; mitral commissurotomy, which did not succeed until the fifth patient and numbered only 5 successes among the first 15 patients; and cardiopulmonary bypass, which succeeded on the first patient but failed on 4 subsequent patients. This list could go on and would include cardiac valve replacement, pacemakers, intra-aortic balloon pumps, arterial grafts, and organ transplantation—these, in the field of cardiothoracic surgery alone.

> These procedures now save thousands of lives each year, but it took time and the courage of countless patients to perfect them. These medical advances took years to come to fruition, and might not have occurred at all, if their initial success rate had been the deciding factor in their development.[57]

The Machine Itself

There was more to this case than simply an organ replacement. For many laypeople, the case symbolized other things, some good, some not. Perhaps the two most dominant images were Barney Clark as the Tin Man from *The Wizard of Oz* (a benevolent, kindly image) and Barney Clark as the unnatural creation of Dr. Frankenstein—an awkward monster who was part machine, part human.

Others feared the momentum of the machine itself and its underlying technology. It seemed to them that American medicine too often went by the slogan, "If we can, we should." Once Clark had shown that the machine could sustain life, it seemed to acquire a life of its own—to be funded, improved, and used in circles expanding outward from Utah to patients across the country.

Still others saw the Jarvik-7 as a metaphor for problems in contemporary medicine. As physician and medical historian Stanley Reiser said, it was a metaphor for ambivalence toward medical technology, something held both in awe and in dread: "The artificial heart is at once a metaphor of concern about unduly sustaining an aging population, the cost of medical care, plunging into technologic creation without adequate thought to consequences, and of an accumulation of means as an end in itself."[58]

For-Profit Medicine

Following Clark's death, Utah's IRB and the FDA delayed further implants until more data could be developed. Claiming he was unhappy with "red tape," DeVries moved to the for-profit Humana Hospital in Louisville, for a freer hand and for reportedly three times his former salary.[59] Humana, which owned 91 hospitals worldwide, agreed to pay for a hundred operations—if successful progress was made. Subsequent recipients were to pay nothing. Humana wanted publicity and hoped that implantation of Jarvik-7s would soon be routine, with Humana as the reimbursed leader and holder of stock in Symbion, Inc., which made the Jarvik-7. NIH spent $250 million developing the artificial heart, but Robert Jarvik was allowed to patent his machines and set up Symbion.

For medical historian and physician Stanley Reiser, the financial conflict of Jarvik and DeVries undermined trust between physicians and patients. If consent was mostly symbolic and trust paramount, then anything which undermined trust was bad.

When physicians get involved with big finance, the stakes and competition increases. In 1976, Willem Kolff formed the fledgling company Symbion, Inc., with four people, including Jarvik and Kolff's secretary.[60] The company limped along for 5 years, but needed to do little because it owned protoypes of artificial hearts, and because research and salaries were paid for by the University of Utah, several blocks away. In return, the university got 5 percent of any sales of any Jarvik hearts and a small amount of stock.

One person working for Symbion, Inc., was Clifford Kwan-Gett, who claims that he, not Robert Jarvik, invented the heart put into Barney Clark.[61] The Australian surgeon claims he made a prototype in 1969, made the superior polyurethane model which replaced the silicone rubber model, and invented the drive-line and seamless diaphragm used on subsequent models. Symbion, Inc., of course held the patents for all these inventions. Kwan-Gett does not want money but recognition in history. Where the truth lies is not clear. (Jarvik later was named "Inventor of the Year" for an electrohydraulic artificial heart, not the device implanted in Barney Clark.)

In late 1981, Kolff went public, looking for venture capitalists to underwrite Symbion's expansion. A struggle for power ensued between Jarvik and Kolff, which Kolff later downplayed as a son rebelling against a father-figure. Jarvik and others squeezed Kolff out of management, but he retained some influence, while Jarvik became president. Needing more money in 1982, Jarvik got $1 million each from Humana, Hospital Corporation of America, and American Hospital Supply. These companies bet on the success of artificial hearts and their reimbursement, hoping taxpayers would have to buy back what they themselves had financed. As one vice president said, Symbion's biggest advantage was that "it had the university as its research and development arm, subsidized by the government."

In April 1987, Warburg Pincus, a venture capital company which had arranged the financing for Symbion, Inc., waged a hostile takeover. Jarvik fought the takeover, lost, and was promptly fired.

UPDATE

In later years, Robert Jarvik became a celebrity. He modeled in ads for Hathaway shirts and was featured in *People* magazine. After being ousted from Symbion, he said he was not interested in practicing medicine anymore. Instead, he intended to work in "grand unification theory in elementary particle physics" as well as "some other kinds of humanitarian [sic] programs."[62] About this time, he divorced and, after knowing her 5 days, married Marilyn Vos Savant, who billed herself as having the world's highest IQ. The two appeared together thereafter on the lecture circuit and on talk shows, billing themselves as "the world's smartest couple." In a joint interview in 1988 and speaking for both of them, Marilyn said that she and Robert believed that they had children from previous marriages "only in a biological sense"—hers, college age; his, school age—and that, "I don't consider either one of us to have children."[63]

After Barney Clark died, Lawrence Altman called Clark's operation "one of the boldest human experiments ever attempted," but concluded that it had failed to prove its worth and, even if it had, would have been one of the most costly therapies available. DeVries said some surprising things: "After the first two days, 95 percent of the issues we were dealing with concerned ethics, moral value judgments, communications with the press—problems I had never thought about."[64]

A few months after Clark died, Kolff predictably defended the artificial heart: "A number of doctors were opposed to the artificial kidney and wrote articles against it. I decided not to respond at all and to ignore it.... I still have the same policy now that people tell us that the artificial heart has no future."[65]

A University of Utah Medical School committee, as well as a committee of the state medical society, investigated Clifford Kwan-Gett's claims and found against him. (The surgeon claims conflict of interest since the university had a financial interest in Kolff's lab.) Chase Peterson became president of the university.

In 1984, nearly 2 years later, William Schroeder became the second recipient of a Jarvik-7. The younger (51 years old) and much healthier (no emphysema) Schroeder lived much longer than Clark, but suffered a stroke after 113 days, probably from a clot formed where the Velcro connectors attached to the remainder of the natural heartwall. In 1985, Murray Haydon became the third recipient and died after 4 months from kidney failure. Jack Burcham lived 10 days after receiving a Jarvik-7. In late 1985, Mary Lund became the first woman to receive an artificial heart—a smaller version of the Jarvik-7—and lived about 10 months. Other artificial hearts were later implanted by Jack Copeland in Arizona and by the Swedish physician, Bjarne Semb, whose patient Leif Stenberg lived 229 days with a Jarvik-7.

The persistent problem with recipients was clots and internal bleeding, both of which could be fatal. After several months, clots always formed on the heart or on its plastic connections. When such clots broke free, they traveled to the small vessels of the brain, lodging there, blocking blood flow, and causing brain damage (strokes). When blood-thinning medication was added to prevent clots from forming, the internal cuts didn't heal and the patient bled to death, so patients either died of clotting or of hemorrhaging. To make things worse, all recipients of the artificial heart showed infections where the artificial heart's drive lines entered the body, and continued use of antibiotics produced resistant infections.

One of the almost insurmountable obstacles of the artificial heart was the degree of freedom from error that was necessary. Early dialysis machines could be successful most of the time, or break down frequently, and the patient didn't die. Early dialysis machines and pacemakers had many problems and there was every reason to expect that artificial hearts would have more. Cardiac pacemakers often failed, yet patients still lived, but when a Jarvik-7 failed, blood loss to the brain produced irreversible damage in minutes. For outpatients who needed to get to medical centers in such emergencies, there would be no hope.

Also, a lot had changed between 1965 and the late 1980s. National medical costs were not perceived to be a problem in 1965, but they became so in the late 1970s and were perceived as uncontrollable by 1985. Medicine could no longer realistically expect to give many people quarter-million-dollar treatments. The number of potential AIDS patients had been recognized and it seemed unreasonable to be spending so much money on artificial hearts for a few when hundreds of thousands were dying of AIDS, with staggering medical bills.

In May 1988, NIH ceased funding artificial hearts. The consensus was that artificial hearts were only justifiable in rare cases as temporary bridges to transplants. DeVries bitterly said that the decision "hurts some really good researchers who have made long-term commitments," but claimed he himself would be unaffected because Humana's funding would continue.[66] Nevertheless, the artificial heart, to many physicians and scientists, seemed like a clumsy thing. One wit once defined an elephant as a mouse built to government specifications. If so, the artificial heart was an erector-set mouse.

Two months later, NIH reversed itself because of pressure from Senators Hatch of Utah and Kennedy of Massachusetts. Before the reversal, funding of $22.6 million over the next 6 years would have stopped for four research centers (one in each senator's state). The two senators threatened to block the entire NIH budget unless the funds were restored. One NIH official said anonymously, "With all that Congressional pressure and the threat of threat of legislation, we felt that the heart institute better eat a little crow rather than risk the future budgets of all the institutes."[67] Which the heart institute did.

By 1989, no one was was implanting artificial hearts as permanent devices. DeVries was incorrect: events did hurt him, as referrals from physicians dropped from 100 a month to almost none (hence, DeVries had few good candidates.) However, Symbion found another use for Jarvik-7's as bridges to transplants. As of the end of 1988, 74 patients had received such transplants and lived at least 30 days.[68] As many also died, waiting.[69]

FURTHER READING

After Barney Clark, ed. Margery Shaw, University of Texas Press, Austin, Tx., 1984.

George Annas, "Consent to the Artificial Heart: The Lion and the Crocodiles," *Hastings Center Report* 13(2):20–22 (April 1983).

Malcomn N. Carter, "The Business Behind Barney Clark's Heart," *Money* (April, 1983).

William Check, "Lessons from Barney Clark's Heart," *Health* (April, 1984), pp. 22–27.

William DeVries, "The Physician, the Media, and the 'Spectacular Case,'" *Journal of the American Medical Association,* 259(6):886–890 (February 12, 1988).

Thomas Preston, "Who Benefits from the Artificial Heart," *Hastings Center Report* 15(1):5–7 (February 1985).

Michael Strauss, "The Political History of the Artificial Heart," *New England Journal of Medicine* 310(5):332–336 (February 2, 1984).

CHAPTER 12

Baby Fae

This chapter discusses the case of an infant named Baby Fae, into whom the heart of a young baboon named Goobers was transplanted in 1984.

HISTORICAL BACKGROUND

Transplants of animal hearts rarely occurred before Baby Fae's operation and had not promised much. Hardy, in 1964, implanted a chimpanzee heart into a 68-year-old man, who lived 90 minutes.[1] Barnard, in 1977, piggybacked a baboon heart next to the dying heart of first, a 25-year-old Italian woman, who lived 300 minutes, and, in another operation, into a 59-year-old man who lived less than 4 days. Starzl and Reemtsma had better luck with simian kidneys, each doing six transplants in the 1960s, but eventually abandoned their projects. Baboon kidneys, at best, only worked for 2 months. In 1975, British cardiologist Yocoub, in events reminiscent of the film *O Lucky Man*, connected veins and arteries of a 1-year-old dying boy to a living baboon, neither of whom lived through the operation.

THE CASE OF BABY FAE

Baby Fae was born on October 12, 1984, at Barstow Memorial Hospital in California, where she was 3 weeks premature at a weight of 5 pounds. When the pediatrician saw that she lacked color, she was transferred to Loma Linda Hospital, a Seventh-Day Adventist facility near Riverside, California, about 60 miles from Los Angeles. There, doctors confirmed that she had a hypoplastic left heart syndrome (HLHS).

In HLHS, the normally powerful left side of the heart and aorta are underdeveloped and too weak to pump blood. HLHS kills 1 in 10,000 babies, almost always within 2 weeks. According to a spokeswoman, Baby Fae almost died on her sixth day. Her parents were told of her dismal prognosis and took her to a nearby motel.

Four days later, Leonard Bailey, a 41-year-old chief of pediatric surgery at Loma Linda and who specialized in developing animal-to-man heart transplants, called the mother to discuss a xenograft. Bailey had been away at a convention when Baby Fae had first come to the hospital. At Loma Linda, the baby's options were discussed with the mother, and Bailey's call surprised the family. Bailey said, "I think they were awestruck that their child might still have the possibility to live."[2]

Baby Fae's mother was a 23-year-old, unmarried, unemployed woman. She and Baby Fae's father had lived together for 5 years, but were separated at the time of Baby Fae's birth. The mother returned to the hospital with 13-day-old Baby Fae, accompanied by the maternal grandmother and a male friend who had been living with the mother since the father had left. The child's father and mother had never married, although they had a previous son together.

The surgeon discussed the operation for 7 hours with the three adults. He showed them a slide show about the operation and the family signed the consent form, which had been reviewed in great detail by Loma Linda's IRB. They were asked to think about the operation for 20 hours, and then signed the consent form again.

Loma Linda Hospital agreed to protect the privacy of Baby Fae's family. The name "Fae" was all the world ever knew of the identity of the child, her mother, her biological father, or her mother's male friend.

On October 26, 1984, Bailey prepared to transplant a heart from a young baboon into 15-day-old Fae. While immunologist Sandra Nehlsen-Cannarella awaited results of final tissue-typing tests, Fae's heart reportedly started dying and her lungs started to swell with fluid. Whether Baby Fae was actually dying is important because Bailey made little effort to find a human heart donor, one of which may have been available (see below).

According to what was now the standard procedure, Fae went on a heart-lung machine, which gradually lowered her blood temperature to 68 degrees. Waiting in the basement was Goobers, a 10-month-old, baby female baboon. Three floors below Bailey's operating room, Loma Linda kept primates in animal quarters. Goobers was purchased from the Foundation for Biomedical Research in San Antonio, whose massive animal colonies include one of 2500 baboons and which supplies many medical centers with primates for research. Goobers was sedated and in 15 minutes Bailey cut out her walnut-sized heart. He then put the heart in saline ice-slush inside a Tupperware container, which was in turn put in a picnic cooler. This rather informal procedure was standard across the country. Goobers never awakened and was killed.

Back in the operating room, Bailey removed Fae's heart and replaced it with Goobers' healthy one. Over the next 4 hours, he connected both transplanted heart and transplanted arteries. Then the heart-lung machine raised Fae's temperature to 98 degrees, and Goober's heart began to beat spontaneously inside Fae.

According to the hospital's spokesperson, a baboon heart was used because a compatible human heart was unavailable. A lack of donated organs from humans has been a chronic obstacle to more transplantation. Patients die every day waiting helplessly for someone who is an appropriate organ-donor to die. If animals could be used as organ-donors, thousands more transplants could be done.

Nine days after the operation, with Fae seemingly doing fine, Bailey enthusiastically predicted that Fae might celebrate her 20th birthday. He predicted that Goober's heart would grow as Fae grew. Eleven days later, Fae died.

ETHICAL ISSUES

Use of Animals

Bailey's attempt generated intense ethical criticism about the use of Goobers. "This is medical sensationalism at the expense of Baby Fae, her family, and the baboon," said demonstrator Lucy Shelton of People for the Ethical Treatment of Animals (PETA).[3] Champions of animal rights protested the use of Goober's heart as unethical because, they insisted, Fae's life was not intrinsically worth more than Goober's. Bailey said animal lovers picketing his campus had ethical sensitivities "born of a luxurious society" and implied that only in California would surgeons have to worry about animal rights: "People in southern California have it so good that they can afford to worry about this type of issue."[4] Moreover, "When it gets down to a human living or dying, there shouldn't be any question" [of using an animal to save a human].

At the time of Fae's implant, philosopher Tom Regan (see Chapter 8) lamented that the operation had "two victims," first, Baby Fae and then, Goobers. Regan argued from his general philosophical view that beings who "have a life" also have a right to life. Regan said Goobers had a biographical life of sorts in that it mattered to Goobers whether she lived or whether her heart was cut out. Arguing from the premise that all primates have equal moral value, Regan condemned the operation: "Like us, Goobers was *somebody*, a distinct individual." For Regan, the crucial moral issue was that Goobers did not exist as Fae's resource:

> Those people who seized [Goobers'] heart, even if they were motivated by their concern for Baby Fae, grievously violated Goobers' right to be treated with respect. That she could do nothing to protest, and that many of us failed to recognize the transplant for the injustice that it was, does not diminish the wrong, a wrong settled before Baby Fae's sad death.[5]

Regan also argued that even if humans had obtained benefits in the past from using animals, it was still wrong. In a possible (but if so, incorrect) reference to the Tuskegee Study, he said:

> In the 1930s, we intentionally gave syphilis to prisoners to trace the disease. Suppose others benefited. It was still wrong. We recognize that there can be ill-gotten gains in the exploitation of human beings, but we

are blind to the fact that this is exactly what we're doing with animals. We are morally inconsistent.[6]

Other animal-rights philosophers emphasized that the difference between Baby Fae and the young Goobers, over their short lives and in their various potentialities, was not as great as that between Baby Fae and an anencephalic baby. Thomasine Kushner and Raymond Belloti, reminding us of the large breeding facility outside San Antonio which raised Goobers, asked in reply if it would be permissible there to also breed severely retarded humans for organ donations. If this is repugnant, they asked, why do we tolerate it for primates more similar to us than severely retarded humans?[7]

Predictably, Baby Fae's mother was unsympathetic to animal rights activists. "They don't know what they're talking about," she said.[8] Loma Linda's director of its Center for Christian Bioethics felt similarly:

> On an ethical scale, we will always place human beings ahead of
> subhumans, especially in a situation where people can be genuinely saved
> by animals. That is the story of mankind from the very beginning.
> Animals, for example, have always been used for food and clothing.[9]

Media Ethics

Although more media attention fell on Baby Fae than any similar recipient of a heart transplant, her family shunned publicity. Some moaners-and-groaners in the press complained about the public's (read: press's) right to know. Bailey held fewer press conferences than the daily briefings by DeVries at Brigham Young 2 years previously. Reporters charged Loma Linda with ineptitude in handling their requests and charged that aspects of the case begged for clarification.

One way of looking at these complaints is that Loma Linda had learned the lesson of William DeVries that it was better to give scant information than to try to satisfy the infinite demands of reporters. Just as many reporters came to Loma Linda as to Utah (more than 300), but they got much less information. This created the inevitable complaints about secrecy.

The media, too, had learned its lessons from the case of Barney Clark. Perhaps never before did the American public receive such accurate, detailed information from other cardiologists and surgeons, about criticisms of Dr. Bailey's attempt and about projected cost. It was one of the first times that the door had opened—for all Americans to see—into the secret room of life-and-death, surgical experimentation.

Informed Consent

A third ethical issue concerned informed consent. Did Bailey carefully describe the alternative Norwood procedure, with a 40 percent success rate by its originator William Norwood, to Fae's parents? Or that it might be used until a human heart was found? Law professor Alexander Capron said,

doubts linger, not only about the adequacy of the information supplied
to Baby Fae's parents but about whether their personal difficulties made
it possible for them to choose freely, and whether the realization that
their child was dying may have left them with the erroneous conclusion
that consenting to the transplant was the only "right" thing to do.[10]

An old saying always evokes knowing smiles among physicians: "Beware
the surgeon with one case." William DeVries suffered criticisms that he only
demonstrated the "clinical feasibility" of the artificial heart, not its "clinical
usefulness." Did Baby Fae's parents understand that their child's operation
might merely demonstrate the former?

As a religious institution, Loma Linda University is not automatically
subject to federal regulations on human experimentation. Only when the
university's research is funded by federal funds does it come under federal
surveillance. According to the hospital, Bailey's research on xenografts was
funded by the Seventh-Day Adventist Church and by donations from Bailey's
colleagues; thus it was not subject to prior, external, federal approval. (Research done on embryos for in vitro research is also funded by private funds
in order to avoid federal regulations, which do not permit such research.) Since
no new drug or device was used in the xenograft, the operation was also not
covered by FDA (Food and Drug Administration) regulations.

Because of the precedent this case would set, the university decided to
subject the operation to prior review by its IRB, which was in place to scru-
tinize other, federally funded research at Loma Linda. This review, over 14
months, was perhaps the most exhaustive internal review by an IRB since the
Utah IRB reviewed the Jarvik-7 for Barney Clark. But was it enough?

One troubling aspect is that Loma Linda refused to make public the informed consent documents signed by the parents of Baby Fae. There were also
newspaper reports of Baby Fae's mother idolizing Dr. Bailey. Most important,
did Baby Fae's parents or the Loma Linda IRB understand that most of the
Bailey's colleagues in pediatric surgery were skeptical of the value of such
operations?

Benefit to Baby Fae: Therapy or Research?

The most important criticism concerned whether the procedure was therapeutic or experimental. Was Baby Fae patient or victim? The answer to this
question came down to another: Did Baby Fae really have a chance to live to
"the best scenario" of being a 20-year-old adult with a baboon heart, as Bailey
claimed? Did she really have a chance to "celebrate more than one birthday
with her new heart"?[11]

In a November 1984 review of xenografts after Baby Fae's case, the editor
of the *Journal of Heart Transplantation* concluded:

> These clinical attempts demonstrated that primate hearts could be
> acutely tolerated by the human body, at least for a few days, but no
> evidence was found to suggest that these grafts could be accepted for

prolonged periods of time with the available methods of
immunosuppression. . . . Using presently available means of
immunosuppression and immunomanipulation, there is no evidence
that a vital organ can be transplanted from one species to another and
result in prolonged survival of the recipient.

From the experimental data and past clinical attempts, there is nothing
to indicate that primate hearts will be tolerated by a human infant for
months or years using today's means to induce and control tolerance.
The Loma Linda surgical team has not informed the medical community, as yet, of any new evidence that might suggest the contrary.[12]

Without this procedure, Baby Fae had probably no chance of surviving a year,
much less of reaching her 20th birthday.

Law professor George Annas called Bailey the champion of the "anything goes" school of experimentation, emphasizing how the two previous
attempts to implant animal hearts in humans were done with little consent
and on similarly vulnerable, similarly poor, patients. Annas emphasized what
standard accounts omitted: that Reemtsma in 1963 had implanted chimpanzee
kidneys into a 43-year-old black man dying of glamerulonephritis and that
Hardy had implanted a chimpanzee heart into a poor deaf-mute who was
dying, who survived only 2 hours, who was brought to the hospital unconscious, and who never consented to the operation. In other words, poor selection of patients and lack of consent marred the operations, which were not
therapeutic but experimental. Annas concluded:

This inadequately reviewed, inappropriately consented to, premature
experiment on an impoverished, terminally ill newborn was unjustified.
It differs from the xenograft experiments of the early 1960s only in the
fact that there was prior review of the proposal by an IRB. But this
distinction did not protect Baby Fae. She remained unprotected from
ruthless experimentation in which her only role was that of victim.[13]

For many people, what was objectionable about the experiment was not
trying a risky operation. Surgery can only know what is impossible by trying.
What was objectionable was that a newborn baby, who could not consent, was
used. The only new developments between Baby Fae's case in 1984 and the
two cases in 1963 and 1964 were the discoveries of cyclosporin and better tissue
matching, but critics say both of these could have used for a xenograft in an
adult—an adult who could have consented to take the risk.

The medical distinction between therapy and experimentation can be expressed in moral terms. In Kantian ethics (deontology), the difference is between
treating a person as "an end in himself" and using him as a "mere means" to
some other goal. As Charles Krauthammer wrote in his essay in *Time:*

Civilization hangs on the Kantian principle that human beings are to be
treated as ends and not means. So much depends on that principle
because there is no crime that cannot be, that has not been, committed
in the name of the future against those who inhabit the present.

Medical experimentation, which invokes the claims of the future, necessarily turns people into means.[14]

In an exclusive interview in *American Medical News*, Leonard Bailey passionately claimed that the operation was intended to be therapeutic:

I have always believed it would work, or I would not have attempted it.... There was always therapeutic intent. My dilemma has been educating the university and the medical profession.[15]

Bailey's comments were made 9 days after the operation, when Baby Fae was still alive and doing well. Bailey implied then that xenografts might be preferable to human transplants. Medical cynics retorted that there is a difference between "therapeutic intent" and "therapeutic probability." Any operation has a "possibility" of being therapeutic; all surgeons can claim that they "intended" their operations to be therapeutic.

Sandra Nehlsen-Cannarella worked as an immunologist with Bailey and agreed that the operation was intended to be therapeutic, arguing that Baby Fae could have accepted the heart if a good enough match had been found, with compatible lymphocytes. She tested for such compatibility in Baby Fae's parents and relatives (weak reaction), lab workers (strong reaction), Nehlsen-Cannarella herself (strong reaction), and three baboons (strong reaction). Baby Fae's reaction to her own blood and tissue was the control. Surprisingly, Baby Fae had a weak reaction to three other baboons, and a "very, very weak" reaction against one baboon—Goobers.[16] From these tests, Nehlsen-Cannarella concluded that she was not fighting across-the-board rejection in xenografts.

Indeed, similarity of blood between human and nonhuman primates has always been considered evidence for common evolution. If so, one would expect that some humans would closely match some primates. Similarly, some humans react strongly against not only some baboons, but also against some humans. One third of humans has a "preformed antibody" against tissue from other humans, and as many as 70 percent of humans have a preformed antibody against baboon tissue. Baby Fae was in the 30 percent minority. Bailey claimed that previous ignorance about human-baboon matching explained Hardy's previous failures in xenografting. But other immunologists and transplant surgeons doubted whether better tissue typing would create more successful transplants.

Finally, Bailey's reason for choosing a baby rather than an adult was not to avoid consent but to avoid immune rejection of the xenograft. An infant's immune system is not fully developed and babies tolerate organ transplants better before their immune systems develop. Bailey also claimed that infants can be given larger dosages of cyclosporin than adults.[17] Thus, to object that new information about tolerance of cyclosporin in babies and improved tissue typing were not big enough advances to try a neonatal xenograft seems odd. Given the success of these advances with adults, what more could the critics want?

Alternate Treatment

William I. Norwood, a pediatric surgeon, had developed a less radical alternative for hypoplastic left ventricle syndrome, and had performed it many times at Children's Hospitals in Philadelphia and Boston. Bailey claims that children did not do well enough after the Norwood procedure to justify performing the operation, but given his extensive efforts to develop xenografts, was he an impartial judge?

Should Bailey have sought a human heart for Baby Fae? Bailey said such hearts were impossible to find at such an early age (under 7 weeks) because criteria for neonatal brain death were problematical ("You can have a flat EEG on a newborn and, yet the baby will survive").[18] Most neonatal transplants come from anencephalic babies. Most such babies do not meet the criteria of most state laws about brain death, and hence, donor-babies must come from the few states with more liberal definitions of brain death.

Second, Bailey claimed most parents would neither accept such brain death in their babies nor agree to be donors for transplants. (This was soon falsified by one of Bailey's own actions—see below). Like William DeVries' comment about Barney Clark, Bailey said the baboon heart was Baby Fae's "only chance to live." Nevertheless, Paul Teraski, director of the Southern California Regional Organ Procurement Agency, said an infant heart had indeed been potentially available the day of Baby Fae's xenograft. Moreover, he added, "I think that they [Loma Linda doctors] did not make any effort to get a human infant heart because they were set on doing a baboon."[19] Bailey had performed more than 150 transplants on animals preparing for such a cross-species operation and it is hard to believe that he wasn't looking for a first case.

Bailey replied,

> We were not searching for a human heart. We were out to enter the whole new area of transplanting tissue-matched baboon hearts into newborns who are supported with antisuppressive drugs. I suppose that we could have used a human heart that was outsized and that was not tissue-matched, and that would have pacified some people, but it would have been very poor science. On the other hand, I suppose my belief that there are no newborn hearts available for transplantation was more opinion than data or science, but it is scientific to acknowledge that the whole area of determining brain death of newborns is very problematical.[20]

An associate surgeon at Loma Linda defended Bailey against not searching for a human heart:

> It would have to be the sort of case where an infant fell out of a crib and was declared brain dead but the heart was okay. Then all these tests would have to be done to insure a proper matching. With Baby Fae, we had five days to do those tests, getting the best possible [animal] donor. With a human heart, we might not have been able to keep the recipient alive.[21]

Costs and Resources

A final ethical issue was rarely mentioned, money. Baby Fae's parents were poor. They had no medical insurance and could not have paid for any alternative procedures. No one ever mentioned this issue, but its importance explains why neither a human heart nor the Norwood procedure was pursued by Loma Linda surgeons. The former costs $100,000 and the latter can cost as much, plus travel costs and lodging in Philadelphia where Norwood practiced. The heart for Baby Fae from Goobers, and the transplant operation, were provided free.

A conspiracy of silence exists in medicine about money and therapeutic treatment. The xenograft was Fae's only chance, not because of medical, but because of financial, realities.

More generally, and as with artificial hearts, critics questioned whether so much money should be spent on so few when so much good could be done for so many others with the same money. Although Loma Linda never revealed the cost of the operation, the research behind Baby Fae's transplant and the operation itself cost perhaps $1 million. Should 500 to a 1000 such transplants be done each year, at a cost of half to one billion dollars, while thousands of babies are born deformed—who might not otherwise have been—because Medicaid will not pay for the $600 amniocentesis for each pregnant mother? (Ironically, a related test, screening of maternal serum for high levels of alpha-fetoprotein—which detects neural tube defects such as spina bifida and anencephaly—would actually decrease the number of anencephalics available for neonatal transplant.)

Should Parents Volunteer Their Children as Research Subjects?

Conservative theologian Paul Ramsey has argued that it is always wrong for parents to volunteer their children as subjects of nontherapeutic research:

> If today we mean to give such weight to the *research imperative*...then we should not seek to give a principle justification of what we are doing with children. It is better to leave the research imperative in incorrigible conflict with the principle that protects the individual human person from being used for research purposes without either his expressed or correctly construed consent. Some sorts of human experimentation should, in this alternative, be acknowledged to be "borderline situations" in which moral agents are under the necessity of doing wrong for the sake of the public good. Either way they do wrong. It is immoral not to do the research. It is also immoral to use children who cannot themselves consent and who ought not to be presumed to consent to research unrelated to their treatment. On this supposition research medicine, like politics, is a realm in which men have to "sin bravely."[22]

Charles Krauthammer cited this passage by Ramsey and agreed with him:

> Baby Fae lived, and died, in that realm. Only the bravery was missing: no one would admit the violation. Bravery was instead fatuously

ascribed to Baby Fae, a creature as incapable of bravery as she was of circulating her own blood. Whether this case was an advance in medical science awaits the examination of the record by the scientific community. That it was an adventure in medical ethics is already clear.[23]

Catholic theologian Richard McCormick disputes Ramsey arguing that parents can volunteer children for "low-risk" nontherapeutic research.[24] His argument is specific to the Roman Catholic natural law tradition in ethics and argues that, because adults should volunteer for low-risk, nontherapeutic research for the general good, infants should also. In other words, the adults should choose for the child not as the child *would* choose as an adult, but as the child *ought* to choose as an adult.

Neither one of these authors accepts a "pluralism" of ethical judgments in ethics and both officially reject a utilitarian justification (although McCormick's view seems implicitly utilitarian). Yet to many people, such a justification is the most natural one. How else will treatment advance for hypoplastic left ventricle syndrome, a congenital defect of babies, unless such babies are subjects of research?

Also, federal regulations require, for operations involving risk to children and where possible, that prior research be done on animals and adult humans: "Research involving risk should be conducted first on animals and adult humans in order to ascertain degree of risk."[25]

Finally, compare Baby Fae and Barney Clark. Both were almost entirely experimental subjects with a remote chance of therapeutic benefit. In one case, an adult man with a lifetime of experience volunteered himself for the experiment. Moreover, he himself was a medical professional. In contrast, Baby Fae was none of these; someone else volunteered her, and she was another possible "victim."

UPDATE

The weight of the medical world eventually came down against Dr. Bailey. The scientific journal *Nature* concluded that "the serious difficulty over the operation...is that it may have catered to the researchers' needs first and to the patient's only second."[26] The Judicial Council of the American Medical Association implicitly criticized Bailey (and DeVries) in coming out with guidelines for cardiac surgery involving xenografts (and artificial hearts), timing its announcement several weeks after the death of Baby Fae (and just after DeVries had operated on William Schroeder, the second recipient of a Jarvik-7).[27] The Council said such research should be part of a "systematic" program and should follow "accepted" standards of scientific research, i.e., it should be done with peer review and randomized clinical trials. Arnold Relman, the senior editor of the *New England Journal of Medicine*, was especially adamant about clinical trials: Unless such operations were compared to similar patients, who received only drugs and other nonsurgical treatments, how would medicine have real evidence that the operations benefited patients?[28]

Using "Brain-Dead" Babies for Other Babies

After animal-to-man organ transplantation failed, Leonard Bailey and Loma Linda turned to using anencephalic babies as "donors." In October 1987, at Loma Linda, Leonard Bailey transplanted into Canadian baby Paul Holc the heart of the anencephalic "Baby Gabrielle" of Canadians Brenda and Michael Winner, who had agreed to keep their fetus alive until birth for the operation.[29] In doing so, they crossed a small line between using donors who had accidentally become brain-dead to keeping alive anencephalic fetuses for "donation."

This action and subsequent ones raised the general question of whether any baby should be used for the good of another and, if so, what were the criteria and social consequences? Had the use of Goobers for Baby Fae opened the gate to use of brain-dead human babies for other human babies with more potential?

One pressing question here was whether such infants really were brain-dead. Critics charged that good criteria do not exist to declare brain death in infants. Moreover, anencephaly is a medical term describing a range of gross, congenital brain deficits—all of which entail no chance of normal brain function—but some of which do not entail brain death.[30] Instead, some conditions of anencephaly are something like PVS (persistent vegetative state) and, as such, infants could survive indefinitely with maximal, supportive care.

Because of this question, critics questioned whether less is being done for anencephalic babies for the good of babies getting transplants:... " By far the most fundamental problem [for Loma Linda's neonatology staff] was trying to sustain an anencephalic's liver, heart, and kidneys without temporarily giving life to its brain stem, the one organ that needed to die for transplant to begin."[31] Putting semianencephalic babies in NICUs paradoxically tended to keep their primitive brain stems alive, while waiting for them to "die."[32]

Critics such as Alexander Capron objected that organ "donation" here was an inappropriate term because no baby had ever explicitly or implicitly consented to the removal of his or her organs. Others did not think a useful distinction could be made between lack of a cerebral cortex and a cerebral cortex which did not work. Physician/ethicist Julius Landwirth said, "I have an uneasy feeling that what lurks behind the anencephalic issue is the vegetative state issue."[33]

One suggestion was to place anencephalics in a special category for organ transfer. Because they were neither dead nor necessarily dying, but because allowing them to die could destroy the very organs which could be transplanted, some ethicists, such as Arthur Caplan, suggested the creation of a new category in brain death laws to allow such transfers. At bottom, this issue broke down into differences about when not to consider a being a person. If

95 percent of anencephalics die within the first week, are they really persons? Critics such as Capron say we must always give marginal persons the benefit of the doubt.

Perhaps 2000 anencephalic babies are born alive in the United States each year, and supporters of Bailey argue that keeping such babies alive for organ transplants benefits everyone. "It's very helpful for the family to feel that some good" can come out of such pregnancies, said William Curran of Harvard.[34]

After 12 unsuccessful attempts to transplant organs from anencephalic infants, Loma Linda University Medical Center halted its program in late 1988. It left open the possibility of pursuing other options.[35]

FURTHER READING

"Baby Fae: Ethical Issues Surrounding Cross-Species Transplantation," Scope Note #5, Bioethics Library, Kennedy Institute of Ethics, Georgetown University, Washington, D.C. 20057.

Dennis L. Breo, "Is 'Baby Fae' Transplant Worth It? Experts Mixed" *American Medical News*, 27(42):1, 41–43 (November 9, 1984).

"The Subject Is Baby Fae," *Hastings Center Report*, 15(1):8–17 (February 1985).

Kenneth Vaux, "Baby Fae and Human Wholeness," *Christian Century* 101(38): 1144–1145 (December 5, 1984).

PART 4

CLASSIC CASES ABOUT INDIVIDUAL RIGHTS VS. THE PUBLIC GOOD

CHAPTER 13

Mayor Koch, Joyce Brown, and Involuntary Psychiatric Committment

For citizens of many big cities in America, being confronted with homeless street people is a tragic part of daily life. Panhandlers ask for money and ex-mental patients roam the streets. One study, in 1988, estimated that the five boroughs of New York City contained 10,363 homeless people using emergency shelters at night, plus 4500 homeless families with three or more people and at least 2000 more homeless people who refused to use the shelters.[1] These homeless people, who are very visible to tourists and city commuters, evoke both compassion and frustration among onlookers.

By 1987, the problem of what to do with such people had become both a national and local controversy. Native New Yorkers and mental health professionals wanted something done. Men with cigars and women in minks, walking by Carnegie Hall on 57th Street in the middle of winter, avoided homeless people sleeping in doorways. Shuttle cars on the subway were taken over at night by the homeless, who stayed awake at night—when life was dangerous—and who slept during the day. Some of the homeless died on cold nights.

In 1987, the New York City administration faced the question: could insane, homeless people just be left "to die with their rights on?" Or could they be forcibly picked up for psychiatric evaluation in a hospital? It might be against their will, but would it not help? Such reasoning led Mayor Ed Koch to strengthen Project Help, which began in 1983 and which evaluated dozens of homeless, mentally ill people for possible psychiatric treatment. The mayor obtained some scarce beds in New York mental hospitals to house the extremely dysfunctional.

The first person picked up on October 28, 1987 was a 40-year-old black woman who called herself "Billie Boggs,"—the name of a prominent New York City me-

265

dia person. "Billie," whose real name was Joyce Brown, had slept a year and half at night on an air grate on the Upper East Side of Manhattan. During the day, she panhandled on the street and muttered to herself. Mayor Koch, who had previously spoken with her on the street, went along with Project Help's decision to choose her as a test case. At the same time, almost a hundred other homeless people were evaluated on the streets, and, of these, 38 were brought to Bellevue Hospital's inpatient psychiatric unit.

After Joyce was evaluated, the mayor was told she wasn't dangerous enough to herself for commitment, to which he replied, "You're loony yourself." Like Koch, most New Yorkers (and certainly, most tourists) felt that the thousands of mentally–ill, homeless people had destroyed New York City's street life. Here, Koch said, was a woman whom compassionate people should help, but who could not be helped because of legalistic quibbles. This case soon attracted national attention because it symbolized a struggle over how far society should go in involuntarily treating the homeless, mentally ill.

HISTORICAL BACKGROUND

Ideology and Insanity

For most of history, the "voices" of schizophrenia were conceptualized as the words of the gods, or other spirits. Julian Jaynes postulated that the first man to have a thought experienced it as an internal voice and was thereby terrified.[2] For Jaynes, mankind's brain evolved to control such "voices" and became bicameral. Schizophrenia's "voices" are then throwbacks to a previous stage of mankind. Plato thought of insanity as one part of the mind dominating the others, (being "unbalanced").[3]

In the Middle Ages, insanity was thought to be caused by demonic possession and exorcists were hired to drive out demons. The insane were sometimes put on a ship ("ship of fools"), which went from port to port, getting food and water, but unable to unload its human cargo. In the 18th century, Philadelphians paid admission to mental hospitals to gawk at mental patients in chains. The gawkers prided themselves on their normalcy. More enlightened treatment was practiced by the Society of Friends, who saw God (not Satan) inside the insane. Such alternative Quaker institutions in 1813 practiced "moral treatment," where patients freely roamed grounds and worked in gardens.

The emphasis on patient rights and treatment characteristic of modern psychiatry came about as an antidote to previous ways of thinking, which saw commitment to mental institutions only as an alternative to imprisonment in jail. Early 20th-century society saw that the insane were not criminals, and needed not criminal, but "therapeutic," justice. Since the insane were not charged with crimes and were presumed innocent, no legal proceedings occurred. Committing psychiatrists theoretically always acted for the patients' best interests.

In the 1960s, two world views clashed over mental patients. Movies such as *Titicut Follies, King of Hearts,* and *One Flew Over the Cuckoo's Nest* dramatized this conflict. Lawyers emphasized patient autonomy, the subjectivity of psychiatric diagnosis, checks and balances, and the coercive squalor of large state institutions. Psychiatrists emphasized benevolence, treatment needs, insanity as mental disease, and dangers of apathy.

Lawyers then allied with the patient rights movement to batter down the locked doors of psychiatric wards. Within psychiatry, heretics such as Thomas Szasz led an internal revolt, claiming that commitment never benefited patients and that it was done chiefly to rid society of strange-acting persons. This psychiatrist questioned whether anyone could correctly define norms of "correct" and "psychotic" behavior. If it was the patient himself, Szasz had no problem, for Szasz saw the proper role of psychiatrists as helping a patient who already had identified his or her problem and who voluntarily sought help. His criticisms came with those who, like "Billie Boggs," did not see themselves as mentally ill and who resisted help.

Szasz's basic position was this. Real disease has a physical cause in the brain, but mental illness is a "myth." So-called mental illness involves problems in living, and such problems are not caused by microbiological lesions. Disease is physical or is no disease at all. Classifying personality disorders as mental illness was especially suspect to Szasz. (Mary Beth Whitehead's "personality disorder" was exactly the kind of diagnosis which made Szasz suspicious, especially because it was made for purposes other than helping Mary Beth.) Psychiatry presumes that homicide, suicide, repeated divorce, chronic hostility, and vengefulness indicate mental illness because it assumes that love, continued life, stable marriages, kindness, and meekness are good. These presumptions are evaluative, not factual.

Hence psychiatry is not value-free and "contains many more value conflicts than medicine in general."[4] Interpersonal relations between all people—wife and husband, colleagues at work, neighbors, citizen, and state—involve stress, conflict of interests, and strain. Much of the resulting disharmony involves conflicts of values, and to pretend that psychiatrists can offer value-free approaches to solving such conflicts is ludicrous: "Much of psychotherapy revolves around nothing other than the elucidation and weighing of goals and values—many of which may be mutually contradictory—and the means whereby they might best be harmonized, realized, or relinquished."

In a similar but slightly different critique, existentialist psychiatrist R. D. Laing viewed insane behavior as an inner mental defense against a brutal, manipulative, terrifying world. So the young girl in *Sybil* develops multiple personalities to distance "herself" from the terrible torture inflicted by her vicious mother. So Joyce Brown's muttering to herself and yelling of obscenities might be interpreted as such a defense (especially because they seemed to increase when rough men came around).

In Rosenhan's famous study, "On Being Sane in Insane Places," several sociologists, psychiatrists, and others voluntarily entered mental hospitals saying they heard a voice (a major symptom of schizophrenia).[5] They then acted normally and no longer mentioned voices. Once labeled as schizophrenic in their medical charts, the staff continued to perceived them so. Ironically, several of the mental patients saw through the impostors when the staff did not.

Deinstitutionalization

In 1972, federal judge Frank Johnson in Alabama ruled in *Wyatt vs. Stickey* that a committed mental patient must either receive treatment or be released. Johnson's decision addressed institutional conditions necessary to ensure minimal treatment for individuals and specified that at least two psychiatrists, 12 registered nurses, and 10 aides had to be present for every 250 patients. While these standards are extremely low, Alabama and many other states had failed to meet them for years. Johnson also required that state mental institutions must provide the least restrictive conditions necessary for their treatment, individualized treatment plans, and freedom to refuse invasive treatments such as ECT (electro-convulsive therapy) and psychosurgery.

Johnson's ruling was a companion piece to the ultimate U.S. Supreme Court decision in *O'Connor vs. Donaldson* in 1975.[6] Kenneth Donaldson was committed in 1943, when his parents asked a Florida judge to commit the 34-year-old man after he was knocked unconscious in a fight with co-workers over politics. When he complained about incarceration, he was labeled paranoid. He later received electroshock treatments. After a few brief visits by nonpsychiatric physicians, and at his father's instigation, he was committed to a state mental hospital. For the next 30 years, he unsuccessfully attempted to be released. During his last 15 years, he never saw a judge, rarely saw a physician, never received treatment, and never had a hearing to re-evaluate his dangerousness. Inside the institution, he was presumed insane, and like Rosenhan's impostors, could not prove himself otherwise.

In 1971, a lawyer helped him bring suit against O'Connor, the superintendent of his institution. The U.S. Supreme Court decided for Donaldson, holding that he could not be held against his will, even if mentally ill, unless he had no means of existing outside the institution. More generally, *O'Connor* said that the two necessary conditions for involuntary commitment were:

I Suffering from mentally illness (being "insane"), *AND*
II Being
    A dangerous to others, *OR*
    B dangerous to self as evidenced by
        1. Suicidal threats
        2. Gross neglect of basic needs

The traditional interpretation of "dangerousness" was imminent risk of harm to body or life (or threats of such) within days or hours. The traditional arbiters were two psychiatrists. Dangerousness to self was eventually stretched to include gross incapacity to take care of one's basic needs. The two necessary conditions both had to be met for involuntary commitment.

With these legal changes, the courts moved rapidly in civil commitment from a medical model in the early 1960s to a patient rights model in the 1970s. Symbolic of this move was the additional requirement (beyond mental illness) of proof of dangerousness to others and the emphasis on least restrictive environments. All states required the first two criteria for involuntary commitment, and two-thirds required the last.[7]

Inmates were then released because individualized treatment could not often be given in state institutions, because halfway homes were less restrictive than large, state-run facilities, and because new psychotropic medications allowed patients to be "treated" as outpatients. In most states, 50 percent of the patients of state institutions were released; in other states, 75 percent.

President Kennedy speeded deinstitutionalization by calling for small, community-integrated facilities rather than large, impersonal state institutions: "Reliance on the cold mercy of custodial isolation will be supplanted by the open warmth of community concern."[8] But communities were hostile, not warm, to having halfway shelters amidst them, and few such shelters appeared.

Tight budgets, psychiatrists seeking less work, and a general distrust of authority in the 1960s combined with court decisions and the Kennedy manifesto to empty mental institutions. Mental patients flooded into communities to live on warm-air grates and to vie for scarce places in understaffed community homes. In 1955, nearly 560,000 patients lived inside state mental institutions, but in 1988, there were only 130,000. Nearly half a million mental patients were "deinstitutionalized" over 30 years. Governments saved monies, the American Civil Liberties Union was happy, and streets suddenly contained bag ladies. Local charities created soup kitchens to feed hungry street people, and instead of being identified as a symptom that deinstitutionalization had failed, were hailed by Reaganites as how government was unneeded.

Deinstitutionalization failed because government funds never came for community homes, because communities rejected local homes; because mental health services were fragmented between county, state, and federal agencies; because of lack of housing, and because the legal pendulum swung toward autonomy of mental patients. In the 1970s, everyone struggled to make a system, which was not a system, work.

In the 1980s, psychiatry revolted. Prominent psychiatrists chastized liberals who resisted committing schizophrenics. Saul Feldman, a former director at the National Institute of Mental Health and a former leader of deinstitutionalization, criticized the profitable ethics of mental health administrators, whom he accused of allowing a new form of segregation: "poor blacks working with other poor blacks while white mental health professionals worked with their own kind."[9] Psychiatrist Paul Chodoff reviewed a decade of deinstitutionalization and concluded that it had failed, that some involuntary confinement was needed to help the mentally ill, and that civil liberties lawyers were often enemies of the insane.[10]

THE CASE OF JOYCE BROWN

Before being picked up by Project HELP, Joyce Brown had been a familiar person to denizens of New York's Upper East Side, an area with the highest per capita wealth in the United States. She had lived through New York City's winter atop an air vent outside a Swensen's ice cream parlor on Second Avenue and 65th Street.

She had lived on the block for a year and a half. One block resident had given her money, only to have it tossed back while she angrily screamed at an invisible man. The homeless woman passed residents on the block with a glazed looks and often muttered to herself. She sometimes sang, "How Much Is That Doggie in the Window?" She was described by a letter-writing neighbor as "full of rage." The black woman disliked black men and cursed them if they walked on her side of the street, but she liked babies in strollers.

Her physical appearance to some suggested mental illness. Her teeth were very unclean, her matted, tangled hair was underneath a bulky, white, knit cap, and the only clothes she had were a striped blouse, beige pants, and a green sweater. She kept sheets and blankets nearby, under which she slept on the air vent.

She panhandled, and each day went to a nearby delicatessen where she bought cigarettes, chicken cutlets, toilet paper, and ice cream. On bitterly cold nights, residents tried to have her picked up, but she resisted. She lived through the winter without gloves. She defecated and urinated in the gutter.

Forcibly brought to Bellevue's emergency room, "Billie Boggs" was injected with 5 mg. of Haldol, an antipsychotic drug, and 2 mg. of Ativan, a fast-acting, short-term tranquilizer. "Billie" also called herself "Ann Smith," said she had lived on the street for 5 years, and said she had no parents or relatives. Once inside, she was taken upstairs to a new 28-bed, locked psychiatric unit on the 19th floor. There, she exercised her right to refuse to take drugs. New York allows involuntary injections only in the emergency room, and before other drugs could be given, a hearing before a judge was necessary. For such hearings, hospitals usually have a designated room inside psychiatric units. Once a person is brought inside such a facility by police or emergency personnel, she does not leave until the hearing concludes.

"Billie Boggs" received a lawyer from the American Civil Liberties Union (ACLU). Both the mayor's office and the ACLU framed the subsequent hearing as a test. City attorney Maureen McLeod argued that the inmate had to be committed because she was endangering herself through self-neglect. The ACLU asked for an injunction to free her.

Judge Robert Lippman presided over the hearing. He was a 51-year-old married lawyer who lived on the Upper East Side, a son of a prominent orthopedic surgeon. Appropriately enough, for 17 years he had worked as a Legal Aid lawyer in the Bronx and was known in the legal community as an advocate for the poor and homeless. He had been assigned to hear mental health cases.

Publicity about the mayor's program caused a sketch of the woman to appear on television. As a result, three women identified her as their sister Joyce Brown, for whom they had been searching for a year and a half. Each sister was married, had worked for years, and lived in what they described as "comfortable homes."

Her sisters revealed Joyce's past to reporters. She had been a "bright, attractive, and happy-go-lucky child" amidst their family in Elizabeth, N.J.[11] Their father was ordained as a Methodist minister, and all the girls had gone to church every Sunday. The sisters emphasized, "behind every homeless person there is a family that just wants to find them and help them."

Joyce Brown graduated from both high school and business school and then worked at several jobs at Bell Laboratories. During these years, the sisters described her as "a big, healthy girl" who wore nice clothes with jewelry and who "always drove around in a new Cadillac." She had no children and never married.

Her sisters said that in her twenties, Joyce Brown became increasingly dependent on heroin and later cocaine. The first signs of schizophrenia often appear in a person's twenties. Joyce proceeded to work for 10 years as a secretary for the New Jersey Human Rights Commission. In 1982, Newark police arrested her for assault. At about this time, her conduct deteriorated. She became less able to support herself and became belligerent. Her mental health and job performance plummeted. In 1985, at age 38, she was fired because of absenteeism. She left her sisters and went to a Newark shelter, but was expelled for assaulting people.

Her sisters admit then tricking her into a psychiatric ward at East Orange General Hospital. There she was judged psychotic and injected with antipsychotic drugs, which she resisted. She was held involuntarily for 2 weeks, and because of assaults on others, was put in restraints in an isolation room.

When she was released, Ms. Brown fled New Jersey and took up residence under aliases on Manhattan's Upper East Side. She did not contact her sisters, fearing she would be recommitted. She avoided shelters for the homeless, believing them dangerous for unattached women. After an abusive phone call from Joyce in Manhattan in July 1986, the sisters spent much of the next year looking for her along Manhattan streets.

Ms. Brown's 3-day commitment hearing occurred 8 days after she was brought to Bellevue. Such hearings are almost always closed to the public, but because of the case's publicity and its potential to set a precedent, Judge Lippman allowed reporters to attend. However, only witnesses who consented had their comments reported.

Four psychiatrists testified for the city that Joyce suffered from chronic schizophrenia; they predicted that she would deteriorate if left on the streets. They testified that she was clearly psychotic and should be treated in an institution. Three psychiatrists countered for the ACLU that she was not psychotic, not dangerous, not unreasonable in her answers, and not incapable of caring for herself on the streets. Psychiatrist Robert E. Gould of New York Medical College said she was living on the street by choice.

At the hearing, Ms. Brown appeared to be an intelligent, articulate person. She called herself a "professional street person" and answered accusatory questions.

Why had she torn up paper money? she was asked. She said she did so only after she had her daily $7 and extra money was forced on her. "If money is given to me and I don't want it, of course I am going to destroy it," she said, indicating she might be robbed if she did not. "I've heard people say: 'Take it. It will make me feel good.' But I say: 'I don't want it. I don't need it.' Is it my job to make them feel good by taking their money?"[12]

Why did she defecate on herself? "I never did," she replied, but added that she had used the streets because no local restaurant would let her use its restroom. "I offered to buy something and they still refused." Why had she used aliases such as "Billie Boggs"? "To prevent my sisters from finding me."

One of the psychiatrists for the city was Luis R. Marcos, a vice president of the city's public hospital system, director of the city's Psychiatric Services, and an advocate of Mayor Koch's program. When challenged about his role, he said, "This is not political psychiatry." Dr. Marcos also stated that Joyce's "self-neglect" was "so severe" that she had to be helped against her will. He noted that being schizophrenic was consistent with being bright and having periods of rationality.

One of Joyce's sisters tried to testify, but was not allowed to do so after the ACLU attorney objected. She had started to describe how her sister's condition had deteriorated over the years. The objection was sustained because it was irrelevant as to Ms. Brown's immediate competency. The sisters resented having family testimony and Joyce's past declared irrelevant.

By the third day, Ms. Brown appeared self-confident. She spoke slowly, deliberately, with assurance, and even smiled a few times at the judge. She told him that Upper East Side passersby chatted with her daily. "They tell me about movies, they tell me about restaurants. They are executives, lawyers, doctors. They are established in their fields. If I asked for large amounts of money, they would give it to me."

ACLU attorney Richard Levy summed up and claimed the city had not proved that Joyce Brown was dangerous to herself or others. "The only evidence the city had is that she goes to the bathroom in the streets," Levy said. "I see that in New York City every day, because there's a lack of public restroom facilities." City attorney Maureen McLeod countered in summation: "Decency and the law and common sense do not require us to wait until something happens to her. It is our duty to act before it is too late."[13]

The Court Finds for Ms. Brown

Judge Lippman found that Ms. Brown was "rational, logical, and coherent" throughout her testimony.[14] He said she "displayed a sense of humor, pride, a fierce independence of spirit, [and] quick mental reflexes." He noted that Ms. Brown met none of the conditions set forth in *O'Connor vs. Donaldson*. He stressed that even if all psychiatrists had said she was psychotic, the city's case had still not met the second condition of dangerousness to others or self.

"I am aware that her mode of existence does not conform to conventional standards, that it is an offense to aesthetic sense," he said. Nevertheless, "she copes, she is fit, she survives." Moreover, "she refuses to be housed in a shelter. That may reveal more about conditions in shelters than about Joyce Brown's mental state. It might, in fact, prove she's quite sane." (New York City shelters are mostly used by homeless men, and many of these men use crack.)

Judge Lippman also complained: "There must be some civilized alternatives other than involuntary hospitalization or the street." He did not invalidate the mayor's program, and even praised it as a step in the right direction. Forced to decide for one side or the other, however, he ruled that the city had not proved Ms. Brown incompetent.

The Next Round

After the hearing, the three sisters insisted Joyce needed treatment. As psychiatrist Robert Gould left the hearing with Joyce's sisters and reporters, he challenged the sisters, "Can't you understand that a lot of people are frightened that the mayor has unilaterally decided to change the statue and pick up your sister?" One sister replied, "The mayor is absolutely right. I have lived with her. You have not lived with her." Gould replied, "Is it possible that your sister doesn't want to live with you because you are so angry?"[15]

Mayor Koch blasted the decision: "If anything happens to that woman, God forbid, the blood of that woman is on that judge's hands." Reminded by a reporter that Judge Lippman had said Joyce was lucid, Koch replied, "This woman is at risk. When she lay on the ground in the rain, in the snow, uncovered—was that lucid?"[16] Joyce Brown's sisters called the judge's decision "racist" and "sexist." They claimed that if the judge's own wife or mother were sleeping on the streets, "he would not stand for it."

But why did Joyce appear so rational in court, the city and her sisters were asked? Bellevue psychiatrists acknowledged that Ms. Brown appeared sane at the hearing, but they claimed she had improved rapidly inside the hospital. Joyce dismissed their claim, retorting that she had never been crazy in the first place. She also objected to being taken into Bellevue like "cattle."

She also claimed that, given her options, it was a rational choice to live on the streets. The sisters dismissed Joyce's claims. "You might be able to survive one winter," one sister replied, "or even two. But you can't survive that way forever."

Following the decision, Ms. Brown had a press conference with her ACLU lawyer, Robert Levy. She said, "I didn't want to play the game before, but now I am...I am going to get an apartment...go back to work, and get my life together." She criticized the city for spending $600 a day on her care: "I could be living at Trump Tower."[17]

Her sisters revealed that after Joyce was hospitalized for schizophrenia in East Orange, they had gotten her declared mentally disabled. As a result, Joyce had received $500 a month in Social Security disability payments, which her sisters said they had been holding for her. Ms. Brown rejected the payments because she rejected the "lie" that she was mentally disabled.

With the mayor's consent, New York City's Health and Hospital Corporation appealed to a five-member New York State Appellate Court, one of whose members stayed Judge Lippman's order. The higher court agreed to an extraordinarily quick date for the hearing, i.e., within 2 weeks. Until then, Joyce would have to remain locked inside Bellevue. Joyce was reported bitter but philosophical about the decision.

During the weeks between hearings, city officials sought and obtained an order to see if she suffered from a genetically caused brain syndrome, lupus cerebritis, an incurable degenerative disease. After negotiations, she allowed a blood sample. The test proved negative, which embarrassed the psychiatrist who had made the grasping-at-straws diagnosis.

Two weeks later, the ACLU argued before the appellate justices that Ms. Brown would not return to the streets but would live in a supportive residence for the homeless. City officials countered that where she would live was irrelevant: "She was not hospitalized because she was living on the streets—" they said, but because "three psychiatrists said she needed medical and psychiatric help." They said she was schizophrenic and should remain in psychiatric care for her own good. Her newfound decision not to return to the streets would not affect the city's decision.

City officials did not claim she was a danger to herself or others. They stressed that the case was not about homelessness but about mental illness. In New York, the homeless tended to be poor, black, or Hispanic. In contrast, Project HELP targeted mentally disturbed patients on the streets, patients who were typically white, middle-class, non-New Yorkers suffering from chronic, undifferentiated schizophrenia.

City attorneys told the five justices that the city could help Joyce. Ms. Brown replied that she did not want help, did not need help, and was entitled to live as she pleased. Having won 11 previous challenges to its commitment programs, the city hoped to win this one too.

While awaiting the decision, Ms. Brown told reporters that she was ready to return to work. "Tomorrow I could sit at a typewriter and take shorthand," she said. "I am not insane. I am homeless." Ms. Brown also said she knew, before the test, that she was not sick from lupus or in poor health, claiming "You have to be good physical shape to survive on the street."

ETHICAL ISSUES

Standards of Commitment

The five appellate justices had to decide if Ms. Brown could be committed under the *O'Connor* standards, and second, whether such standards were morally deficient. Because the legal issue was clear-cut (favoring Ms. Brown), ethical issues drove legal moves in this case.

In its argument to this court, the city used the moral argument that the traditional legal standard allowed too much risk of harm. Personal liberty had been valued too highly and such an orientation ultimately harmed the mentally ill.

The city's argument hung on two points. First, it argued that the mentally ill would "eventually" come to harm if simply left alone. If Joyce Brown stayed on her spot, hurling insults at tough men and sleeping unguarded, she would eventually get attacked.

Not everyone thought this was a good argument, including Joyce Brown and Judge Lippman. After all, she had already lived a year and a half there and seemed to have come to no harm.

The city's other argument bypassed the first and appealed directed to humanitarian motives. The state had the ancient right of *parens patria* ("parent of the country"), which originated from English common law where the king had a royal prerogative to act as guardians for incompetents. In modern law, state attorneys general exercise the same right in bringing anti-trust suits on behalf of residents.

Exercising this ancient right of guardian, the city argued that people like Joyce Brown were deteriorating. It was degrading and unmerciful to let them continue to live without help. To say society cannot help them—because otherwise it would violate their rights—was to value personal liberty more than sanity, more than health, more than life itself. The city noted that while these appeals were occurring, three homeless men had been found frozen to death in Central Park.

Charles Krauthammer, a well-known liberal essayist who writes often for *Time* and *New Republic*, supported the city.[18] He argued that Joyce should be committed, not for her dangerousness, but for *helplessness*. For every insane person committed who protested, he emphasized, hundreds did not protest and appeared to like warm beds and regular meals.

The Limits of Altruism to Strangers

A persistent ethical dilemma of civilized life concerns how much any person should do for strangers who appear to be in need. Few people are completely indifferent to such face-to-face meetings; few people do not debate what they should do. Krauthammer argued that the ultimate solution for people such as

Joyce was more facilities and staff. To implement this solution, Krauthammer urged higher taxes. In justification, he noted a dilemma of modern life: "To expect saintliness of the ordinary citizen is bad social policy," but "society must not leave the ordinary citizen with no alternative between ignoring the homeless and playing Mother Teresa. A civilized society ought to offer its people some communal act that lies somewhere in between, such as contributing to the public treasury to build an asylum system to care for these people."

Civil libertarians charge Krauthammer with missing the two big problems. First, what if no real treatment exists? As Szasz says, for whom is incarceration then a good? Second, if a person is either legally free or not, which way is it going to be? Who bears the onus of proof—patient or psychiatrist? Who determines who is "suffering" enough, despite their protests to the contrary, to be locked inside psychiatric wards? How broad should commitment laws sweep? Yes, Ms. Brown could be forcibly treated by broadening commitment criteria, but how many abuses would thereby be allowed? How many people like Joyce enter mental hospitals not by well-meaning but by ill-meaning relatives? Isn't this what Barbara Streisand portrayed in *Nuts*? How many psychiatrists use medication, "time out rooms," restraints, and continued commitment, not as treatment, but as punishment for patients who thwart their wills?

Responding to the kind of claim Krauthammer and the city made, three authors argued in a legal journal that:

> Most of us profess to believe that there is an individual moral duty to
> take care of a senile parent, a paranoid wife, or a disturbed child. Most
> of us also resent the bother such care creates. By allowing society to
> perform this duty, masked in medical terminology, but frequently
> amounting in fact to what one court has described as "warehousing,"
> we can avoid facing painful issues.[19]

Autonomy, Paternalism, and Diminished Competency

Many philosophers, physicians, and legal scholars have discussed the conditions under which paternalism might be justified. "Paternalism" in medicine is to treat adult patients as incompetent children who do not know their best interests. One test of justified paternalism is that the condition was temporary and that the person herself later agreed with it. A suicidal patient may later be glad he's not dead. In cases like Joyce Brown's, it would have been impressive if city psychiatrists had brought forth any patient who was previously forced to undergo psychiatric treatment and who was now gratefully sane.

The American legal system tends to treat mental patients as if they were either totally autonomous, and hence deserving to be free, or totally dysfunctional, and hence deserving of mandatory treatment. Many authors argue that this is a false dichotomy which harms the patient, especially in medical settings. Competency is not a black-or-white issue but one of degrees.

Psychiatrist Virginia Abernethy argues that "disorientation, mental illness, irrationality, or commitment to a mental institution are not conclusive proof of incompetence."[20] She discusses Ms. A, a highly intelligent, very independent woman who lived alone in a large house, with six cats, in a garbage-strewn room heated by a wood fire. After a fire in her house, Ms. A was hospitalized, found competent, and released. When winter came, a concerned social worker investigated, and he found her feet black, ulcerated, and bleeding. When he tried to get her to go with him to a hospital, she ran him off with a shotgun. Police later came and forcibly hospitalized her, where surgeons wanted to amputate her feet for gangrene. Ms. A refused, and psychiatrists commenced evaluations.

A few years previously, her feet had also blackened and she had recovered. Psychiatrists interpreted her hope for another recovery as denial of her prognosis. Surgeon tried to get her to say she wanted to live, so they could operate. She refused, avoiding their questions. Ms. A tried to avoid the Hobson's choice of either letting surgeons amputate or appearing to be in psychotic denial, but she was ultimately not to win. "Her rejection of the two-choice model became the grounds finally, for concluding that Ms. A was not competent to refuse amputation."

Psychiatrist Abernethy analyzed the psychodynamics of this process. First, a false aura of medical emergency "pervaded the psychiatric consultations and judicial process." Second, "Ms. A herself was quick to anger and regarded most interactions with medical personnel as adversarial." Third, Ms. A's anger created anger in those evaluating her competence: "Professionals who think of themselves as altruistic, or at least benevolently motivated, may be particularly sensitive to hostility because they feel deserving of gratitude." Abernethy says her colleagues are outcome-oriented and cannot tolerate watching a patient self-destruct in the name of autonomy, even if the self-destruction is from an underlying disease which they ultimately cannot stop.

Like Ms. A, Joyce Brown nurtured hope that she was not schizophrenic. Both women regarded psychiatrists as enemies who wanted to treat them against their wills. Abernethy notes that "hope (disbelieving the physicians' pessimistic prognosis) is not a criterion of psychotic denial." Both women were also admitted to be generally competent, but were charged with a "focal incompetence," i.e., a specific incompetence to make decisions about their own psychiatric treatment. "The criterion of a focal delusion is dangerously liable to error because a patient can easily be seen as delusional in an emotionally charged interchange, when in other circumstances he addresses the same issue appropriately."

Abernethy emphasizes that the logic of commitment for incompetence is a two-edged sword. If the incompetent cannot consent to refuse treatment, how can they be competent to consent to treatment? In the majority of cases, consent of incompetents is allowed for admission and rarely challenged. Abernethy concludes, "Competence is presumed and does not have to be proved. Incompetence has to be proved (by those who wish to commit.)"

What's the Real Issue Here?

City officials claimed that Joyce Brown's homelessness was a side issue, but her ACLU lawyers disagreed: "The Joyce Brown story has captured the issue of the homeless that a lot of people have been trying to deal with for years."[21] The real problem, they implied, was how to get homeless people off the streets, not how to best treat the mentally ill. They suggested reopening the public baths America had during the Depression and using condemned housing as temporary shelters. Sounding like Szasz, they said that similar problems didn't come up about schizophrenics who stayed out of good neighborhoods. Incarcerating the homeless "for their own good" was just a cheap solution and a paradigm of psychiatric sin. Building homes for street people was much more expensive.

On a talk show about this issue, one respondent said he had been working 15 months in Manhattan as a home health aide. He made $4.50 an hour and brought home $130 a week. Just to rent a room—with no stove, no sink, and no refrigerator, not in Manhattan, but along a nosy, overhead "subway" line somewhere—would cost him two weeks' pay in security ($250) and one week's take-home pay ($130) in rent each month. He bemoaned the fact that he couldn't save the security or the (paid-in-advance) rent on what he took home (subway fares alone were $1 each way). Worse, he worked for New York City, which required him to live within its five boroughs, where he could not find affordable housing.

It's important here to separate different ethical issues. The danger of Joyce Brown's kind of homelessness (a single women sleeping on exposed sidewalks at nights) differs from the danger of budding schizophrenia. The danger the city often emphasized came from being homeless and living on Manhattan streets, not from being mentally ill itself. The city's argument seemed to be: Manhattan streets are dangerous to sleep on. No one but the insane would sleep there. Therefore, those who do so are insane. Therefore, we should commit—whom? The homeless? Or just the insane homeless? But what does being homeless have to do with committing the insane? Shouldn't an insane woman in a middle-class suburb be committed against her will by the same standards as a homeless woman? Aren't legal rights about "equal justice for all?" The city's argument both cut too broadly (in including all the noninsane homeless) and missed the mark, in begging the question of whether Ms. Brown was in danger because she was mentally ill. Only dangers to self from mental illness satisfied legal criteria of commitment.

On one talk show, a member of the audience said to Joyce, "but a woman of your obvious intelligence, why would she be happy to spend the rest of her life on the street?" Joyce replied:

> I didn't say I was going to spend the rest of my life on the street. I'm not a career homeless person, I have skills, I'm very intelligent, I am employable, but at that particular time that was my choice. I had a

limited choice and that's what I choose to do. And I'm a 40-year-old woman, I didn't commit a crime while I was on the street.[22]

Potential for Abuse

Shortly after Joyce Brown was picked up, she was defended in the *The New York Times* by her ACLU lawyer Robert Levy and the New York psychiatrist Robert Gould.[23] They emphasized possible abuses of involuntary round-ups, handcuffing, forcible injections of medication (as happened to Joyce), and confinement in locked wards. Moreover, they stressed, Ms. Brown had been examined at least five times previously and had been found not to require involuntary hospitalization. Indeed, nearly half of the 215 people brought to emergency rooms by Project HELP were found not to require involuntary hospitalization.

In 1972, the U.S. Supreme Court threw out a vagrancy law in Jacksonville, Fla., under which vagrants had been jailed without hearings or due process. No such law existed in New York. Nevertheless, after hearing about the Brown case, one Queens Democrat said homeless people refusing to go to shelters should be "accommodated overnight in a cell" for their own protection.[24] To some people, these remarks illustrated the dangers of the mayor's program.

Gould and Levy emphasized that to allow "preventive detention based solely on nebulous predictions of future self-destructive behavior" would invite abuse. They raised the spectre of "totalitarian regimes" which would use psychiatry for political control. When confronted with such accusations, Mayor Koch replied, "This is not political psychiatry! This is not Russia! We're trying to help this woman!"

Compassionate Treatment, Not Punishment

A. M. Rosenthal, former editor of *The New York Times* turned columnist, saw Joyce Brown "almost every day" from his Second Avenue apartment, and claimed Mayor Koch was attempting to get therapy for Joyce, not rounding up a political dissident.[25] The city wanted to be compassionate and got its hands slapped for trying. For Rosenthal, the Brown case symbolized a case of modern ethics where the law seemed helpless. Her commitment was not arbitrary, because psychiatrists had evaluated her "in the street." An arbitrary program would use only secondhand reports or biased reports of neighbors. Joyce got a hearing and legal counsel at Bellevue. That the case received publicity showed that the legal safeguards worked. The mayor's program, Rosenthal concluded, "is an attempt to help, not a program of incarceration."

The director of the psychiatric unit at Bellevue agreed. David Nardacci, a 32-year-old psychiatrist, said he had chosen to be a physician, "not a lawyer." As such, he was more concerned with helping people such as Joyce Brown than tiptoeing around legal pitfalls.

Embarrassing the Rich

The ACLU retorted that Rosenthal ignored three facts: Ms. Brown did not want to leave, she was never proved dangerous, and she embarrassed the rich by her presence. New York City had thousands of people like Joyce Brown (America has hundreds of thousands). Why was there no similar outcry about the others? Why no letters to *The New York Times* about those in the Bronx?

A citizen visiting from a Communist country was shocked when he saw the homeless all over Manhattan and reflected that the opportunity to pursue happiness was no good without the means to pursue it. "When I walk up Park Avenue and I see people...living in the streets, I say to myself, 'This is not a fair society. That should not be in a society so incredibly rich as the United States.' In this poor country, "no one lives in the streets. No one."

ACLU's executive director Norman Siegel said, "In sweeping up the homeless, the mayor is attempting to place these people out of sight and out of mind and hide the crisis from the public consciousness." Once Joyce was gone, how many of her former Upper East Side "neighbors" would inquire about her condition? Siegel claimed that Project HELP targeted people for pickup who lived in areas seen by tourists and inhabited by the rich. New York City's Mental Health commissioner confirmed that patients had been picked up in such areas, not because of tourism or selectivity, but because the homeless went to rich areas for safety and successful begging.

Limitations of Psychiatry

In his ruling, Judge Lippman mentioned that he could place little faith in psychiatry because the four city psychiatrists and the three ACLU psychiatrists who had testified were equally qualified, yet had dramatically disagreed. From such testimony, the judge concluded, "it is evident that psychiatry is not a science amenable to the exactness of mathematics or the predictability of physical laws."

A classic generalization is that about one-third of schizophrenics can function well on medication as outpatients, another third do well on medication within institutions, and, unfortunately, little can be done for the last third, who deteriorate and must be institutionalized. Some psychiatrists now say that only 10 to 20 percent of schizophrenics fall into the worst category. More pessimistic psychiatrists think that true cases of schizophrenia are never cured; at best their symptoms are abated and the progression of schizophrenia is halted.

Other psychiatrists would bridle at this portrayal. They point out schizophrenics who were dysfunctional, but who gained years of ability (or at least minimal function) after being made to take medication. After being stabilized, such patients achieved freedom from delusions. If they regularly took their medication (an important condition), they could even return to life outside an institution. Psychiatrist Paul Chodoff defends limited involuntary commitment:

> But is freedom defined only by absence of external constraints? Internal physiological or psychological processes can contribute to a throttling of

the spirit that is as painful as any applied from the outside. The "wild" manic individual without his lithium, the panicky hallucinator with his injection of fluphenazine hydrochloride and the understanding support of a concerned staff, the sodden alcoholic—are they free? Sometimes, as Woody Guthrie said, "Freedom means no place to go."[26]

Indeed, people suffering from paranoid schizophrenia can undergo amazing changes. One such schizophrenic believed that the grounds crew mowing lawns were communicating with themselves in secret motor language about his faults. After weeks of medication, he began to doubt his former bizarre beliefs. After more weeks on medication, he really wasn't sure. Still later, he admitted his belief was probably false. Finally, after more medication, he concluded one day, "How did I ever think that?" Chemicals can change a person's thoughts over time, even his deepest thoughts about himself. Since some schizophrenia might be either caused by, or manifests in, chemical disturbances of the brain, this result is not surprising.

U.S. News and World Report contributing editor Harold Evans agreed, saying Joyce had lost "the rational freedom of choice offered by medicine that can alleviate mental anguish and paranoia."[27] Thus part of the debate about Joyce's case concerned differing opinions about psychiatry's ability to help schizophrenics.

Harm and Benefit to Joyce Brown

Charles Krauthammer said that ethical questions boiled down to not whether people like Joyce Brown were likely to harm themselves, but whether they were suffering. Columnist Ellen Goodman agreed—Joyce should be taken off the streets before she died on the streets "with her rights on."[28] These writers thought that it should be enough to convince a judge that the mentally ill were in distress and that medication would help. But was it really so straightforward? To say that commitment is justified to end suffering assumes first, that a person is really suffering, and second, that psychiatric commitment could ease the suffering. But could involuntary psychiatry, involuntary medication, and involuntary therapy help Joyce? In a locked, in-patient unit? In a large institution such as New York City's Creedmore?

In a locked unit, Ms. Brown might harm herself while being forced to take antipsychotic medications and tranquilizers. The long-term "side effects" of such medications can be as bad as the disease. Administration over years of antipsychotic drugs such as neuroleptics creates *tardive dyskinesia* in 10 to 25 percent of patients. This condition is impairment of power of voluntary movement, is untreatable, and continues in two-thirds of patients even when medication stops.

Francine Cournos, Ms. Brown's court-appointed psychiatrist, was the most likely psychiatrist to be impartial. She found that Ms. Brown suffered from "serious mental illness" and would benefit from medication, but would suffer more from forced treatment. Commitment might destroy her fierce independence (as happened to McMurphy in *One Flew Over the Cuckoo's Nest*). What Joyce feared most was commitment to an in-patient unit like the one at East Orange Hospital.

Psychiatrists tend to think that schizophrenics "benefit" from losing their inner voices and living a medicated life. But "benefit" and "harm" are terms which, above the level of basic needs, are defined by a person's life-plan and self-conception. To say Ms. Brown must be treated to accept someone else's idea of a "benefit" is to accept a shaky kind of paternalism. As Livermore, Malmquist, and Meehl noted:

> When faced with an obviously aberrant person, we know, or we think we know, that he would be "happier" if he were as we are. We believe that no one would want to be a misfit in society. From the very best of motives, then, we wish to fix him. It is difficult to deal with this feeling since it rests on the unverifiable assumption that the aberrant person, if he saw himself as we see him, would choose to be different than he is. But since he cannot be as we, and we cannot be as he, there is simply no way to judge the predicate for the assertion.[29]

Moreover, if there is "internal pain" in patients, as psychiatrists imply, why don't patients want to get rid of it? Is it permissible for psychiatrists to explain that patients don't want to get rid of pain "because they're crazy"?

More generally, wouldn't exactly the same kind of paternalism justify removing cigarettes and alcoholic drinks from psychiatrists? Is it superstitious or enlightened to single out nondangerous mental illnesses for paternalistic intervention?

Harm to Others

A few years before this case, Juan Gonzalez, a homeless person suffering from symptoms like Joyce's, went berserk with a sword on the Staten Island Ferry and killed two people. As a result, people clamored for greater incarceration of the mentally ill who were "potentially dangerous." This argument is often used to justify temporarily holding someone thought to be dangerous, for a "cool down" observational period.

Gonzalez had, in fact, been picked up for just such an observational period. Although judged paranoid schizophrenic, he was judged not imminently dangerous to others and discharged. One of the few statements about which most psychiatrists, lawyers, and judges agree is that predicting dangerousness is very, very difficult.

UPDATE

Legal Results

Joyce Brown lost on appeal. The appeals court ruled 3 to 2 that Justice Lippman had incorrectly ruled that the city had not provided evidence for commitment and had placed too much emphasis on Joyce Brown's testimony rather than that of psychiatrists who predicted she would harm herself. Two dissenting justices vigorously disagreed.

The three justices noted that a very high standard of proof was required in this case—the "clear and convincing evidence" standard—not the weaker, "preponderance of evidence" standard. Paradoxically, the majority concluded that the city had met the high standard.

The court, in an unusual move, reviewed detailed testimony in the case, especially that of a social worker who said she personally observed "fecal matter" on the sheets in which "Miss Boggs" wrapped herself. The appellate court also reviewed the testimony of one Dr. Mahon, who claimed Joyce had told him that she often defecated and urinated on herself. The court found "that the evidence presented in this case clearly and convincingly demonstrated Ms. Bogg's past history of assaultive and aggressive behavior."[30] (Why the Appellate Court referred to her as "Miss Boggs" was unclear.)

The majority showed no sympathy for Ms. Brown's lucidity in court. It discounted this as due to "a week of hospital treatment." (Ms. Brown had in fact received no medical treatment.) Mayor Koch reacted, "Up until this moment, the only treatment has been care, loving, a safe environment. Now we will seek to treat her medically."

The two dissenting justices roared that the city's argument could be "narrowed to one claim," which was that "she is dangerous to herself" because "she is likely to provoke others to do injury to her." They found that commitment to prevent such possible harm was "an extreme remedy" and "somewhat offensive." They were dismayed that their colleagues had dismissed Justice Lippman's assessment of Ms. Brown's lucidity in court: "Yet if the court's [Lippman's] judgment of her mental condition is to be completely ignored, then what was the purpose of the hearing in the first place?" Finally, they stressed that in Joyce Brown's six prior hospitalizations, disinterested psychiatrists had unanimously concluded that she was not dangerous to herself.

The city still had to get a court order to medicate Ms. Brown. One month later, on January 19, 1988, a state judge ruled that she could not be given drugs against her will. Bellevue Hospital promptly released her, saying there was no further point in holding her. The ACLU appealed the original commitment decision to New York's highest court, the Court of Appeals, which declined to hear the case because it presented "no novel, constitutional or substantial case for this court to review."

Altogether, Ms. Brown was held 84 days. One city councilman noted that the city spent more than $42,000 for her stay at Bellevue and suggested that in this case "the mayor's ego got in the way of what was right." After her release, Joyce held forth:

> I was incarcerated against my will...[I was] a political prisoner. The
> only thing wrong with me was that I was homeless, not insane. You
> just can't go around picking everyone up and automatically label them

schizophrenic. I'm angry at Mayor Koch, the city and Bellevue. They held me down and injected me.... They took my blood against my will.

I need a place to live; I don't need an institution.

People are treated differently just because of your economic status, [because of] what you look like and where you live....

I was mistreated, mentally abused, and I will never, ever, forget this.[31]

Other Events

When New York City officials planned their pickup program, they envisioned that people such as Joyce Brown would stay for a few weeks in psychiatric hospitals and then be moved into community facilities, where they could live under supervised conditions much as they had done before. When the people were actually evaluated, however, they turned out to be far sicker than had been expected. Far more permanent places were needed in psychiatric hospitals than had been predicted.

Because of years of limited funding to balance the gigantic New York medical budget (worsened by AIDS), such places were unavailable. By 1988, lack of such beds was a crisis in New York. Budgets had been cut years before in releasing patients, staff had been fired, and legislators had spent saved monies on other projects. The gates of deinstitutionalization had opened and saved money, and now no one knew how to get the money and patients back.

Joyce Brown was released to live in a nonprofit hotel for women. She received several job offers and worked temporarily as a secretary in the ACLU office. Interviewed there, she said, "I was supposed to have deteriorated within 3 or 4 days [once out of Bellevue]." A reporter said she then noted with a smile that 3 weeks had passed and, "I'm fine. I'm working."

Indeed, in the first quarter of 1988, Joyce became something of a celebrity. She dined at Windows on the World restaurant atop the World Trade Center and was congratulated there by waiters. She received half-a-dozen movie and book offers. She shopped at Bloomingdale's, Saks Fifth Avenue, and Lord & Taylor. Her shopping sprees were paid for by *The Donahue Show* and *60 Minutes*, both of which aired shows on her case. She seemed to flourish with attention.[32]

On her television appearance on *The Donahue Show*, a hostile immigrant claimed he had found a job, and bought a house "in just 25 years," and wondered why Joyce couldn't, too. He said, "You're an intelligent woman, how come you're homeless? I'm sure you can find a job." Joyce replied, "Right now I'm trying to get a job. Mr. Donahue, do you need any help around here?" (the audience heartily laughed).

Joyce also lectured to students at Cardozo and Harvard law schools under the title: "The Homeless Crisis: A Street View." Reflecting on these developments at the time, she said, "It looks like I have been appointed the homeless spokesperson."

Her sisters resisted giving her the accumulated money from the disability checks, which Joyce had finally decided to accept. They said they would release the money when the ACLU lawyers ceased "manipulating her" for their political purposes.

Nevertheless, not everything ended well. Her roommate at the hotel said Joyce had a lot of anger inside and frequently talked to herself. One day while walking to work, she was heard muttering racial obscenities to herself. Joyce dismissed these things as misinterpretations due to her habit of singing popular songs to herself. In mid-March, she was seen begging on a Times Square street, where she shouted obscenities at passersby. When asked how she was doing, she insisted, "I'm not insane."[33] In May 1988, she was admitted to a hospital for dangerously high blood pressure, medication for which she had always refused. In September, she was charged with possession of a small amount of heroin and two hypodermic needles.[34] As a result, Charles Krauthammer (and others who had sided with Mayor Koch) felt vindicated.[35]

In a poll during June 1989, 59 percent of New Yorkers said they would be willing to pay $100 more per year in taxes to help the homeless.[36] The poll found that, in 1985, only 62 percent saw homeless people in their neighborhoods or on their way to work, but in 1989, the figure had jumped to 82 percent. With the election of mayor coming in November, New Yorkers identified homelessness as the third most crucial issue (behind crime and drugs) on which they wished the next mayor to focus.[37]

FURTHER READING

Virginia Abernethy, "Compassion, Control, and Decisions about Competency," *American Journal of Psychiatry*, 141(1):53–58.

Paul Chodoff, "The Case for Involuntary Hospitalization of the Mentally Ill," *American Journal of Psychiatry*, 133(5) (May 1976).

Saul Feldman, "Out of the Hospitals, Onto the Streets: The Overselling of Benevolence," *Hastings Center Report* 13(3) (June 1983).

Charles Krauthammer, "How to Save the Homeless Mentally Ill," *New Republic* (February 8, 1988), pp. 22–25.

J. Livermore, C. Malmquist, and P. Meehl, "On the Justification for Civil Commitment," *University of Pennsylvania Law Review*, 117 (November 1968).

CHAPTER 14

Preventing Undesirable Teenage Pregnancies

This chapter discusses ethical issues in preventing pregnancies among female teenagers. It focuses on a case made famous by a film from the Joseph P. Kennedy, Jr., Foundation in which a 15-year-old girl named Bertha, from West Virginia, was prevented from having children. This happened after she was labeled retarded. The chapter begins with a history of past abuses in eugenics in attempting to limit the freedom of Americans to procreate.

A SHORT HISTORY OF EUGENICS

Before scientific genetics, popular ideas about genetics influenced domestic politics around the world. In the late 1880s, Charles Darwin's cousin, Francis Galton, created the term "eugenics" (good birth) for his ideas about improving humanity. Galton thought that famous people were the most "fit."[1] The famous liked the theory, for obvious reasons.

Most champions of eugenics were racially biased. The ensuing ideology of *Social Darwinism* claimed that the most fit races had emerged from the struggle for existence in evolution. Blacks were predicted not to survive into the 20th century because they were biologically unfit for competitive survival with the white Aryan race (see the discussion of 20th-century racism in medicine in Chapter 9).

Social Darwinism was never a sophisticated theory and almost immediately contradicted itself. If the Aryan race was destined to emerge triumphant, why worry about the breeding rates of *lower* races? If lower races were destined to die out because they were cursed with defectives, why sterilize them?

Phrenology, a popular notion of the late 19th century, held that the size and shape of the head determined intelligence and character. It is still popular among some novelists who write as if character can be inferred from a person's face or physique. About this notion, George Eliot wrote in *Middlemarch*:

286

"so much subtler is a human mind than the outside tissues, which make a sort of blazonry or clock-face for it."

In the 1880s, cell nuclei were found to contain chromosomes. Around 1900, chromosomes were found to carry genes, and Gregor Mendel's laws were rediscovered. Men such as Karl Pearson and Charles Davenport popularized crude genetics, and magazines advocated both "eugenic marriages" and sterilization of the unfit. Eugenic organizations popped up worldwide, especially in Germany, Japan, South America, Italy, Austria, and Scandinavia. As historian of science Daniel Kevles write, "the center of this trend was the American eugenics movement. Its headquarters was at Cold Spring Harbor on Long Island, N.Y. and its leader was Charles Davenport."[2] Although many people identify modern eugenics with Nazi Germany, it was in heterogeneous America that eugenics was most publicly championed. Politics, popular culture, and scientists declared that America's "breeding stock" was declining through interbreeding of unfit races.

Shocked by the numerous progeny of the Irish, Italians, and Greeks, descendants of Mayflower immigrants saw a Malthusian doom approaching. Catholic ethnic groups bred copiously, and anti-Catholic sentiment grew. The beginning of the 20th century was a time when a few great families, largely English, Swiss-German, and Dutch, controlled great wealth, and saw "contamination" of America's purity in the interbreeding of their children with Jews, Irish, Orientals, blacks, Italians, Turks, and anybody else who did not come from where their ancestors emigrated. These people tended to control the ideas of the time through universities and magazines. William Hearst and Theodore Roosevelt thundered against immigrants from the Orient invading the United States. Henry Ford in the 1920s ran for president partially on the platform of ridding the country of the "Jew bankers," whom he accused of first forcing America into World War I, and later, of causing the Depression.[3]

The upper classes were unanimous that the unfit had no right to have children. Famous New York urologist William Robinson proclaimed:

> It is the acme of stupidity to talk in such cases of individual liberty, of the rights of the individual. Such individuals have no rights. They have no right in the first instance to be born, but having been born, they have no right to propagate their kind.[4]

This kind of thinking brought forth fruit in the Supreme Court in 1927.

The Case of Carrie Buck

The floodgates of sterilization in America opened with the case of Carrie Buck, a supposedly retarded girl who was a daughter of another supposedly retarded woman, Emma Buck. Carrie had a mental age of 9 years according to a crude IQ test, and her mother tested at 8. Both at the time and now, female inmates often become pregnant after visits with guards or relatives. Carrie, a 17-year-old girl was pregnant before her commitment and gave birth to her daughter, Vivian, inside a state institution in Virginia. The institution's director wondered if Carrie could be sterilized, so that Vivian would be her last child.

Virginia officials asked Harry Laughlin, an influential geneticist who worked at Cold Spring Harbor, to decide whether Carrie's retardation was hereditary. Laughlin did not visit the women, but used the report of a social worker who said Carrie had a strange "look" about her. Based upon these items and the low-tested mental ages of Carrie's mother and grandmother, Laughlin declared that Carrie "lived a life of immorality and prostitution," and that the three Buck females belonged "to the shiftless, ignorant, worthless class of antisocial whites of the South."[5]

A court order for sterilization of Carrie was appealed to the U.S. Supreme Court, which upheld the legality of sterilizing Carrie Buck in 1927 by a vote of 8 to 1. Justice Oliver Wendell Holmes wrote the opinion in *Buck vs. Bell*, and deliberately used the strong phrase, "three generations of imbeciles are enough."[6] Holmes championed science as a guide to public policy and emphasized that the public good in sound genetics outweighed the individual rights of the retarded to procreate, concluding that, "the principle that sustains compulsory vaccination is broad enough to cover cutting the Fallopian tubes."

Unfortunately, "sound genetics" was more complicated than Davenport or Holmes understood. At the time, several basic genetic truths were poorly understood, including the fact that genes could be recessive, so that normal people could have defective children. Eugenics, in 1927, mistakenly assumed that each trait was inherited through a single gene, e.g., if a person had 378 traits, he or she had 378 separate genes. Eugenicists also incorrectly assumed that there was a specific, inheritable, trait for retardation. Finally, they were ignorant about mutations and chromosomal breakage, and hence incorrectly believed that if all retardates remained childless, retardation could be eliminated from the gene pool.

Then and today, it is often difficult to determine exactly what is an inherited trait. It is difficult to separate nurture from nature. Psychologists debate whether intelligence scores are due to hereditary or environment. Retardation is now known to be caused by many factors, including nonhereditary causes such as maternal alcoholism and lack of stimulation due to poverty.

An example of such bias occurred when Charles Davenport decided that prostitution was caused by a gene for "innate eroticism."[7] He also believed that poverty and criminality were hereditary. All these biases flourished because of ignorance about exactly what was inherited and what was not. These controversies still thrive today, e.g., in the 1980s, Harvard psychologist Richard Herstein argued that criminality ran in certain families and suggested a genetic link.[8]

Another truth poorly understood in 1927 was that defective people could have normal children. If a defect came from mating two recessive genes, and an affected child didn't mate with another carrier, any resulting child would not have the disease. An example was Vivian Buck, the only daughter of Carrie Buck, who before dying of an intestinal disorder at 8, was considered bright by her teachers and was doing well in school.

The American Eugenics Movement's Apex: 1900–1935

From roughly 1900 to 1935, the eugenics movement influenced American legislation. Many geneticists supported the movement in its earliest years, but as the century approached the Depression, most geneticists dropped out, abandoning the movement because of its racism, its zealous "religious" nature (emphasizing the perfectibility of man), and its assumptions contrary to emerging facts in genetics. By 1935, geneticist Hermann J. Muller lamented that eugenics was "hopelessly perverted" into a cult for "advocates for race and class prejudice, defenders of vested interests of church and state, Fascists, Hitlerites, and reactionaries generally."[9]

In Germany between 1934 and 1937, 225,000 people—mainly "mental defectives"—were sterilized against their will. The Germans were more systematic, secretive, and biased by racism in their selection than Americans, but similar sterilizations occurred in both countries.[10] Indiana, in 1907, first required mandatory sterilization of the retarded and criminally insane, followed soon by 30 other states. A board of experts ultimately decided who would be sterilized. In the 1930s, mandatory sterilizations peaked. People believe these sterilizations occurred mostly in the deep south or Appalachia, but in fact, California led other states, performing nearly a third of the nation's total, and Indiana was third (Virginia was second).[11] Altogether, over 36,000 Americans were involuntarily sterilized by 1941. People were often sterilized for the vague condition of "feeblemindedness" or because of being born into big families on welfare.

Leading geneticist J. B. S. Haldane said, at the time, that "many of the deeds done in America in the name of eugenics are about as much justified by science as were the proceedings of the Inquisition by the Gospels."[12] Eugenic populists hoped to perfect humanity through selective breeding, but population genetics showed that a regression to the mean would occur, prompting Haldane to remark, "An ounce of algebra is worth a ton of verbal argument."[13] Moreover, the number of generations needed to eliminate a defect was much greater than anyone had expected. Not understanding the difference between having a trait and merely carrying a nonexpressed gene, eugenicists failed to understand that reducing the frequency of a defect from 1 in 100 to 1 in 1000 might take 22 generations. To reduce it to 1 in 1,000,000 might take hundreds of generations. Nor did they understand that spontaneous mutations occurred.

Besides mandatory sterilizations, the most important legacy of the American eugenics movement was the Immigration Restriction Act of 1924. This act, hailed by champions of American eugenics as its greatest triumph, assumed that Orientals, Poles, Africans, Italians, Greeks, Irish, and eastern and southern Europeans were the inferior peoples, whereas the superior stock was assumed to be English, Dutch, Scotch, Scandinavian, German, and possibly, French (if not Catholic). The act was eagerly signed by President Calvin Coolidge, who as vice president had declared, "America must be kept American. Biological laws show . . . that Nordics deteriorate when mixed with other races."[14] In lobbying for the act, the phrase "American's modern melting pot" was first used, but in contrast to its later honorific usage, at the time it was pejorative. The subsequent act created quotas according to country of origin, and it became very hard to immigrate to America from an "inferior" country. The Statue of Liberty is often presented as an historical symbol of freedom, but thousands of the world's "teeming masses" arrived to see it after 1924, only to be turned away and sent back home.

Other legacies of American eugenics were the linked, false assumptions that race determined behavior and that race was a biological kind or a subspecies. Irish, Italian, Poles, black, Jew, and Arab were seen, not as political, religious, or ethnic generalizations, but as biological types. Julian Huxley and A.C. Haddon argued in 1935, in attacking Nazi eugenics promoting Aryan racial superiority, that race was not a uniform, biological type but a mixture of many peoples. They wrote that "the word *race* should be banished, and the descriptive and noncommittal term *ethnic groups* should be substituted."[15] Similar attacks occurred on the notions that Poles, Irish, and blacks were naturally promiscuous (i.e., promiscuity was a genetically determined trait) or that members of such groups "naturally" liked certain foods or whiskeys. What was crude was the belief, despite the lack of any evidence, that genes influenced such highly specific behaviors, as well as the hasty generalization that all people from a certain area (Ireland, Africa) had the same genes.

A measure of the degree of bad science inherent in this eugenics was that World War I was held by eugenicists to be eugenic, by others to be dysgenic. Dysgenicists argued that the best male stock went off and died. Their opponents pointed out that the remaining men had the choice of the best women. Dysgenicists rebutted by arguing that the available women would marry inferior men to avoid spinsterdom. As might be imagined, few champions of eugenics were women. Talk of dysgenics frequently reflected male fantasies and biases. Champions of eugenics uniformly saw themselves as part of the "most fit" breeding stock.

The Depression discouraged many advocates of eugenics. When the "most fit" lost their jobs and fortunes, they failed to believe they had failed the test of survival. Traditional eugenicists could either accept inferiority or give up their beliefs. Most gave up. In the meantime, genetics became more scientific and discredited many of the simplistic ideas of eugenics.

In the 1960s in Montgomery, Ala., two black teenage girls were sterilized after they had signed a consent form for sterilization. Their Fallopian tubes were then cut. They later claimed, along with their mother, that they hadn't understood what they had signed. When they sued, they claimed that physicians had coerced them and had done so because they were black girls on welfare. The case caused national controversy when other women on welfare reported similar pressures.

BERTHA'S CASE

The subject of this case is Bertha, who grew up in in the 1960s and 1970s in a very poor family in the rural section of Virginia in the Appalachian mountains. Bertha's mother bore 10 children. Bertha's father worked in a gas station and in 1969 earned $70 a week. Bertha was the oldest female child. Her impoverished mother appeared overwhelmed with 10 children, and consequently, Bertha often tended to the younger 8 children. (Bertha had one older brother.) From this experience, Bertha formed a desire to have her own children.

Bertha was the subject of the film *Bertha,* financed by the Joseph P. Kennedy, Jr., Foundation.[16] (Quotations from Bertha or film commentators are from this movie.) The film was originally commissioned as a movie about ethical issues in sterilizing the retarded. Bertha was one case among several which were given to producer Ann Michaels to study. The actual movie was more ambiguous than originally intended because it didn't seem that Bertha was retarded. Thus, the movie was also about stopping unmarried teenage pregnancy. However, once the label of "retarded" was put on Bertha, it stuck as her chart was handed from one professional to the next. The film illustrates the problems of such labeling.

Bertha's family lived atop a steep hill outside town and, during the harsh winter in the mountains, the trail down to school was difficult. Bertha and her siblings were acutely self-conscious about being poor around children whose families were not on welfare. She said:

> We got some neighbors. They don't like us because we were poor people. You know. We wasn't rich and sophisticated like them, so they didn't like us. There wasn't much I could do about it. Just stay and live with it. I mean, like to me, I was just as good as they were. I just didn't have what they had. They called us "coodies," "fleas," you know—I guess 'cause the way we looked. We didn't have nice clothes like they did. They would start—as soon as we got on the bus—teasing us. I was always glad when school was over and I could go home and not have to listen to it.

As a result, Bertha and her siblings became truants. Bertha stumbled over reading and was illiterate. Because of this, she was held back year after year, and her classmates made fun of her large size. In the euphemisms of education, Bertha was an "underachiever" who was rejected by her "peer group" and who received "social promotion," starting in the third grade and continuing at least until the seventh grade. But on many days, Bertha said her teachers told her, "There's nothing we can do for you. Go out and play." So she did.

Bertha's problems increased as she entered her midteenage years. As she grew older, she stayed away from school more. She and other truants would often spend the day at an abandoned ice-house. Eventually, Bertha and her sister were placed in foster homes so that they would attend school. Bertha wanted to stay at her parents' house and didn't like staying at the foster home.

At age 15, Bertha was a cute, social, friendly, white woman. At one of her foster homes, an attempt may have been made by a foster father to molest her. Allegeny County Director of Social Services Barbara Hammond heard about the attempt and temporarily placed Bertha in a state institution before another home could be found. During this time, Hammond heard about a program for birth control at the Kennedy Institute in Baltimore and brought Bertha there. Bertha was intent on having children and Hammond feared that if Bertha conceived, the child would be taken away from her. If this had been done, Hammond said, it would have been "the worst thing in the world for her." Bertha reluctantly agreed to go to Baltimore to avoid living in the foster home.

After taking tests at Baltimore, Bertha was diagnosed at Johns Hopkins as mildly retarded with an IQ of 68. The test result and label of "retarded" were controversial, because Bertha appeared unmotivated in taking the tests and because the test scores may have been influenced by her inability to read. In the film, made 4 years later when Bertha was 19, Bertha has excellent social skills and seems quite able to take care of herself. The producer and film crew were very impressed with Bertha's intelligence.

At Johns Hopkins, an intrauterine device (IUD) was inserted in Bertha against her will. The official justification was to "protect her," but upon hearing this justification, Bertha asked, "What are you protecting me *from?*" She was told, "You might otherwise get pregnant" and Bertha replied, "So?"[17] Bertha did not believe that her own good consisted in being "protected" from conception.

An IUD was inserted, instead of sterilizing Bertha, to temporarily limit her reproductive ability. Insertion of an IUD was reversible by retraction, but cutting her Fallopian tubes was not. Pediatrician Colin Gordon said that the professionals in the adolescent unit at Hopkins thought they were "buying time" for Bertha.

The IUD was inserted in Bertha because it was thought likely that she would have retarded kids, or kids on welfare, or kids without a father. As the female psychiatrist says in the film, "We thought this was an opportunity to do some preventive work." Pediatrician Colin Gordon concurred, "I thought the suggestion of an intrauterine device was a reasonable one."

Bertha intensely disagreed with the decision. In the film, she argues with (the late) William Hershey, the social worker who arranged for her IUD. She objects to the insertion of the device against her will and she objects to the "retarded" label.

After the IUD was inserted, Bertha returned to her small town in West Virginia. The Kennedy Foundation finished the movie and Bertha returned once to Baltimore to see the final version. She then returned to West Virginia, still angered at having an IUD inside her. According to Eunice Kennedy Shriver, who introduces the film, the IUD "was later removed at her [Bertha's] own request."

ETHICAL ISSUES

The ethical issues of this case are two quite different kinds: those involving labeling someone as "retarded" and those involving rights of people to have children. We will first focus on issues regarding retardation and then turn to the more general issues about rights to procreate.

Justified Paternalism to the Retarded

Philosopher Robert Neville argues that it can be to the good of a mildly retarded person, such as Bertha, to be sterilized. If she can enjoy sexual activity, but cannot be allowed to participate in such activity without sterilization, or cannot handle the responsibilities of parenting, then sterilization is good for her. However, Neville adds an important qualification: "if they prefer nonsterilization, then society should respect that choice, whatever other compensatory restrictions it requires (such as no sexual activity)."[18] Unfortunately, Neville does not explain how to "respect that choice" and implement the "compensatory restriction" of no sexual activity.

Neville also raises the question of "who decides" what is best for the mildly retarded person. He answers this question: "I suggest that this decision is a broad social one, which should be as informed as possible by experts in all relevant fields, including mental retardation and ethics." Ironically, he does not mention the decision of the mildly retarded person herself. Because Bertha sees her own good as being a mother, the questions in this case are whether motherhood is really in Bertha's good, and if so, whether it is morally permissible to bring a child into the world under less-than-ideal conditions.

Test Worship

The mildly retarded vary greatly in capacities, and many generalizations about them are erroneous. Each person must be evaluated on his or her own merits. Perhaps 5.25 million American fall under the "mildly retarded" label with Stanford-Binet IQ ranging from 52 to 68. Especially in this group, abilities greatly vary, and in it, retardation is sometimes due to poverty.

Perhaps the most important issue of all is that Bertha received a 68 score on the Stanford-Binet IQ test—one point under the cutoff for the normal range at 69 and the highest possible score for a mildly retarded person. Nevertheless, the mental health professionals at Johns Hopkins accepted the accuracy of the test. Psychologist Shirley Mark says that although Bertha's social skills belie her score, her other abilities were lacking, such as her ability to interpret the meaning of stories (where she scored as an 8-year-old). Such professionals appreciated the significance of the difference between the highest score in the retarded range and the lowest score in the normal range, but nevertheless decided Bertha was retarded.

In the film, Bertha asks social worker Bill Hershey, "Just because I can't read—does that make me retarded?" He replies, "Whether you were or were not retarded when you took the tests that we used—the Stanford-Binet and other psychological tests—you *acted* like you were." Psychologist Shirley Mark concurred: "This [IQ score] is primarily due to the way her nervous system, her brain, has developed."

In this case, great meaning rested on a score of 68 rather than one of 69. One justification of inserting the IUD into Bertha rested on the assumption that Bertha was retarded. Why? Because few people attempt to coerce sterilization on similar young women with low but normal IQs.

All in all, it is difficult to believe that lack of stimulation in the home, plus Bertha's own lack of motivation, didn't contribute to Bertha's score of 68 and not 69. If so, then at a later day, and after greater education and with more motivation, Bertha could have tested in the normal range. If so, one major justification for insertion of the IUD vanishes, and the real reason seems have been because Bertha was likely to become an unwed mother on welfare.

Is Mental Retardation a "Morally Relevant" Trait?

At one point, Bertha asks social worker William Hershey, "How would you like it if they fixed it so *your* daughter couldn't have kids?" He avoids the question by replying, "They couldn't because they'd have to have my consent to do so." Bertha replies, "Right! And you didn't have *my* parents' consent." Bertha continues by asking, "What right did you have to fix me so I couldn't have kids?" To which the social worker replies, "I could sit here and say we didn't have the right." This raises the question of whether, if she was indeed retarded, should Bertha be treated just like any other girl or should she be treated in a special way?

Philosopher Barry Hoffmaster discusses a dilemma of advocates for the mildly retarded.[19] On one hand, such advocates want, for the mildly retarded, rights as for normal people. For example, Article 1 of the Declaration of General and Special Rights of the Mentally Retarded says, "The mentally retarded person has the same basic rights as other citizens of the same country and same age." Yet as Hoffmaster observes, Article 6 in the same declaration says, "The mentally retarded person has a right of protection from exploitation, abuses, and degrading treatment." This last, claimed, right implies that the retarded are not treated as if they have the same rights as others and need special rights.

Rosalind Pollack Pechchesky, a professor of political theory, argues about women such as Bertha that: "Involuntary sterilization is an invasion of a woman's bodily integrity and identity for ends that usually accommodate the needs of others in disregard of her own needs, and that preempt her bodily self-determination."[20] But the key question is: is Bertha just like other women or does her borderline retardation mean she needs help being a mother? If so, does Bertha need what Hoffmaster calls "special rights"?

Psychiatrist George Tarjan (in the film) says that whatever is done to Bertha should be the same as is done to similar nonretarded girls. For Tarjan, equal cases should be treated equally, and being on the edge of retardation doesn't qualify as a morally relevant difference for different treatment. But Hoffmaster retorts: how can such borderline retardation not count in a decision about social policy, if Bertha requires special help?

Isolating the Undesirable Trait

Suppose everyone agrees that a certain trait is undesirable. Even so, we do not know that other, valuable, traits are not linked to it. For example, the gene for hemoglobin S is found in carriers of sickle cell anemia, which appears now to be an undesirable trait. But the same gene in years past protected its black possessors from dying of malaria. Similarly, the dominant eye cancer of retinoblastoma may be closely associated with intelligence.

What is a desirable trait is partly a function of a culture, a particular time in history, and a point of view. Massive physical strength is more desirable in frontier than in computer societies. Female fecundity may be advantageous in siring a pedigreed line, but disastrous for the mother herself. Having hemophilia may not be so bad if one is born royal.

Eugenics and Justice

The implementation of any just eugenic policy may be difficult. In the past, some programs focused on *negative* eugenics (eliminating undesirable traits from the gene pool) whereas others focused on *positive* eugenics (improving the gene pool). Regardless of which approach is used, the genetically disadvantaged would seem to be the ones who will be discouraged from procreating. Philosopher John Rawls argued that justice maximizes the welfare of the least well-off group, to which the genetically disadvantaged would seem to belong.[21] Libertarians emphasize the primacy of liberty above all other values in politics, and a eugenics policy cannot be implemented and still give women the liberty to conceive with whom they please and to have as many children as they want.

An objection to a policy of sterilizing those with "high genetic risk" is that society does not sterilize others at above average risk for being poor parents or who have above average risks of having defective children. Why not sterilize young women or young men who are alcoholics, manic-depressives, psychotics, or drug addicts? As genetics identifies markers for hereditary disease, more women will be eligible for similar eugenic sterilization. Why single out a woman merely one point away from the normal range of IQ, and why single out women from welfare families? Why single out just one category?

Unmarried Teenage Pregnancy

According to the Alan Guttmacher Institute, a nonprofit organization which tracks population trends, over a million teenage American girls become pregnant each year, a figure that remained constant between 1984 and 1988.[22] In other words, 1 in 10 teenage girls in America becomes pregnant each year. Of these, about half give birth. About half of those who give birth are under 18.

Bertha's Good

Bertha appears not to have been retarded. She was nevertheless prevented from having children. This raises the second general issue of whether it is right to prevent any teenage girl from having children. One subquestion here is whether such a pregnancy would be in such a teenager's self-interest.

Social worker Barbara Hammond emphasized that Bertha "needed desperately somebody to love and something to call her own." She emphasizes that if Bertha had given birth to a child and if it were then taken away from her, "it would have been very bad for her." So the question of Bertha's good also involves asking what would harm Bertha. Hammond says, "she wouldn't have been allowed to keep her child" if she became pregnant, and if that was true, preventing pregnancy in Bertha would be right. However, the premise could be challenged that she shouldn't keep her child.

On the other hand, even if Bertha's good requires a "child of her own," it does not follow that allowing creation of this child is morally right or good social policy. Moral questions arise when another person is affected, and Bertha's child would certainly be such a person.

Encouraging Welfare Mothers

Bertha's family was on welfare (Aid to Families with Dependent Children [AFDC], Food Stamps, and Medicaid). Had Bertha had children, she would likely have been an AFDC mother. Bertha herself later went on welfare. Some Americans resent paying taxes to support generation after generation of AFDC families. Because of this, women from such families are often encouraged to undergo sterilization, especially after several teenage pregnancies. This was undoubtedly the major reason why Bertha got an IUD. Psychiatrist Sharon Howell said, "If this pattern was continued, her children would be in the same situation as she was."

According to the Census Bureau, in 1960, there were 3.1 million AFDC recipients and, in 1980, there were 11 million, which is over 300 percent growth. In 1985, 322,821 white teenagers gave birth, as did about 60,000 Hispanic teenagers. Of this total, 50 percent were unmarried. Of the 140,000 black teenagers who gave birth, 126,000 were unmarried, 14,000 were married.[23] Moreover, and for all pregnant mothers under age 20, almost 40 percent again became pregnant within 2 years.

According to a study by ABC News, it was still true in 1989 that 1 in 10 American teenage girls became pregnant. Of these, half decided to keep their babies. Most of these were young (31,000 under the age of 15), urban, poor, and had poor academic skills. According to their research, the babies of such teenagers in 1987 cost America $19 billion a year in welfare payments for AFDC stipends, Medicaid, and food stamps, or $19,000 per baby. "Just say 'No' isn't working," reporter Carole Simpson concluded.[24]

Some scholars such as Charles Murray believe that the creation of this large group was partly an unintended result of the programs of Lyndon Johnson's "Great Society" legislation.[25] These programs included Medicaid, food stamps, a great expansion of Aid to Families with Dependent Children (AFDC), and expansion of basic welfare benefits. Also, rules changed in welfare programs to eliminate work requirements and to penalize mothers with live-in, unmarried fathers (a rule which encouraged men to leave). This net effect has been called the "feminization of poverty," because men are so often missing.

The moral dilemma here is acute. Like Bertha, and whether they are pink or brown, many of these children will grow up without fathers and in poor families. Life on welfare is not easy: for an unmarried mother such as Bertha who has no other income and who has two children, monthly payments range from $633 a month in California to $118 in Alabama (in Bertha's West Virginia, it is $239).[26] With such meager sums, people have difficulty renting housing, much less feeding and clothing three people.

Is there nothing society can do to prevent this? Must it just watch generations of women in vicious cycles of poverty, beginning with multiple teenage pregnancies?

Good of the Child

We have seen the Paradox of Existence before. How can we say that it is bad for a child to be born into a welfare family when the alternative is not to be born at all? When some such children become successful?

One distinction is between the good of this child and the good of a group of children. All other things being equal, it's better to have money than not. All other things being equal, it's better to have two parents than one. All other things being equal, it's better to have parents who have the self-respect of work than the usual humiliations of welfare. Shouldn't rational public policy encourage these value judgments?

Who's a Good Mother?

As in the Baby M case, the central issues in this case concerned the qualities of a good mother. Regardless of Bertha's exact IQ score, she did not have a high IQ and was poor. She seemed uninterested in relationships with boys and to have regarded men merely as things temporarily needed to create children. In this situation, should Bertha be a mother? Should a child be brought into the world who will be unlikely to ever have a permanent, live-in father?

Psychiatrist Sharon Howell of Johns Hopkins thought Bertha might be good in some areas of mothering, but doubted her "sense of follow through" abilities, e.g., to buy food for the kids and prepare it. Psychologist Shirley Mark said Bertha was "surprisingly good" in the "little social areas," and could be a permissible mother if she had help from other people.

Bertha's sibling Norman, a year younger, strongly disagreed with this assessment of his sister's mothering skills. "Bertha was our mother. Bertha practically raised us. Everywhere Bertha went, the [other eight] kids went." Social worker Barbara Hammond agreed, noting that when she intervened in the family, when Bertha was 12 or 13, Bertha was already acting like a mother. "She seemed to take responsibility around her own home as far as the other children." Bertha also emphasized that she had already raised kids: "The rest of 'em were little and, you know, it was really my responsibility to get up and do it. It was just something that had to be done. It was hard, yes, I must admit it, but I did it. I didn't complain." In the film, Bertha seemed more qualified than her own mother to raise children. Indeed, Bertha had already taken over for her mother in many of the jobs in raising a half-dozen small children.

In 1988, half of new mothers returned to work within months after birth. Half the country's kids are now raised during the day at "cradle-rock," day-care centers, and kindergarten. In elementary school, they wait until parents get off work in after-school care or at home as latchkey kids. Are kids born to a stay-at-home mother on welfare who desperately needs children any worse off than latchkey kids?

The issue is becoming a general issue in medical ethics, as numerous cases arise which judge some women to be bad mothers. Sue Miller's *The Good Mother* raised this question, as did the similar Parrilo case in 1989.[27]

Mandatory Sterilization

Insertion of the IUD in Bertha was intended to be reversible and temporary. In the past, society has sterilized women against their will. Sometimes people talk about doing so again, so it is helpful to briefly look at modern China.

China today limits couples to one child. Those who conceive again are sent to "education centers" where they stay until they agree to an abortion. The Chinese goal "for the fifth of humanity that it commands" is for no couple to have more than one child. This goal has already been moderately successful in nondemocratic China (versus the failures of democratic India) because of the social-control techniques perfected by Mao "to a high, if Machiavellian, art during the four decades of his rule." An anthropologist who lived in China writes:

> How this [only one birth per couple] will be accomplished is diabolically simple. "The licensing of first births" was how one birth control worker privately described it to me. "Every brigade will be given an annual quota of babies," she explained. "Newlyweds who wish to have a child must apply to the commune family-planning office for a birth permit. To receive this, they must meet two conditions: they must fall within their brigade's yearly quota, and they must agree to have only one·

child. If they go ahead and have the child without a permit, they will be violating the birth control regulations. Their baby will be a 'black market person, ' no grain, oil, cloth, or other ration coupons will be issued, and the parents will have to pay a monthly fine of 20 rmb." Couples who conceive a child without first obtaining a birth permit will be ordered to attend birth control meetings, at which they will be pressured to accept the one-child limit and sterilization.[28]

Abortions by caesarean in the third fetal term and female infanticide occur in some places where the first child was not male. These formal and informal administrative structures in China—from tough national leaders to village officers—work to change behavior in ways unimaginable in America. A Chinese medical professor visiting America, who watched the film *Bertha* and who discussed this case, could not understand how a girl like Bertha could be "allowed" to get pregnant. Despite visiting here several times for many months, he had not understood the depth of the average American's reproductive freedom and how her daily life was not controlled by her parents and peers. Similarly, when the author visited China in 1988, he was astonished at how much social control exists over the most intimate details of a Chinese citizen's private life.

The Chinese are extreme, but even they do not drag women from their homes into clinics, tie them down as they struggle to be free, and surgically invade their bodies. That is the real extreme. American policy between 1950 and 1980 is nearer the opposite extreme in valuing reproductive freedom, but not so liberal as that of some Scandinavian countries.

This large freedom also grounds the controversial right to abortion. In China, people starve if too many babies are born, so that the public good requires great limitations on reproductive freedom. Wealthier America has so far been able to grant maximal freedom and not have children starve, allowing most Americans to decide for themselves that the way to economic success is through small families.

A Right to Have Children

At one point, Bertha accused social worker Bill Hershey: "What right did they have to fix it so that I couldn't have kids? I'm a human being. I should be able to have kids. Right?"

In opposition, philosopher Hugh LaFollette champions licensing parents, arguing that people can be harmed by bad drivers, polluting industries, reckless hunters, marriage between close relatives, and incompetent professionals.[29] Because of the possibility of real harm, LaFollette argues, these activities are regulated by the state. Similarly, children can be harmed by having bad parents. (Note: LaFollette does not define "bad" as being "poor," a rich person can be unsuitable for parenthood.) Practical difficulties aside, no theoretical difficulties arise from regulation per se, and as China shows, the practical difficulties may not be as insurmountable as once thought (most Chinese couples, in fact, only have one child).

A United Nations study released in 1989 showed that 'the United States had the highest teenage pregnancy rate among all developed nations.[30] Almost 10 percent of American females between 15 and 19 became pregnant, versus 1 percent in Japan. Even the Netherlands, known for its liberalism in many areas, had only a 1 percent rate.

Licensing parenthood would emphasize that the state, if it has the obligation to pay for a child's food, clothes, and medical care, has a right to decide who should have children. Such a proposal must have teeth, however, similar to the willingness of China to make life rough for a teenager who conceives without a license. In China, an unapproved pregnancy results in the loss of income for the family. Not only does the family not get extra money for the extra child, but a monthly fine is imposed. The child may not be allowed to enroll in school and the grandparents may be penalized. The parents also may lose the chance to get a raise at work or a promotion.

Many Americans are reluctant to cut such children off from societal support—from school lunches, from free baby food and food stamps, and from free medical care—because they feel that doing so will ultimately cost society more. Consistent application of such a policy would have to withstand a charge of callousness.

In *Bertha*, a group of experts cannot even begin to agree about how to prevent poor girls like Bertha from having children. In this film, resident William Bartholome said he saw unmarried teenagers like Bertha "every day," at a clinic in downtown Baltimore, who wanted to get pregnant to "have something of their own." (Baltimore has traditionally had one of the country's highest rates of teenage pregnancy.) Bartholome asked, "What should I say to such girls?" Arthur Dyck seems to advocate letting girls like Bertha have maximal freedom to conceive. Bartholome angrily retorts that if he does that, Bertha will be "less free" with a kid than with an inserted IUD. A touchy Dyck replies nervously, "Do you think that you can just simply say, on the face of it, that for Bertha and others like her, and for persons that age, that she's made a mistake?" Bartholome replies: "To have a baby? At age 15? With her judgment and capability and financial income and support and job? *Hell yes*, it's a mistake!"

Bartholome is then challenged by Mary Robinson, executive director of the Martin Luther King Parenting and Child Center, who asks him, "Why?" Bartholome gets angry and asks her, "For a 15-year-old, unsupported girl to have a baby is not a mistake?" Mrs. Robinson does not want to come out and agree, but Bartholome asks her how she can be a director of a parenting clinic and not emphasize that such behavior is mistaken. Mrs. Robinson prefers to blame "society" for not helping teenagers.

Eunice Kennedy Shriver retorts that everyone should be able to have children. If this right is taken away, she says, a girl's "reason for existence" may be taken away. She says the community has an "obligation" to provide basic family clinics, schools, part-time work for mothers such as Bertha, and good reading clinics for children if they can't read.

Mrs. Shriver furthermore says society can't rely on the judgment of a 15-year-old about whether she wants an IUD and thinks it wrong that such girls have the choice to have an IUD inserted. "When you're 15 years of age, you're too young to get IUD or contraception," she says. She wants parents involved, but when the physician says that parents often won't get involved, she retreats like Mrs. Robinson to saying that the "solution isn't to pop a few (birth control) pills into such girls." Instead, she wants to get (an undefined) "community" involved. Bartholome retorts that this is a "cop-out."

Sex Education and Teenage Pregnancy

The disagreement of the above people mirrors a larger, continuing disagreement, in our society about these issues. Indeed, can people even agree about where to *begin* to attack the problem? One logical place to begin is in providing information about contraception and in providing contraception itself. But parents disagree mightily about the wisdom of this.

Providing such information and contraception clearly works in some countries. Holland is famous for not only decriminalizing mercy killing but also for decriminalizing prostitution, access to sexually explicit materials, and for giving teenagers access to contraception at early ages. Anthropologists have surveyed cultures around the world and divided them into sexually liberated, moderate, and repressive, America is regarded by them today as a sexually repressive culture.[31] In some ways, America takes a severe, even Puritanical attitude toward sexuality (including homosexuality—see Chapter 16) yet it has ten times the rate of teenage pregnancy of Holland. Why?

One answer is that America takes an encouraging approach toward sexuality on soap operas, in movies aimed at teenagers, on music/television networks, and in advertising directed at teenagers. Messages bombard teenagers about sex, encouraging them to believe that sexual activity will make them mature and that decisions to become sexually active are their decisions alone. Partly as a result, in the age group of 15 to 19, 80 percent of boys have had sex as have 43 percent of girls.[32] Sexual scenes on soap operas or in movies are not preceded by men putting on condoms. The million teenage pregnancies each year, and 1.6 million abortions, are not popular subjects in the above media.

Faced with the success of countries such as Holland, and the staggering numbers of teenage pregnancies, some inner-city schools in America attempted to set up clinics in the schools to provide contraception. What happened was that some parents vociferously opposed these plans, fearing that children who were not sexually active would become so when they obtained contraception. These battles were often very emotional, pitting groups of parents against each other. Different schools had different results, with some clinics reducing teenage pregnancy, while others never opened.

Similar differences lay behind other disputes. In some communities, the social stigma against unmarried, or teenage, pregnancy (or both) has lessened. As a result, tough questions arise: Should pregnant girls, or teenage mothers, be allowed to go to their senior proms? To participate in graduation ceremonies? To work in day-care centers where they are role models? To counsel younger girls? Does toleration at some point become encouragement?

Such discussions, like others on this subject, usually end in a paralyzing stand-off. People want to decrease unmarried teenage pregnancies, but some don't want to give teenagers contraception. Others don't want to sound moralistic and paternalistic about such matters, but really don't have a workable alternative. The cycle of teenage pregnancy may at bottom be a crisis over the correct ranking of values and willingness to stand up for them in public policy.

EUGENICS, TEENAGE PREGNANCY, AND SOCIETAL VALUES

This chapter began by discussing the excesses of the eugenics movement at the beginning of the 20th century. Because of these excesses, as well as because of Hitler's eugenics program, eugenics has become a discredited idea in American political life. As a result, the idea of forceably preventing someone from having a wanted pregnancy has also become discredited. This legacy has helped bequeath contemporary America an ineffective policy in stopping teenage pregnancy, especially such pregnancy among poor, unwed girls.

UPDATE

Barbara Hammond is still director of Social Services for Allegheny County, Va. According to Hammond, the IUD caused endometriosis in Bertha. Because of this, Bertha became sterile. She eventually married. Bertha still lives in her hometown. She, and at least some of her 9 siblings (her older brother and one of her sisters), live on public assistance.

FURTHER READING

Daniel Kevles, *In the Name of Eugenics: Genetics and the Uses of Human Heredity*, Knopf, New York, 1985.

Hugh LaFollette, "Licensing Parents," *Philosophy & Public Affairs* 9(2): 182–197 (1980).

Donald Mood, ed. *Responsibility, Rights & Welfare: The Theory of the Welfare State*, Westview Press, Boulder, Colo., 1983.

Stephen Mosher, *Broken Earth*, Free Press, New York, 1983.

Charles Murray, *Losing Ground: American Social Policy: 1950–1980*, Basic Books, New York, 1986.

Robert Redmon and Joyce Bermel, "Risk-Taking for a Minor Birth Defect: Commentaries," *Hastings Center Report*, 11(2):25–26 (April 1981).

CHAPTER 15

Nancy Wexler and Genetic Markers

As many as 15 million Americans may suffer from moderate to severe genetic disease.[1] Perhaps everyone carries at least some disease-causing genes (are "heterozygous") which could be passed along to children, and which could result in a disease if a carrier child mates with another carrier to produce a "homozygous" child. According to the definitive list by McKussick (updated daily, and available on-line), over 2200 hereditary disorders are "established," another 2100 "suspected."[2] (The main reason that they are only suspected and not established is not lack of scientific knowledge but a lack of families to confirm the tests on rare conditions.)

Many of these genes are recessive, meaning that a child will have the condition only if two (heterozygous) carriers mate and produce a homozygous (affected) child. Moreover, perhaps every family has someone who, if not a potential victim of genetic disease, has a susceptibility to diseases which are linked to genetic causes, such as alcoholism, cancer, or coronary artery disease.

Furthermore, genetic diseases cause over a third of medical care for children under 18 in acute-care hospitals. Also, from every 100 successful human fertilizations, only 35 babies are born, partially because genetically defective pre-embryos do not implant on the uterine wall.[3]

HISTORICAL BACKGROUND

Genetic Screening Programs in the 1960s and 1970s

In the early 1960s, well-intentioned reformers revived negative eugenics when prenatal predictive tests made it possible to identify newborns suffering from PKU (phenylketonuria). PKU is a recessive genetic disease causing retardation due to an excess of phenylalanine, an amino acid. Identification of birth of PKU babies allows mothers to put babies on special diets and prevent retardation.

Tests for PKU were cheap and easy. More importantly, PKU could be treated by modifying the diet, so that normal children then developed. If not diagnosed until after symptoms appeared, PKU always caused retardation. What better justification for mandatory screening could there be? Most states subsequently required PKU screening.

One reviewer of genetic screening notes that PKU screening was "in many ways a type case of the kinds of difficulty encountered by all mass screening procedures, which frequently turn out to be less perfect in practice than had been hoped when they were instituted."[4] Subsequent studies showed that the diagnostic test was not reliable and that normal babies, who were erroneously thought to have PKU, could be harmed by altering their diet as if they had PKU.

Despite such problems, PKU screening saved thousands from retardation, targeted a specific deficit, and possessed a known remedy. If all screening was so specific and for such a treatable condition, genetic screening would be routine today.

Screening by Jacobs in 1965 found that some men with an extra Y chromosome were inmates of penal and mental institutions. Some newborns were subsequently tested and followed to see if XYY caused antisocialness. However, some researchers felt they should intervene, but worried that disclosure would bias any results. Critics said different solutions to these problems invalidated the project.

Screening for carriers of a genetic disease, who may pass the gene on to their offspring, but never suffer symptoms themselves, should be distinguished from those afflicted with the disease. Screening for carriers occurred in the 1960s for Tay-Sachs disease. Ashkenazic Jews in the United States have a 1 in 30 chance of carrying the gene for Tay-Sachs disease, a lethal, neurological disease developing around 6 months of age. Tay-Sachs is carried by a recessive gene. A cherry-red spot in the bottom of a baby's eye is virtually a definitive diagnosis. Children almost never live to school age.[5]

Like PKU, a simple and cheap test allowed screening for Tay-Sachs. Unlike PKU, no treatment existed for Tay-Sachs, and the test had to be done on a fetus, which had to be aborted if the test was positive. (If a couple would not consider abortion, the test was not done.) The screening was only a partial success. It failed because some people at risk opposed abortion and because others feared being stigmatized by being identified as carriers.

In screening for carriers of sickle cell anemia, authorities failed to think through the possible repercussions. Sickle cell anemia, a blood disorder which often is fatal in childhood, is a recessive disease carried by 1 in 11 American blacks. Unlike PKU or Tay-Sachs, sickle cell disease manifested a variable clinical course. Importantly, some diseased individuals led nearly normal lives. Like Tay-Sachs, the "treatment" in screening was abortion. No real cure existed. Moreover, unlike Tay-Sachs, but like PKU, some misdiagnosis occurred. Thus, abortion alone was offered as "treatment" for a positive prenatal diagnosis of a condition which might or might not be serious.

The public subsequently confused carrying the sickle cell gene (heterozygous) with having the disease itself (homozygous). Some laws required mandatory screening for carriers of sickle cell, but treated carriers as if they had the disease itself. Some heterozygotes were denied medical insurance or fired. (People later similarly confused having HIV, human immunodeficency virus, with having AIDS.) Protests from the black community defeated the programs, and state laws faded into limbo. Sickle cell is now known as a paradigm of how *not* to set up a screening program.

It became possible in the early 1970s to screen for the chromosomal aberration of Down syndrome. Pregnant women over age 35 routinely get tested today. Indeed, it is malpractice for an obstetrician not to suggest it for women over this age.

One in 22 Caucasians carries the CF (cystic fibrosis) gene. A test for genetic markers for heterozygotes and homozygotes for CF has recently been discovered.[6] If one carrier (heterozygote) procreates with another, each child has a 25 percent risk of this disease (being homozygous). Although one child in four would be affected in a hypothetical family, heterozygote parents with four children may have none, one, two, or even three homozygous children. CF makes victims suffocate on thick, excessive mucus in their bronchi. It may not show symptoms until the teenage years, when adolescents must be held upside down and thumped on their backs to loosen secretions for postural drainage. Sportswriter Frank DeFord described this deterioration in a book about his CF child—later made into a television movie.

Susceptibility screening is also possible for cholesterol, lipids, and HLA-antigens. Some genes appear to be linked to certain diseases, e.g., to some cancers and to multiple sclerosis. Prevention might occur by early intervention, such as by identifying hypercholesterolemia to prevent later heart attacks. However, discrimination might also occur by employers seeking to minimize medical costs by screening prospective employees.

NANCY WEXLER'S CASE

This chapter focuses on the case of Nancy Wexler. Specifically, it examines her decision about being tested for a marker for Huntington's disease.

Nancy Wexler was born in 1946. Today, she is a clinical psychologist waiting to find out if she has a time bomb among her genes. Her mother had suddenly felt strange symptoms begin at age 58. A physician diagnosed Huntington's disease (or simply, "Huntington's"). For this terrible disease, there was neither treatment nor cure. Because the disease was dominant, Nancy and her sister Alice were also each at 50 percent risk. Over the next decade, the two Wexler girls and their father watched as their mother became emaciated and catatonic. Her condition mirrored the final years of folk singer Woody Guthrie, father of Arlo Guthrie, and portrayed briefly in the movie *Alice's Restaurant*.

Over 100,000 Americans with an afflicted parent are at risk for Huntington's. Almost all affected people are white, except for one large black family around Baltimore. About 20,000 to 25,000 people presently suffer from Huntington's. Some genetic diseases such as Down syndrome start at birth, but Huntington's typically begins during a person's third to fifth decade. The people who are diagnosed as having Huntington's usually have children before they know that they are affected.

Victims of Huntington's have been treated poorly in the past. The defect came to America around the time of the Mayflower from three affected males who left their small English village of Bures in 1625, including the ancestor of Long Island physician George Huntington, who first described the disease in 1872.[7] The disease was called "St. Vitus' dance" or "Huntington's chorea" (dance) because of the victims' strange grimaces and erratic twisting of limbs. As a result, seven female descendants of the original three Englishmen were thought to be witches, and one was burned at Groton, Conn. in 1692. Some of the Salem witches probably had Huntington's. Because their distorted movements were said to resemble those of Jesus on the cross, witch-hunters (strangely!) inferred that the women worshipped Satan and were being tortured by God.

Huntington's is a severe, progressive, neurological disease in which neurons rapidly shed in the caudate nuclei region of the brain. Average age of onset is 36. The disease progresses through roughly four 5-year stages. At first, small losses of muscular coordination come, then changes in personality, making victims angry, hostile, depressed, and sexually promiscuous (probably due to loss of neurons from the frontal lobe). The second stage brings slurred speech, grotesque facial distortions, constant muscular jerkiness, clenching and unclenching of fists, staggering, falling, and involuntarily flailing of the limbs. Nancy Wexler says that: "Gradually, the entire body is encompassed by adventitious movements. The trunk is writhing and the face is twisting." In this stage, victims often lose their jobs. The third stage brings incontinence, severe mental deterioration, and dependence on others at home or in institutions. In the last stage, victims stare blankly ahead and never move. Although onset of the disease varies, by age 65 it is completely "penetrant" (i.e., every homozygote is affected).

Huntington's is a bad possibility for Nancy Wexler to contemplate. Another woman at risk says, "being at risk for Huntington's is almost as fundamental to my identity as being a woman."[8] For people who know they have it, it's much worse. Over 25 percent of its victims consider suicide, 10 percent carry it out.[9]

As Nancy Wexler points out, Huntington's victims during the first stage do not lose memory and can recognize relatives. "Huntington's patients know their family and they know what's happening to them," Wexler says, "So in a way, it's worse than Alzheimer's."[10] Patients may become frustrated at being unable to tie a shoe and fly into a rage. Later, they may be ashamed and become depressed.

Nancy Wexler and the Search for a Genetic Marker for Huntington's

In 1969, Milton Wexler, a Los Angeles psychoanalyst and Nancy's father, started the Hereditary Disease Foundation in Santa Monica, Cal. Nancy had earned a Ph.D. in clinical psychology, and her older sister Alice had earned a Ph.D. in history. In 1976, after teaching psychology at the New School for Social Research in New York City, Nancy became president of this foundation. She then played a crucial role in promoting research on Huntington's. She attended symposia where patients and their families were studied. Researchers were motivated after seeing both the devastation in patients at case-conferences and also upon talking to the at-risk Nancy Wexler—described as "so intelligent and vital." As one article about Wexler and her work said:

> So she found out everything she could. She studied genetics. She organized patients' groups. She helped start a brain collection program so that the brains of Huntington's victims would be available for research. She lobbied Capitol Hill for research funds. She convinced a wide variety of scientists such as molecular biologist David Housman of the Massachusetts Institute of Technology to study Huntington's. Soon she was a driving force in the Huntington's community.[11]

The first step in finding such a marker was to find a large number of people in a single family tree where Huntington's had been inherited. Blood would be taken from each member, a genetic analysis would be carried out, and geneticists would visually examine tiny bits of the genetic map to see if some bit of DNA was only found in Huntington's victims. But the first step was to find such a large family. One family in Iowa was found, but only about 30 members participated—not enough for a full study.

In 1972, a Venezuelan psychiatrist discovered a large number of carriers descended from a single Huntington's ancestor. All of them lived in the village of San Luis along the shores of Lake Maracaibo in Venezuela. Here was the necessary concentration. In 1981, Nancy Wexler led an expedition there. Her sister Alice, with a Ph.D. in history, researched ancient records to determine how the original ancestor Maria Concepción Soto had received the gene. It looked as though a European sailor had jumped ship there in the early 1800s and then conceived 14 children with Maria. Because no birth control was available, and because families in this area were large (10 + children), by 1981 Maria had between 2000 and 3000 descendants. Of them, 100 had Huntington's and 1100 others were at 25 percent or 50 percent risk.

Once the team arrived. Nancy Wexler played another key role in the research. The natives were reluctant to allow skin biopsies and to give blood. Wexler, through an interpreter, explained that she too was at risk for "le mal" (the evil), had undergone these procedures, and that they all shared a common ancestor. This encouraged participation.

Getting the blood samples and skin biopsies back to the United States on time proved difficult. Some Huntington's families lived far away from the nearest big city and the samples had to reach American researchers within 48 hours. Keeping things in order also created headaches. For example, the family tree in Wexler's office included over 3000 descendants and was more than a hundred feet long.

A Genetic Marker Is Identified

After successfully locating a family of descendants in which to "map" the hereditary pattern of the Huntington's gene, Wexler and geneticists then had to actually find the bit of genetic matter which caused Huntington's. In 1979, Wexler's Hereditary Disease Foundation held a workshop about using recombinant DNA techniques to find a genetic marker linked to Huntington's. She then said, "A lot of people were skeptical—it sounded like science fiction." Wexler had already lobbied Congress and obtained some funding in 1977.

Two years later, James Gusella used techniques of recombinant DNA to look for a DNA marker in the genetic karotypes (blueprints) of the Venezuelan families. Gusella had a hunch where to look from his previous study of Iowa families, but he still planned to take 5 to 10 years to find any marker. Each human cell contains 46 chromosomes, and inside each chromosome is an enormously complicated double helix of interwoven DNA. Each of these 46 strands of DNA is composed of combinations of four chemical bases in around 3 billion pairs (one bit on one each side of the helix). Put differently, a chromosome is a macromolecule composed of repeating nucleotides. The pattern of these four nucleotide bases in this double helix is a person's genetic code. Somewhere inside these 3 billion pairs, a scant 100,000 sequences of base pairs are genes. Gusella had to find these genes, and then force them to reveal which small sequence carried Huntington's.

One of Mendel's laws holds that genes without alternative forms (i.e., without "alleles") mix independently of each other in reproduction. However, small bits of genetic material close together on the same chromosome may be inherited together in 50 percent of cases and are said to be "linked." Genetic linkage is a major exception to Mendel's law of independent assortment.

Linkage was little studied for decades, but has recently dominated medical genetics because of great advances, which compare to previous medical breakthroughs such as the germ model of disease. Five general technologies were brought together to achieve recent advances: computers, banding (marking) studies of chromosomes, somatic cell hybridization, isozyme analysis, and recombination of DNA molecules with restriction enzymes.

Gusella had great luck in his linkage study and found a marker (G8) for Huntington's on the far tip of the short arm of chromosome 4. A *marker* is a bit of DNA linked with the targeted, pathological gene. Because the larger marker is easier to find than the very small gene causing the targeted disease, the marker can be used to predict the disease. Gusella's discovery meant that the search for the Huntington's gene itself could be restricted to the tip of chromosome 4, i.e., to less than 0.03 percent of the human DNA. The next step is to identify the gene with which the marker travels. Gusella said in 1983 that "we're still 3 to 5 years away from finding the gene—unless there's another lucky break."[12]

Gusella, Susan Naylor, and geneticist Michael Conneally received primary credit for the scientific discovery.[13] Nancy Wexler was listed as a principal codiscoverer. Mrs. Marjorie Guthrie had organized clubs for Huntington's descendants and had an indirect role in the discovery.

Genetic Markers

Probably 4000 diseases are inherited in the well-known ways of Mendelian inheritance.[14] Many more diseases, such as cancer, manic-depression, and schizophrenia may involve genetic cofactors. Until recently, nothing could be done for such diseases except ameliorate symptoms. The underlying genetic pathology, expressed in every cell, could not be known. Today, the discovery of genetic markers is changing all this. Such markers, using blood tests and family histories, can predict who is carrying a dormant genetic disease.

Similar techniques have identified markers for some kinds of manic- depression (chromosome 11, tip of short arm), hemophilia, familial Alzheimer's (chromosome 21), retinoblastoma (an eye cancer), PKU (phenylketonuria), Duchenne muscular dystrophy, Gaucher's disease, and cystic fibrosis. Markers are also tentatively associated with several forms of cancer and heart disease.

A Test Is Developed

People at risk for Huntington's live with a genetic sword of Damocles over their heads, constantly wondering if a stutter, spill, or stumble marks the beginning of the disease. Wexler says, "You become aware of all kinds of things you never noticed before—little muscle jerks in bed, or clumsiness. I remember dropping a carton of eggs and thinking, 'Oh, no! Is this the beginning?'"[15] Nancy says that not a day goes by when she doesn't think about having Huntington's.

By the fall of 1987, a test was developed to detect Huntington's. It is not an "orphan test," i.e., it requires blood (DNA) samples from both sets of grandparents and both parents. Common misconceptions are first, believing that the test is an orphan test and second, believing that the test itself proves Huntington's (a family history must prove a case). The test can be 97 percent accurate (but in 3 percent of cases, the marker does not "travel" in heredity with the Huntington's gene). The test can also be only 75 percent predictive, depending on the pedigree and what is known.

ETHICAL ISSUES

A Right to Know

To many people, it seems obvious that those at risk have a right to take the test and be told the results. Nancy Wexler believes this. Such information, affecting the literal core of every cell, must be made available to the person whose cells they are.

If people do not know, childbearing decisions will be based on uncertain information in two ways. First, children may not be born because parents may erroneously fear the disease. Second, children may be born with the disease when parents hope they lack the disease. Either way, tragedy occurs.

Inhumane to Tell?

Huntington's cannot be cured or ameliorated. A positive test will tell Nancy Wexler that she will likely die an early, terrible death. Isn't it inhumane to tell someone this and not be able to offer any treatment? Wouldn't it be better to wait until some positive treatment could be given? Nancy Wexler's father thinks so.

The President's Commission emphasized that if the test was given, counseling should be guaranteed ("A full range of prescreening and follow-up services...should be available before a program is introduced.")[16] This has not happened. Is a person's right to know so strong that he can exercise it, even if no help is available?

The right-to-know argument works best for negative results. If results are positive, some victims will say that they wish they hadn't taken the test. It is easy for champions of individual autonomy to avoid the question of what will be done for the person who tests positive, but the question must be faced. Will people with positive results just walk away and "deal with it" by themselves?

Perhaps the most humane thing about the test is that it is not 100 percent accurate. Some uncertainty allows for hope of error. A 4 percent risk of recombination exists, i.e., the material marked by the probe may recombine in sexual reproduction with some other gene. Even if such uncertainty could be eliminated, perhaps it would be better to keep it. But if the purpose of giving the test is to prevent affected children, or to plan for future care, then allowing uncertainty allows denial. This raises a key ethical question:who is the test for? The person at risk? Society? Possible children? Recall that a conflict of goals of screening was a key problem in previous programs.

In the initial study (described below), most people taking the test already were past childbearing age. This suggests that the test primarily was not for eugenic purposes. Moreover, scientists in this study found that, "Persons found to have high probability of having the Huntington's disease gene were shocked by this outcome and had more difficulty coping with it than we had expected."[17] The early evidence implies that society should be extremely careful about revealing devastating news when it can do nothing about the effects of such news.

Some people would here reply, "Sure, why not?" We already allow people to know about having HIV (causing AIDS) and about cancer, both of which can lead to death. Besides their newness, what's so different about genetic diseases? Are people making an unjustified exception for Huntington's?[18]

A Duty to Know?

If there is a right to know, isn't there a right *not* to know? If so, such a right may be complicated. In one case presented to a large medical class, a man decided not to take the test and discussed his reasons. These reasons were honored, the class ended, and the students started to file out. Suddenly a female voice cried out from the back of the room, "What about me and the kids?" It was the man's wife.[19]

She wanted to plan their future. If her husband was positive, she would be taking care of him. In the second stage, Huntington's victims become highly promiscuous and have been described as interested only in constant, "animalistic" sex. She probably wondered if she could take that. Savings would be needed for medical and custodial care. It might be still possible to purchase life insurance. Huntington's makes relatives suffer as much as the victim. Should the husband have been pressured to take the test? Does he have a a duty to do so for his family? Whether Nancy Wexler should take the test would be more complicated if she were married, or had children, as does Arlo Guthrie.

A compromise is to bank descendants' blood and family histories of relatives at the International Research Roster for Huntington's Disease in Indianapolis, Ind. If someone dies unexpectedly or before any symptoms appear, his or her blood can be tested postmortem. This plan—for some—may be too little, too late, since children will usually have been born.

Because the test requires family histories, other family members must donate blood for testing. Some family members have refused to do so, even when promised that they would not be told the results. Some people say that such family members have a moral duty to donate blood for such testing. If there's not a strong duty to help members of your own "blood," when is there?

If relatives refuse to donate blood, the delicate question arises of how far counselors can bend the truth. Suppose an intergenerational person, Fred, refuses the test because he doesn't want to know his fate. Suppose Fred's father and son take the test and are positive. Then Fred, too, is positive. It would be difficult for Fred not to learn this and for his "right not to know" to be respected.

Similarly in testing fetuses, there is no such thing as only testing the fetus. A positive fetus reveals a positive parent (this is also true for testing for HIV). In the example above, the wife could test a child to find out if her husband was positive.

What if the husband is positive and won't tell his children? What if a genetic counselor knows this? As his children approaching childbearing age, the counselor might agonize when an at-risk child becomes pregnant and refuses to take the test. Would the child test if she knew her father was positive? If so, the counselor might break the parent's confidentiality. To many people, the good of preventing a Huntington's child outweighs the harm of the violation of privacy, especially where there is a strong sense that the father had an obligation to reveal his disease to his adult children.

Finally, there is the problem of unexpected results. A positive result for a child and negative results for both parents reveals that the husband is not the father of the child. Similar problems occur for a recessive disease where only the mother is a carrier or for incompatible blood types. Genetic tests may also reveal unexpected conditions such as XYY syndrome or testicular feminization (a condition where a genetic male seems female due to undescended testicles and low testosterone levels). In taking genetic tests, people may learn more than they expected.

Preventing Suicide and Paternalism

People who are positive for Huntington's often consider suicide. Nancy Wexler does not think this weighs against using the tests: "suicide is not unreasonable. It's not so awful that we can't discuss it or consider it."[20] Johns Hopkins neuropsychologist Jason Brandt opposes thinking about suicide, arguing that such ideation is caused by depression, which he says is "treatable."[21] He subscribes "to the school which says one must choose life over death." One Australian psychiatrist says that Huntington's patients should only be submitted to the burden of truth that they can carry.

In the literature of medical genetics, it is usually assumed that suicide after a positive test would be a bad thing, that such suicide should be prevented at all costs, and that those who say they might commit suicide should not receive the test. Nancy Wexler replies that "for some of my friends who have Huntington's disease, knowing that they can commit suicide, gives them a certain sense of control. They want to feel that if it gets too bad, they can have a way out. They can do something."

The suicide question needs to be faced squarely. Physicians and psychologists are trained only to prevent suicides. The patient's condition may reverse itself, they are taught, or it may be "treatable" in future years.

Lack of a real option of suicide may force Huntington's victims to kill themselves early. If they cannot count on physicians to help them later, they may have to kill themselves now.

Researchers conducted a pilot program to see if they could predict who would try to commit suicide after getting positive results. Victims predicted to kill themselves would either not be told or would have counselors intervene intensely. As Jason Brandt says, "We'll stop doing the test if we see we're doing more harm than good." His statement assumes that committing suicide counts as "doing more harm."

At a conference in Salt Lake City in 1986, scientists debated whether the new test should be made available. Arthur Beaudet of Baylor College of Medicine accused his colleagues of unjustified paternalism in blocking release of the Huntington's test. He said, "I think we can trust people to make these decisions. I'm not so convinced we researchers should be dictating how the technology gets used."[22]

Surprisingly, perhaps, Nancy Wexler was less sure. "We have to understand that the day you tell someone he has this gene, his life and view of himself change forever. We're worried about the potential for suicide."[23]

Do They Really Want to Know?

Can people who agree to the test really understand what they are doing? One counselor for Huntington's says, "When people say they want this test to find out if they have the gene so they can make decisions, they really want to find out that they *don't* have it. The trouble is that 50 percent of them do. And there's no way to prepare them."[24] Nancy Wexler agreed.

Previously, most at-risk people (63–79 percent) claimed they would take the test, but later, some changed their minds. This occurred for two reasons. Some people were convinced they would not be positive and were taking the test only to prove this. Since they had a 50 percent chance of really having it, they were in denial, and had not really prepared themselves for positive results. Once counseling broke through their denial, they decided not to take the test.

Some people do not know themselves and cannot predict what they will do. In the first pilot study of the Huntington's test, "participants found to be probable gene carriers reported being surprised or shocked by the test result."[25] They said they had not really expected to have the lethal gene. That is an important result.

Some researchers suggest a benevolent white lie: the "good news" or "no news" option.[26] Because results can be indeterminate, a person testing positive has no way of knowing if he is really positive or is merely indeterminate. The drawbacks of such white lies are that they foster distrust of physicians and may result in the gene being passed to children.

Employment Screening

Some companies have screened applicants for genetic susceptibility to asbestosis or to lead poisoning. A 1983 Office of Technology report found that 18 companies already screened applicants, and by 1988, another 60 planned to do so.[27]

In general, confidentiality is a good because it allows a person to exercise control of his or her life. As the power of government grows, especially through computerized information and surveillance techniques, rights to privacy become more important. The President's Commission championed a right to have the results of genetic tests held confidential.

Several national companies, e.g., Medical Information Bureau of Boston, tell insurance companies about applicants who are risks.[28] Two concepts of medical insurance conflict here: making profits versus sharing risk. In sharing risk, everyone pays premiums to help pay the costs for those who become sick. In England, Canada, Australia, and Europe, employers have no motive to find out Huntington's test results, but in for-profit systems, they do. Patients testing positive for Huntington's or HIV are then excluded from the risk pool.

Children of any Huntington's victim have a 50 percent risk. With other genetic diseases, insurers can calculate odds that children will be affected. When a parent gives insurers information about genetic inheritance, she gives information which may affect the availability and cost of medical insurance for her children. When positive test results come from the nursery and parents file for insurance, they may not realize what they are revealing.

Already, it is crucial to control the scope of who receives the test results. Many large institutions, such as the military, universities, and large companies, "self-insure" themselves. The institution itself passes along losses by increasing premiums to employees. The military screens for the HIVvirus to exclude recruits. Other companies may not be motivated to keep test results confidential, especially if key employees are involved. A positive test result may keep a young executive off the fast track, prevent a young physician from being accepted in a medical group, or prevent a student with cystic fibrosis from being accepted at medical school.

One legal issue concerns conflicts between confidentiality and rights to know. Courts have ruled that relatives cannot be compelled to be tested for bone marrow or organ transplantation, even when lives of kin are at stake. Even imminent death cannot legally compel a person to be his brother's keeper. Such legal precedents indicate that the courts will not force relatives to participate in genetic tests.

Finally, it would seem that confidential test results should be revealed against a person's wishes only when some great public good was at stake. If a person was an airline pilot and beginning to suffer Huntington's, and if he refused to retire after private discussions, then his condition might be ethically revealed.

Children and the Test

Another issue concerns testing young people. Testing a teenager might have enormous effects on a population already highly suicidal. Children merely at risk for Huntington's already agonize about going to college and spending their parents' money. How much more intense such concerns will be for those who are certain they have Huntington's.

A related issue concerns premarital testing, which may come up during teenage years. Could hiding results be grounds for legal annulment? Do prospective spouses have rights to know about risk of Huntington's, as well as the reality? Or does marrying "for better or for worse" preclude such knowledge?

In Utero Testing

Feelings run high about the ethics of giving such tests to fetuses. A mother who already had two children with cystic fibrosis (CF) underwent amniocentesis and was relieved to discover that her third child had very little chance of having CF. "I couldn't bear bringing another child into the world with cystic fibrosis," she said.[29] That attitude angers of Brian Scully, a New York physician specializing in treating CF children who said that taking such a prenatal test is like telling victims that "it would have been better for all of us if you had not been born."[30] Dr. Scully's remarks are echoed by some organizations of parents of Down syndrome and spina bifida children. For most people, however, a test to avoid having a baby with CF is a test they want to take.

UPDATE

James Gusella's work was published, in 1984, in the prestigious journal *Nature.* Two years later, Watt et al. of Oxford's Medical Genetics Unit criticized Gusella for not giving them the test.[31] The English scientists had collected 300 cases in 140 families, and wanted to do the test on at-risk relatives. Watt cited canons of scientific replication of results and suggested that *Nature* not publish studies of researchers who would not release their tests. He argued, "If Wasserman had published his test for syphilis, which was far from reliable, in a way which delayed its application, neurosyphilis might now be more common than Huntington's chorea." Watt pointed out that many patients and their families must have been distressed by false positives and false negatives, "and there were probably a few suicides" because of mistakes. Nevertheless, "In no field of effective medicine can techniques be applied without casualties." Watt et al. closed by suggesting that Gusella was really withholding information "to allow a monopoly of further research or development."

Gusella replied that he welcomed confirmation of his results, but stressed that presymptomatic clinical tests were premature because "there is considerable precedent in genetics" where "mutations at two or more separate loci result in the same phenotype."[32] If a second locus caused Huntington's in some families, "predictive testing for them using the G8 marker would be no better than guesswork."

Six months later, Gusella published a note in *Nature,* saying his team had now estimated that the risk of a second loci was at most 10 percent.[33] That figure was low enough to proceed with clinical testing for people such as Nancy Wexler. However, Gusella emphasized, the first step would be a controlled clinical trial.

Three medical centers in northeast America offered the test for Huntington's in early 1987. Subsequent actions of those at-risk did not match their words. Previous surveys predicted that between 60 percent and 80 percent of them would take the test, but of 1500 people at risk in New England, only 32 signed up for preliminary genetic counseling, with 18 actually taking the test.

In 1986, Nancy Wexler said she would take the test: "My feeling was that the advantages of knowing, even if the answer was yes, outweighed the disadvantages."[34] And given her place in the development of the predictive test, and her own risk, she may have been the most informed person in the country to make the decision.

In May 1987, Diane Sawyer interviewed Nancy and Alice Wexler for *60 Minutes*:

DIANE SAWYER: Did you think you'd get the test if they ever had one?

NANCY WEXLER: I was positive I would. Unquestionably. It *never* occurred to me that I wouldn't.

DIANE SAWYER: And all of a sudden when you have the option, you're not so sure?

NANCY WEXLER: I wasn't so sure. Exactly. I even said to people, "When the test is actually here, a lot of people are going to change their minds." It never occurred to me I would be one of them. That wasn't in the book.

ALICE WEXLER: I would like to know if I don't have it, but I absolutely don't want to know if I have it.

NANCY WEXLER: This is absolutely the hardest choice I've ever made in my life.[35]

At the end of the show, Diane Sawyer asked Nancy Wexler, "Will you take the test?" and "Is there a right answer?" Nancy Wexler said, "I think for each person there's a right choice."

Dr. Wexler now thinks that people who take the test to end uncertainty may be fooling themselves. If the result is positive, the question won't be, "What if?" but "When?" And for her, there looms the worst possibility of all: both she and her sister could test positive.

Their father, psychoanalyst Milton Wexler, opposes either of them taking the test. He argues that with a 50-50 chance of each daughter having the disease, one of them will probably test positive. Why, he says, would he want to know something which would destroy the three of them? In a daughter who tests positive, he says, such knowledge is a "potential for madness."

Nancy admits there are lots of bad outcomes: "If I found out that I was free of the disease, but Alice wasn't, I'd die." In thinking through the consequences of taking the test, Alice Wexler says she tries to imagine the "unimaginable," i.e., that she is positive, which she admits she has not really done. As she tries to imagine sitting at her own desk and knowing she had this lethal gene at work in her, she says,

> If you have the certainty that you have the gene, and if you have the certainty that you're going to die this absolutely miserable death over many years, I'm not sure it's possible to keep on living. To use the knowledge constructively. I'm sure I wouldn't. I think I would be devastated by it.

Diane Sawyer then asked, "So some hope is better than possible bad news?" Alice replied, "Hope is better than despair."

RELATED ISSUES IN CLINICAL GENETICS

Gene Therapy

The predictive marker test for Huntington's is the first step down the road to developing genetic therapy. It is possible that, once the strands of DNA causing Huntington's are identified, scientists might try to change that DNA to prevent Huntington's. Even if such therapy had unexpected consequences, almost anything would be better than the final stages of Huntington's.

In discussing such genetic therapy, two kinds of therapy are frequently confused. *Somatic* therapy, the first and least controversial kind of such therapy, attempts to alter the disease-causing genetic material of a particular individual while leaving him or her otherwise the same. It is much like ordinary medical treatment. *Gametic* therapy, in contrast, alters the hereditary genetic material of individuals and those of their descendants, who inherit changed genetic material. The latter, but not the former, is "genetic engineering."

Skeptics doubt that geneticists presently know how to do gametic therapy without inadvertently causing problems as bad as the ones they want to eradicate. To this critique, others reply that some dominant genetic conditions are so terrible that almost anything would be better. Moreover, they say, such dire predictions sound like those a priori criticisms made against in vitro fertilization.

Scientists have already reported promising results in somatic therapy in animals in normalizing hypercholesterolemia in livers of animals, opening the door to trying similar therapy on humans. Victims of Lesch-Nyhan disease, a terrible progressive neurological disease causing babies to eat their own flesh, will likely be the first candidates for somatic gene therapy.

Pre-Employment Susceptibility Screening

In 1988, a front-page story in *The New York Times* reported the discovery that 50 percent of colon-rectal cancers had a genetic predisposition.[36] It was the first real evidence that some cancers were genetically based.

In the same year, commercial biotechnology firms were busily developing simple test kits for physicians to use on patients. Such screening was not only for genetic diseases, but also for susceptibility to diseases, such as cancer, linked to genetic factors. This development raises ominous possibilities, as noted by well-known geneticist Marc Lappe:

> In 1997 it might be common for a physician to give patients a battery of DNA probe tests as part of an intake procedure. Such a panel of tests would likely include susceptibility markers....Predictive testing would almost certainly appeal to the physician charged with performing the intake screens on prospective applicants to an HMO—or to General Motors for that matter—...and thereby enable the employer to take

appropriate "remedial" measures—such as not employing them [job applicants] in the first place.[37]

One defect of such tests is that they ignore the variability of the expression of the genotype in the individual phenotype.

In 1988, scientists reported on a breakthrough in doing such testing in a physician's office:

> British geneticists are performing amazingly simple tests to tell families whether they carry potentially deadly genes, and if imperiled babies will be born normal. "For the carrier tests, all someone has to do is rinse out his mouth with water," said Robert Williamson of St. Mary's Hospital and the University of London. "The water washes out enough cells from the inside of his cheek for us to retrieve DNA [deoxyribonucleic acid] and tell him within hours whether he carries the gene for cystic fibrosis, sickle-cell anemia, or thalassemia.[38]

Although such tests can only be done now for families where the disease has shown up, i.e., it's not an "orphan test," the researchers hope for such a test in a few years.

Preliminary Results

In March 1988, a study reported on 46 adults at risk for Huntington's who decided to take the predictive test.[39] Of these people, 19 were like Nancy Wexler and changed their minds after counseling. One person could not have the test done because his family was too small to allow adequate testing.

Of the remaining adults, four tested positive on the basis of the genetic marker, 5 others already exhibited Huntington's according to neurologic tests, making a total of 9 positive results. Seven people had negative results. Results for the rest were unavailable. All 9 positive patients reported "intermittent depression," but none were "hospitalized."

In 1989, Nancy Wexler said she had not taken the test because she now felt happy, and knowing she was negative wouldn't make her *that* much happier. But knowing she was positive would make her *very* unhappy.[40]

Arlo Guthrie has also decided not to take the test. He feels he has "escaped the trauma" which killed his father. He lives today with his wife and four children in western Massachusetts. Does he regret having children without knowing his status? No, he says, "Life is more important than learning about diseases. . . . I could've said I don't want to 'inflict pain and suffering' . . . [but] life is wonderful! There's a *lot* to live for."[41]

Nancy Wexler agrees. To people who want to be tested so they can decide, say, whether to go to law school, she says, "Go to law school! Develop your mind! What are you going to do if you're positive? Spend the rest of your life waiting to be a patient?"[42]

FURTHER READING

Joseph Fletcher, "Ethical Aspects of Genetic Controls," *New England Journal of Medicine*, 285:776–83 (1971).

Daniel Kevles, *In the Name of Eugenics: Genetics and the Uses of Human Heredity*, Knopf New York, 1985.

Gina Kolata, "Alcoholic Genes or Misbehavior?" *Psychology Today* (May 1988), pp. 34–37.

Charles McKay, "Ethical Issues in Research Design and Conduct: Developing a Test to Detect Carriers of Huntington's Disease," *IRB: A Review of Human Subjects Research*, 6(4):1–5.

Margery W. Shaw, "Genetics and the Law," *Encyclopedia of Bioethics*, Free Press, New York, 1978.

CHAPTER 16

Mandatory Testing for AIDS

Perhaps no modern disease raises so many ethical issues in medicine as does AIDS. Susan Sontag points out that AIDS has reinstated a "premodern conception of disease" in contemporary civilization, one where people are not sure how they get sick, what the sickness is, or whether physicians can do anything about the disease.[1] Moreover, "AIDS, like cancer, leads to a hard death." Heart disease is a "soft" death, like the ennobling tuberculosis of the Romantics. It does not rot the flesh or produce stigmata, as do AIDS and cancer, which transform the victim into one of "them."

This chapter's historical section surveys social reactions to past plagues and how other diseases have stigmatized their victims. It also gives a brief chronology of contemporary knowledge about AIDS.

HISTORICAL BACKGROUND

Plagues in History

The bubonic plague, or the Black Death, was caused by the bacillus *Yersinia pestis*, which came to man via bites of fleas, which in turn were transported by rats on ships and over land. The causative agents remained unknown for 500 years. The plague's more virulent, respiratory mode of infection made discovery of its true cause more difficult and made physicians reluctant to come near its victims. Daniel Defoe's *Journal of the Plague Year* about the epidemic of 1665 in London said "it is scarce credible what dreadful cases happened in particular families every day. People in the rage of distemper, or in the torment of their swellings, which was indeed intolerable, running out of their own government, raving and distracted, and oftentimes laying violent hands upon themselves, throwing themselves out at their windows, shooting themselves...."[2]

During this time, medicine accepted astrology, which held that plagues came from the conjunction of Saturn, Mars, and Jupiter. Plagues of the time seemed to be associated with earthquakes, which in turn released sulfurous miasmas. In this account, there was one small grain of truth, for miasmas surrounded sewage, which in turn attracted rats and their fleas.

Medicine might teach one thing, but everyone else saw the hand of higher powers. Plague was the curse of the Evil One, or God's punishment for exceptional sin. Either way, only God could end the disease. Men were pitiless sinners deserving nothing and must suffer to atone. In one procession, the pope himself crawled on his stomach through the mud, begging forgiveness for mankind's sins. In the 14th century, people marched from town to town, whipping one other (and thereby spreading fleas). As the Pulitzer-prize winning historian Barbara Tuchman wrote:

> Organized groups of 200 to 300…marched from city to city, stripped to the waist, scourging themselves with leather whips tipped with iron spikes until they bled. While they cried aloud to Christ and the Virgin for pity, and called upon God to "Spare us!," the watching townspeople sobbed and groaned in sympathy. These bands put on regular performances three times a day, twice in public in the church and a third in privacy. Organized under a lay Master for a stated period, usually 33 days to represent Christ's years on earth, the participants were required to pledge self-support at 4 pence a day or other fixed rate and to swear obedience to the Master. They were forbidden to bathe, shave, change their clothes, sleep in beds, talk or have intercourse with women without the Master's permission. Evidently this was not withheld, since the flagellants were later charged with orgies in which whipping combined with sex.[3]

But this noted historian says one group would not admit sins. Their persecution satisfied the need for a scapegoat. The Jews were blamed, and the "Toledo conspiracy" was hatched. Several Jews were tortured into confessing that they had left Toledo, Spain, carrying small cloth bags (actually containing the Torah) and had poisoned wells of European towns. It mattered little that the plague felled towns where Jews had never visited.

In addition, Tuchman writes, the usual rumors circulated that Jews kidnapped Christian children, killed them, and drank their blood in secret ceremonies. Jews at this time were easily identifiable by their distinctive clothes and hair (following traditions still followed by Orthodox Jews today). They were different, "other," un-Christian. They had to wear cloth yellow badges shaped like a head of horns to symbolize their work with Satan (in later concentration camps, they wore similar cloth pieces).

When the processions of flagellants reached the Jewish quarter of cities, Jews inside would often be killed. On January 9, 1349, in Basel, Switzerland, "several hundred" Jews were burned on an island where they had been herded inside a wooden settlement. In Strasbourg, Germany, 2000 Jews were taken to open graves, where all were killed (except for those who converted to Christianity on the spot).

In such times, courage was rare. Physicians who tended the sick died at very high rates, sometimes approaching 80 percent. As a consequence, many physicians decided their calling was elsewhere.[4] In Camus' *The Plague*, a sick Father Paneloux reluctantly feels he must trust in God rather than in physicians—for he had previously claimed that the plague was God's punishment for sinners—and so he pays the ultimate price in death.

Victims of Hansen's disease (leprosy) have always provoked fearful reactions. As they walked, victims had to wear cow bells which rang to warn others away. The Hansen's bacillus is only transmitted by prolonged exposure over many months, usually among family members, and enters through the skin or mucosa of the upper respiratory tract.[5] It incubates 3 to 5 years before showing lesions.

Similar reactions occurred in America's three great cholera epidemics. In 1813, Americans blamed wanton prostitutes, lazy blacks, drunken Irish, and the dirty poor for cholera. Sickness was due to low character. The wealthy fled to the countryside (and unknowingly, to clean water), proving that the virtuous did not succumb. Ministers praised God for bringing down cholera to "cleanse the filth from society." President Andrew Jackson opposed a national day of fasting to cure the disease, and ministers asked what else could be expected from such an atheist.[6]

The Lord supposedly operated through disease to punish the guilty and through miracles to reward the virtuous. The view was defended with no attention to logical consistency or ordinary observation, since some of the best people died, some of the worst, flourished.

In 1849, physician John Snow noted that victims in London lived in houses served by one water system and not another, and concluded that cholera spread via contaminated water. Snow's views had no effect on the epidemic of 1849. By 1862, when the third great cholera epidemic hit America, the enlightened were thinking along public health lines, but were not strong enough to prevent the normal toll of death. Not until the germ theory of disease was accepted by physicians in the 1890s and not until public health laws were passed, did cholera epidemics cease in America.

In the early part of the 20th century, victims of syphilis were treated as pariahs. In New York City, infected patients were kept on special wards so as to not infect others.[7]

Contemporary History

Recent years have witnessed three well-publicized threats to the public health besides AIDS. Government and media responded mightily to each of these threats, in contrast to government's later lack of response to AIDS.

In 1976, after an American Legion convention at a Philadelphia hotel, veterans returned home and suddenly started to die. The disease was of mysterious origin, infectious, and killed many of its victims. It was later learned that *Legionnella* bacteria had existed all along in nature and had probably killed 10 to 20 percent of past cases of unclassified pneumonia. Patients with Legionnaire's disease were not blamed for bringing it on themselves and were not widely feared. After the first deaths, the government spent $9 million to investigate causes of Legionnaire's disease.[8]

In 1978, some American women suddenly became dangerously sick from a mysterious cause. The Centers for Disease Control, or CDC, investigated toxic-shock syndrome and the television stations followed its progress with almost nightly reports. A cause was identified in 1980 in a neurotoxin produced by staphylococcus, which grew in new material in superabsorbent (especially Rely) tampons.

In October 1982, poisoned Tylenol capsules appeared. The CDC and the FDA spent millions of dollars and hundreds of thousands of work hours to discover how the capsules were poisoned. It was finally judged that one person had tampered with some packages. Within weeks, new tamper-resistant packages appeared. Moreover, and as a result, millions upon millions of dollars are now spent every year so that most over-the-counter drugs and toiletries are tamper-resistant (in order to please skittish customers). In all, seven people died from poisoned Tylenol capsules.

In June of 1981, the first medical report was published documenting three cases of the mysterious "homosexual cancer" which had been rumored to have killed dozens of gay men.[9] One month later, 108 cases were reported, with 43 deaths. Within another month, more people were dying from this disease than from the combined total of toxic shock syndrome, Tylenol poisoning, and Legionnaire's disease.

Nevertheless, the American government and its medical representatives did virtually nothing. AIDS afflicted different kinds of people—victims who were gay, people of color, drug users, and prostitutes. If 100 white housewives had mysteriously died in 1981, massive federal programs would have immediately started.

Spread of HIV in America

At the end of 1980, some physicians already suspected that the mysterious "gay cancer" was a lethal infectious organism, but there was no real evidence. Physicians began making requests from CDC for experimental drugs to treat *Pneumocystis carinii* pneumonia (PCP).

After CDC described these three cases of unexplained PCP in young gay men in June of 1981, it exhaustively interviewed sexually active gay men to see if substance abuse had destroyed their immune systems. It concluded that the only major risk factor was number of sexual partners.

Gay sex was postulated to be spreading some deadly disease, but this postulate was politically sensitive. Hostility to gay men was prevalent and reporters feared increasing it. Within the gay community, stances were intensely debated. As Larry Kramer portrayed himself in *The Normal Heart*, he worried that over 100 gays had died and no one was doing anything. He suspected that sex in bathhouses might be spreading the disease, but his suggestions were dismissed by gay men as Puritanical. After all, Jerry Falwell wanted to shut down bathhouses. Bathhouse owners spent big money in gay newspapers calling for sexual freedom.

Three months after CDC's July report of 108 cases of AIDS, it reported that babies of drug-addicted mothers in the Bronx seemed to have the "gay cancer." In July 1982, 1 year after the first cases, CDC formally defined acquired immune deficiency syndrome (AIDS). There was also a kind of "pre-AIDS" or "junior AIDS," called AIDS-related complex (ARC).

AIDS Terminology

The above history discusses some facts about AIDS which were not known during the early years (1981–1985) of research on AIDS. Researchers did not know until years later that AIDS was caused by a virus, that the virus had a very long incubation, that the virus could be spread in blood, and that viral infection was often fatal.

AIDS can be defined as the tip of a four-stage pyramid. The base consists of people engaging in at-risk behavior. The second level consists of people who test positive for antibodies to the human immunodeficiency virus (HIV). (The issue of "false positive" tests is discussed below.)

A person may have the virus for at least a year without forming detectable antibodies (a Birmingham nurse who got HIV through a needle-stick took 13 months to develop antibodies). A person may then test positive to HIV but remain asymptomatic for years. Normally, the body fights off dozens of infectious agents each day. But when symtoms such as swollen lymph nodes or night sweats develop, it is an indication that the person's immune system has begun to weaken, allowing opportunistic infections to invade. If the person develops serious opportunistic infections, the disease is considered to have progressed to the next stage: ARC. Physicians can treat many opportunistic infections of ARC, and some new drugs, such as AZT, slow the destruction of the immune system. A person may have ARC for many years. Only when the immune system is completely compromised is the disease classified as full-blown AIDS.[10]

By 1990, over 100,000 people had contracted AIDS. That figure does not include numbers of persons with ARC or HIV. Of these people, about 60 percent were dead, and the rest had a life expectancy of 2 to 3 years. By 1990, over 60,000 men had died from AIDS—more than the number of men who died in Vietnam.

In 1981, real facts about AIDS were hard to find and everything was very confusing. An excellent book about AIDS, Randy Shilts's *And the Band Played On*, first explained this confusion and documented the politics of AIDS research. Many of the details in this history are from Shilts's book.

In 1981, three CDC physicians had hypothesized that a new virus-borne epidemic had begun, that its cause was a virus which could cause the new specific cancers, and that massive new monies were needed. This was controversial because it would not be proven until 2 years later, in 1983, that a virus could cause even a rare cancer, and this proved nothing about most cancers. The name of the man who proved that there was a viral link was Robert Gallo.

In 1982, average survival in AIDS after immune weakening was 2 years. No adult AIDS patient achieved prolonged remission. In 1982, physicians in New York and California were seeing hundreds of new cases. Worse, the incubation period was unknown, and CDC guessed it could be as long as several years, which implied that millions could become infected.

That AIDS was spreading in 1982 became clear to CDC. By the 1970s, people could fly anywhere in the world in 15 hours, even from central Africa to America. In western countries, a new acceptance of drugs and sexuality between 1960 and 1980 had led to gay bathhouses and the sharing of intravenous (IV) drugs.

AIDS seemed to be transmitted by sharing needles among intravenous drug users. Between 1981 and 1987, the New York metropolitan area had 50 percent of American IV drug users and 82 percent of AIDS cases from IV drug usage.[11] People there went to drug houses where powdered drugs were diluted in water, heated in a bottle-cap "cooker," and sucked into a syringe attached to a needle. Blood was withdrawn from a vein into the syringe, where it was mixed with the drug before being reinjected. The same "works" (needle, syringe, and "cooker") would be rented by a series of customers and contaminated with small particles of blood.

AIDS was also transmitted sexually, especially in intercourse which ruptures sensitive anal membranes and transmits the virus into the bloodstream. Anal-receptive sex seemed to spread the virus in gays, as did heterosexual sex among people with poor hygiene and open genital sores from herpes, syphilis, and cuts.

A female's breast milk could also transmit the virus, especially to babies. "Blood, sex, and breast milk" were the routes of transmission. HIV is a fragile virus, killed by bleach or soap and water, and needs warm protective substance (blood, mucus, semen, or breast milk) for transmission from internal substances of one person to internal substances of another.

AIDS and the Blood Supply: A Failure of Mandatory Testing

In the summer of 1982, worries began about possible transmission of the causative agent of AIDS in donated blood. If it could be so transmitted, AIDS might kill thousands. In January 1983, representatives of the American Red Cross, commercial blood banks, hemophiliacs, pharmacy companies, and gay activists met together, but could not agree to screen blood for AIDS.

Although blood could not have been screened in 1982 for HIV, it could have been tested for hepatitis, which would have eliminated perhaps 80 percent of the HIV-infected blood. CDC proposed doing so, but was argued down. Opponents countered that screening blood would be expensive, would "quarantine" gay blood, and would be succumbing to hysteria, because no hard proof existed that AIDS was either caused by a virus or blood-borne. In October 1982, Irwin Memorial Blood Bank (serving all San Francisco hospitals) reported a proven, blood-transfusion case of AIDS. In May 1983, after several such cases in hemophiliacs, Stanford University Hospital's blood bank broke ranks with other hospitals and started screening. Irwin Memorial did not follow.

That summer, on July 17, 1983, Health and Human Services Secretary Margaret Heckler held a national televised press conference and confidently said: "I want to assure the American people that the blood supply is 100 percent safe....The blood supply is safe both for the hemophiliac who requires large transfusions and for the average citizen who might need it for surgery."[12] Dr. Joseph Bove, chairman of the FDA's committee overseeing blood transfusion, blamed existing concern about contaminated blood on "the overreacting press."

Secretary Heckler's assurance was shameful, as was her confident prediction in 1983 that a vaccine against AIDS would be available in 2 years. Neither was based on fact. Today, as many as 80 percent of hemophiliacs are HIV-positive. These mistakes made Americans skeptical of political appointees responsible for their health.

By March 1984, CDC counted 73 cases of transfusion-related AIDS, 24 in hemophiliacs (the first in Birmingham). The same Joseph Bove, now a spokesperson for the blood bank industry, dismissed fears of transfusion-related AIDS as irrational: "More people are killed by bee stings."[13] In May 1984, Irwin Memorial began screening its blood for hepatitis, 1 year after Stanford's hospital had done so. In anticipation of the new ELISA screening test, Irwin Memorial stored samples so it could later notify patients. By September 1984, CDC counted 80 cases of transfusion-related AIDS, 188 of transfusion-related ARC. Joseph Bove suddenly changed his views.

In January of 1985, a San Francisco woman who was both a prostitute and an IV-drug abuser tested positive for HIV. Heterosexuals became worried. Proof that heterosexuals tested positive for HIV accelerated release of the ELISA test in February 1985. Gay groups feared discrimination and opposed the test. Irwin Memorial immediately began testing in March 1985. The new tests reduced the risk of transfusion-related HIV in San Francisco from 1 to 440 to 1 in 1,000,000.

Almost 3 years later, in 1987, Irwin Memorial Blood Bank announced that between 1977 and 1983, at least 1 in 100 of its transfusions of blood were HIV-positive. It notified 30,000 former patients from 1984 that they should be tested, that it had already discovered 191 people who tested HIV-positive and 69 full-blown AIDS cases, and that a "minimum of 2,000 HIV-positives would be discovered." (It could not notify those patients who had become infected before 1984 and for whom it had not kept blood samples.) Los Angeles' Cedars-Sinai Hospital notified parents to check 900 babies who had received blood between 1980 and 1985.

Altogether, probably 1 million units of HIV-infected blood were transfused between 1982 and March 1985. That more did not develop AIDS reflects the fact that some people get many units of blood and the high mortality of medical interventions for which people get blood transfusions. Because of the age at which many people undergo serious surgery, because such surgery often occurs for likely terminal conditions such as pancreatic cancer, and because trauma victims in the emergency room are often too injured to live, perhaps half of those who received infected blood were dead of unrelated causes before they had a chance to develop antibodies to HIV, and perhaps two-thirds were dead before they could develop symptoms of AIDS. These facts explain why there are not presently thousands of cases of AIDS among postsurgical patients. However, given the long incubation period (possibly a decade), it is difficult to know how many people were infected.

1987: The Big Chill

Before 1987, the official medical and liberal view about AIDS was that irrationality was running wild, that evidence only indicated that 10 percent of those with HIV would get AIDS, and that the privacy of gays should be protected at all costs. By the end of 1987, things had changed.

In June 1986, 100 epidemiologists, statisticians, researchers, and immunologists met at the Coolfront Conference Center in Berkeley Springs, West Va. The prestigious Institute of Medicine and the United States Public Health Service (USPHS) made predictions for each year from 1987 to 1992. They predicted that by 1992, 179,000 Americans would die from AIDS (almost three times the number who died in Vietnam). In 1992, and barring some cure, another 91,000 would be dying of AIDS. Their projections for the early years have so far been accurate. Indeed, some government estimates place the numbers far higher.

Newspapers had already described so many "what if" scenarios that the new projections were ho-hum. Most writers had previously repeated the optimistic line that only 10 percent of HIV-positives would develop AIDS. However, in 1986 at the Coolfront conference, the projections dramatically jumped: at least 25 to 50 percent of those testing positive were predicted to develop AIDS. Virologists had hoped for "a hump," after which chances of developing AIDS would lessen in HIV-positives.[14] Instead, more and more people who tested positive would get AIDS, and with enough time, all might get it.

Ominous news also came in early 1985 from the new ELISA tests. In the late 1970s, blood of California gay men had been saved for studies on the hepatitis B vaccine. For the first time, solid data about HIV infection came out, indicating that half to two-thirds of these gay men were HIV-positive. Projections of HIV-positive Americans jumped, from 400,000, to 1 million, to 1.5 million. These estimates assumed 750,000 American IV-drug users and relied on Kinsey's estimate that 4 percent of American males (2.5 million) were exclusively gay and that another 5 to 10 million men had occasional gay sex.

Projections were somewhat uncertain, first, because not all states required reporting of HIV-positive cases and second, because the 1986 estimate of HIV incubation of 4.5 years was a median depending on individual variations, state of immune health, and dosage of exposure.

AIDS-Gate

Reporter Randy Shilts's *And the Band Played On*, in 1987, argued that prejudice against gays retarded AIDS research. Shilts said that federal scientists, physicians, and Reagan appointees resisted reports that HIV was lethal and infectious. Shilts blamed bureaucrats, gay leaders, reporters, and physicians for "letting" AIDS kill gay men. To most federal officials, AIDS in the early years wasn't important, whereas saving money was. Some bigots even hoped that AIDS would go away after killing most gays and drug addicts.

Shilts charges that Robert Gallo coveted the Nobel prize and that he prevented anyone else from surpassing him in AIDS research. Worse, Shilts charges that France's Luc Montagnier in fact discovered HIV, that Gallo actively prevented scientific reporting of Montagnier's discovery, that Gallo tried to grab credit by reinterpreting HIV to be a member of the family of viruses Gallo had accidentally discovered, that Gallo manipulated patriotic feelings of American researchers to turn against Montagnier, and finally, that Gallo obtained a sample of Montagnier's virus from CDC and claimed it for his own.

In an extraordinary incident in the history of science, a compromise was worked out between the American and French governments. Gallo was held to be a "codiscoverer" of HIV because he supposedly figured out how to keep the virus' cell line alive. Privately, American scientists pointed out that Gallo had patented his cell line in America, so that the French could make no money in the big American AIDS market without his help. In one incident reported by Shilts, Gallo presented an electron-microscopic picture of his sample of HIV. Such samples normally vary in the same strain by 6 to 20 percent in structure. Shilts reports that Gallo's sample differed by less than 1 percent from Montagnier's—an unheard-of coincidence—and that the scientists present realized that Gallo's sample was the same as Montagnier's.[15]

How much of this is true is unclear. Years after Shilts's book appeared, on television Gallo is still called "America's premier AIDS researcher." Shilts still believes that Gallo is an eloquent, charming egomaniac whose quest for power retarded AIDS research. A Presidential AIDS Commission concluded in 1988 that the government's AIDS research (headed by Gallo) lacked coordination and leadership.

This is tragic. Here is a disease which had 100,000 cases by 1990, with nearly 300,000 cases predicted by 1993. Yet the government still had not begun a coordinated attack with a real leader.

The Famous Get an Infamous Disease

Roy Cohn, Senator Joe McCarthy's lawyer, tried to disguise his diagnosis of AIDS in 1985. AIDS is often disguised in notices as "pneumonia" or "cancer," and has hence been underreported. A great cultural shock came in 1986 when actor Rock Hudson was discovered to be dying of AIDS. With that news, America took another step away from perceiving AIDS as only a disease of deviants. The all-American hero of *Giant* and countless movies with Doris Day—a man with rugged, he-man looks and macho physique—had died of AIDS. President Reagan's personal physician said that only after Rock Hudson died of AIDS did the president express interest to him about this new disease. Other famous men who died of AIDS include clothes designer Perry Ellis, Washington Redskins pass-receiver Jerry Smith, Terry Nolan, cofounder of the National Conservative Political Action Committee, gay physician and Olympic decathlete Thomas Waddell, pianist Liberace, and the first black television anchor, Max Robinson.

MANDATORY TESTING FOR HIV

One of the first opportunities to test for AIDS arose over donated blood between 1983 and 1985, when the opportunity was not taken. In March 1985, with the arrival of the cheap, reliable ELISA test, authorities began testing. Such testing was *mandatory* in that all blood was tested. People with a positive test were notified, and in states where reporting was required, results were forwarded to state authorities.

Whether and how to test for HIV will be an ethical issue for many years. Proposals abound for premarital testing, preadmission testing in hospitals, preinsurance testing, and pre-employment testing (including the Armed Forces as employers). Such testing creates passionate, conflicting opinions. On one side are those who resist any mandatory testing at all, and on the other, those who wish to test all Americans. The arguments below discuss the goals of such testing, whether such testing reflects prejudice, and whether it would work.

ETHICAL ISSUES

In the discussion below, arguments favoring mandatory testing for HIV are first examined, followed by arguments against mandatory testing.

ARGUMENTS FAVORING MANDATORY TESTING

Lessons from the Blood Supply

Conservatives in public health derive an important lesson from the failure to test blood between 1983–1985, and argue as follows. In the early years when AIDS mysteriously appeared, civil libertarians and gay activists intimidated blood banks into not screening, and as a result, thousands of people became HIV-positive. Even if donors did not want to know themselves, they had no right to donate in ignorance of their HIV-status.

Confidentiality for gay men was not more important than human lives, and fears about confidentiality were groundless. Sex researchers William Masters, Virginia Johnson, and Robert Kolodny emphasize that no scandal has occurred from the years of screening since March of 1985, even though thousands of people have been identified.[16] They say that the lesson of the blood supply is that society must screen whenever possible.

Contact Tracing and Expanded Testing

Medical ethicist Ronald Bayer of the Hastings Center was being interviewed in 1985 on a national talk show. He outlined the problems about confidentiality and discrimination against HIV-positive individuals. With equally grave tones, he emphasized how cases would mushroom in future years. At this, his host asked in exasperation: "If I understand you correctly, you're saying that millions of people will become infected and die, but because of concerns about prejudice and confidentiality, we have to just let it happen?" Bayer reiterated that education could slow HIV's spread—a view also stressed countless times by public health school dean, June Osborne, in various national media.[17]

The above position seemed fatalistic to many people. In 1989, a survey of entering college freshmen found the vast majority were dissatisfied with this "testing is ineffective" position. Are the freshmen correct? Can society really do no effective testing to prevent the spread of HIV? Are motives to test only prejudicial? Are any legitimate? Isn't testing about saving lives, not exposing people with secret lives? Should society really just stand back and say, "Nothing else can be done"?

Moreover, should society assume that most people, upon learning they are HIV-positive, are really likely to go on infecting others? Even if only 25 percent of people change their behavior, a 25 percent decline in the spread of HIV, multiplied over many people, is a significant decrease. If as many as half of those testing HIV-positive change their ways, things would be even better.

Finally, the arguments that mandatory premarital testing won't work generally are made by civil libertarians. Faced with these arguments, champions of testing say society must have enough will "to do what is necessary" to save lives, i.e., to do things which would be ethically repugnant to obtain lesser goals. Rights of individuals were abused in the past for bad reasons, e.g., in the McCarthy era and in the quarantine of Japanese-Americans during World War II, but simply because past mistakes occurred, it does not follow that drastic measures are never justified. Mandatory testing is nowhere near as drastic as is quarantine or job discrimination.

Masters, Johnson, and Kolodny advocate that both sex and drug contacts should be traced. So does Congressman William Dannemeyer, who wrote, "It is absurd and unwise public policy to trace persons with a nonfatal venereal disease and counsel them about the risks of transmission but to fail to take the same prudent steps with persons who may have acquired or carry a 100 percent fatal disease."[18]

There is nothing new about contact tracing. Public health officials have become quite sensitive and skilled in doing it. No reason exists why the same could not be done for HIV-positive cases. One strong argument for such tracing is as follows. Many people are in denial about their possible condition. Just as women do not want to do breast self-examinations for possible cancer, so people with possible exposure to HIV would rather not know. Contact tracing breaks though such denial and motivates action. It also creates guilt about possibly infecting someone new.

According to the tough-minded view of Masters, Johnson, and Kolodny, the problem is not mandatory testing but not going far enough. They write that "if implementation of effective prevention strategies is delayed by a mistaken belief that this epidemic is now under control or by a single-minded preoccupation with individual autonomy, many millions of lives will be needlessly lost."[19]

Discovering the Incidence and Rate of Spread of HIV

The above sex researchers emphasize that no one really knows the true incidence of HIV and its true rate of spread to heterosexuals. Mandatory testing, they say, would at least establish accurate data.

Because no one else had any data, these sex researchers went out to find their own data and discovered some controversial results. They did not randomly sample heterosexuals, and to accuse them for not doing so is to miss their point. They emphasize that in past breakouts of sexually transmitted diseases such as herpes, 5 percent of the population accounted for 50 percent of new infections. Moreover, the incidence of such diseases correlated with the number of sexual partners. Members of the "study group" of heterosexuals (200 men, 200 women) had at least six sex partners each year over the previous 5 years. Previous studies indicated that fewer than 5 percent of Americans under 40 met this criterion. Additionally, members of the subject group could have no history, since 1977, of using drugs, blood transfusion, or homosexual sex. To get 430 such subjects (30 for backup), over 2000 singles had to be interviewed. To get a more national representation, subjects came from not only New York and California but also from St. Louis and Atlanta (50 men and 50 women from each city).

Four hundred monogamous heterosexuals were the control group, selected initially from a thousand persons married at least 5 years, then from the 568 of these who avowed fidelity over these years, and finally culled from the 485 who were "highly confident" of their partner's fidelity. (Even with all this care, one married man was HIV-positive.) The controls came from the same cities and met the same exclusionary criteria as the study group.

For women in the study group with more than 12 partners a year (for each year during the previous 5 years), 14 percent were HIV-positive. For the same group of men, 12 percent were HIV-positive. Overall, and in the less-active majority of the study group with 6 to 12 partners per year, 7 percent of the women and 5 percent of the men were infected. In New York, 10 percent of the women in the study group were infected.

Such data appear to indicate that the spread of HIV among heterosexual Africans is a good predictor *only for the small percentage of Americans who are extremely sexually active with multiple partners.* Of the 200 men in the study group, none regularly used condoms and only 6 of the same 200 women regularly asked male partners to do so. Africans in AIDS-infected areas have unprotected sex each week with several partners, especially the hundreds of thousands of prostitutes and the millions of men who patronize them.[20] Because of this number of different sexual partners, because of the prevalence there of other diseases weakening the body such as malaria, shingles, and syphilis, and because of frequent sores on genitals of Africans, the African experience is closer to the previous norm for gays than the norm for heterosexual Americans.

In February 1988, CDC's James Curran said there that were nearly 2000 cases of AIDS classified as due to heterosexual sex.[21] The vast majority of these came from having sex with a drug-using partner. For the average heterosexual, the danger is small of getting HIV from sexual activity. CDC estimates that one act of sex with a person with unknown HIV status has a risk of HIV infection of 1 in 5 million without a condom, 1 in 50 million with a condom. If a partner has a negative HIV test and condoms are used, chances of HIV infection jump to one in 5 *billion.*

So the sex researchers' data has uncertain implications. Yes, HIV can be acquired heterosexually, especially by not using condoms and having sex with partners who take risks. But whether HIV will soon be "epidemic" among heterosexuals depends on how much sex occurs and with whom.

New York City veteran public health officer Anastasia Lekatsas believes that most men lie about how they became HIV-positive. She dismisses other studies by social scientists who use easy-to-use questionnaires, rather than nondirective interviews which take hours and which gain the trust of each man (as Kinsey did too in his pioneering studies).[22] She claims that 99.5 percent of cases of HIV-positive men who claim they became infected through heterosexual intercourse, in fact used drugs or were bisexual. Of 15,000 AIDS cases in New York City by 1988, only 8 men are listed as having became HIV-positive from a woman (and Lekatsas "has doubts about 7 of them.") It is not that HIV-positive men necessarily lie, but it's possible that those who patronize prostitutes, often inebriated, don't realize they're having sex with men who are transvestites or transsexuals. Indeed, in having quick sex with some of these prostitutes in cars, some customers may not realize they're having anal sex.

Expanded Testing Once More

Masters, Johnson, and Kolodny advocated mandatory testing for HIV for pregnant women, for hospital admissions between ages 15 and 60, for premarital applicants, and for prostitutes. They argued that pregnant mothers should at least be given the choice about bringing a baby into the world with a 40 to 50 percent chance of having HIV. In prehospital admissions, testing would document the spread of HIV. Moreover, HIV-positive patients may have adverse reactions to certain vaccines. Patients with ARC or "pre-ARC," with possibly compromised immune systems, should be kept away from patients with infectious illnesses.

Masters, Johnson, and Kolodny dismiss objections that people will avoid marriage to avoid the tests, that violations of civil rights outweigh the benefits of mandatory testing, and that too many false positives will occur. They argue:

> First, it is interesting to see that no one is insisting that the blood supply shouldn't be screened because of the problem of too many false positives. Yet the percentage of false positives in screening blood donors is precisely the same as it would be in a mandatory HIV testing program (because exactly the same laboratory tests with exactly the same sources of error would be used). Second, as the prevalence of HIV infection increases in the general population, as it inevitably must do over time until a vaccine is found, the relative number of false positive tests will decrease. This general principle of screening programs is of particular importance because the need for mandatory premarital testing will be even more acute if the prevalence of infection in the general population becomes considerably higher than it is today. We are afraid that this is exactly what is going to happen. Playing ostrich in the face of this reality is not going to save lives or diminish the anguish in our world—in fact, it will have precisely the opposite effect.[23]

In response, it can be argued that their point about false positives in the blood supply is misleading. So what if extra blood is disregarded because it is falsely positive? This is very different from falsely telling a pregnant women or engaged man that she or he has HIV.

Quarantine: A Goal of Mandatory Testing?

Tough-minded people sometimes contemplate quarantine of those who test HIV-positive. It is important to think through such measures and to understand the problems. First, the number of people who test HIV-positive presents logistical nightmares. Perhaps 2 million Americans are infected. Where would they go? Which state would become the "AIDS camp?" How would they be guarded? Would visitors be allowed? Who would prevent rich inmates from making bribes? If those with HIV are quarantined, and if they perceive this to be unjust, why should they refrain from sex before they're quarantined? Will the 2 million foreign tourists be screened each year?

Second, quarantine would require compulsory testing of every American, and each would have to be retested each year for new infections. Third, the quarantine of people with HIV might be indefinite. It is not clear if people with HIV will ever be noninfectious. Until there is a safe, cheap vaccine which could be given to sexually active people, those who test HIV-positive might have to stay in insolation forever.

Third, many of these people would become sick. If quarantine occurred in some rural area, expensive hospitals would have to be built and would require physicians and nurses. The quarantined patients would lose their jobs and, hence their medical insurance (most people get medical insurance through their jobs). As such, government would have perhaps 2 million unemployed people with HIV who would require expensive medical care in an area without such care.

Still, quarantine might be selectively used for individuals who cannot refrain from spreading the virus. Several states have reactivated "Typhoid Mary" laws to isolate such individuals. If a person is compulsively or wantonly spreading the lethal virus through indiscriminate needle-sharing, prostitution, or casual sex, society must preserve life and isolate him or her.

However, more generally, when people adopt the perspective of quarantine, it seems justified only for immediate, life-threatening situations. People without HIV are not threatened by being around HIV-positive people and can safeguard themselves simply by not having unsafe sex and not sharing needles. The blood supply is already screened. Thus, most people are not in danger from those with HIV and quarantine is both unjustified and, ultimately, based on unfactual premises.

Finally, quarantine imposes great harm on people: the quarantined Japanese-Americans during World War II experienced ruined careers, lost real estate, and had their patriotism questioned. They suffered great assaults on their dignity and rights to lead normal lives. In retrospect, the possible danger from possible Japanese-American spies did not justify the quarantine. Similarly, quarantine of HIV-positive people today is not justified.

Tatoos

William F. Buckley, Jr. first proposed, in the mid-1980s, putting permanent tattoos on HIV-positive people. Such a plan might indeed warn some people of the possible dangers.

However, such a proposal has problems. People vary in skin color. People vary in how they get HIV. If such a tattoo were placed near the genitals, it would not help drug users. At the very least, a tattoo would need to be placed on the face, or two tattoos would be needed.

Such tattoos would subject bearers to great social stigma. In addition to likely suffering from ARC and AIDS, those with tattoos would suffer more harm. Such a policy could be conceivably justified, but it would have to meet two stringent conditions. First, strong evidence would be needed that such tattoos would—in fact—prevent acquisition of new HIV infections. Evidence is needed about why people take risks of becoming infected with HIV, why, and what (if anything) deters people from taking such risks. Second, an argument would be needed that the additional harm to victims—

from discrimination, stigma, and lack of self-esteem—is overcome by gains in saved lives.

Finally, putting such tattoos on people would discourage most people from being tested—it would be like, if you went to the clinic and got a positive result, you would be held down and branded. And what if it was a false positive?

ARGUMENTS AGAINST MANDATORY TESTING

Decriminalizing Homosexuality

Perhaps the root issue of all ethical issues about AIDS concerns the morality of homosexuality. Voluntary testing for HIV would improve, and mandatory testing would be less needed, if homosexuals could not be arrested for their sexuality and if people could not be fired for homosexuality.

Many people argue that homosexuality is neither unnatural nor immoral, just as heterosexuality is neither unnatural nor immoral. What is immoral is hurting others, not sex. If certain forms of sex involve hurting others, then harm has been done, just as when certain college sports can involve hurting (exploiting) students. What is wrong is the harm, not the context of the harm. Sexuality involves private life and is therefore not the concern of the government or police. Must not some part of life be private and separate from public life?

Perhaps the root ethical question is whether hostility toward homosexuals manifests *prejudice*. Almost as soon as the first victims appeared, Jerry Falwell blamed gays for AIDS. Other clergy blamed gay men for spreading the virus by "promiscuous sodomy." The national secretary of Moral Majority wrote that, "If homosexuals are not stopped, they will in time infect the entire nation, and America will be destroyed—as entire civilizations have fallen in the past."[24] The head of the Southern Baptist Convention said God created AIDS to "indicate his displeasure with the homosexual lifestyle."[25] Monsignor Edward Clark of St. John's University in Queens claimed that, "If gay men would stop promiscuous sodomy, the AIDS virus would disappear from America."[26] Patrick Buchanan once said, "The poor homosexuals—they have declared war upon nature, and now nature is exacting an awful retribution."[27] When babies and hemophiliacs came down with AIDS, people distinguished between "innocent" victims and "other" (i.e., gay, and drug-using) victims.

Critics retort that gays were not innocent because they knew that practices such as anally receptive intercourse and oral/anal contact ran risks of hepatitis, syphilis, and gastrointestinal diseases. Moreover, they claimed, gay men were neurotic about sex, focusing on quantity rather than quality, on sex rather than love and commitment. For such critics, AIDS was a predictable consequence of the past sexual behavior of gays.

Against this view, scholars have argued that gay sex has been a fact in civilization since before the time of Jesus. Bisexuality was popular in ancient

Greece, and many famous Greeks then preferred male lovers. Famous people have been gay or bisexual, including Socrates, many of the Roman emperors, including Hadrian (of "Hadrian's Wall" fame), probably Michelangelo, King Fredrick II, playright Tennessee Williams, and novelist Gore Vidal.[28] Christianity vigorously attacked homosexuality after the 12th century, but before then was much more tolerant.[29] In his 1950s study, Alfred Kinsey found that 37 percent of white male adults had had sex with another male to orgasm—indicating that many men disguise their gay experiences.[30]

Is Testing a Prejudicial "Purification Rite"?

Some critics see a much darker purpose behind mandatory testing, especially mandatory premarital testing (required in Illinois and Louisiana). Some thinkers see such testing as a symbolic "purification ritual" where the cultural response to AIDS goes far beyond the danger to public health. HIV carriers represent "dirt" which must be "cleansed" by the system: "dirt" represents chaos and disorder. Such "dirt" must be cleansed by symbolic ritual, creating not only a physical but also a spiritual cleansing. It matters not that nothing really happens as a result of such rituals, that no new cases of AIDS are prevented, or that innocent false positives are harmed. What is important is an impression is created that something is being done to identify the "unholy." Philosopher Richard Mohr agrees:

> Mandatory AIDS antibody testing laws are social purification rituals
> through which, by calling for sacrifices of and by the dominant culture,
> that culture reaffirms the sanctity of compulsory heterosexuality and
> rededicates heterosexuality's centrality and controlling place in society.
> The imprecatory counterpoint of such sanctification is the degradation
> of gays, even though in part for social convenience and moral salve, the
> laws make no mention of them.[31]

He adds a bit later:

> When a government uses coercion to express a society's deepest values
> and establish or rededicate them as sacred, there will be no stopping it
> however odious and immoral its acts, for these values are already come
> to be embedded in a pre-institutional social knowledge which serves as
> a lens through which all else is judged.

Critics retort that Mohr confuses antigay prejudice with anti-AIDS efforts, as well as confusing promoting heterosexuality with promoting public health. Moreover, the ideas of dirt and purification were not entirely metaphorical because the blood system was in fact once contaminated with the lethal HIV virus.

Much of this argument depends on whether mandatory testing would actually prevent spread of HIV, so that the final answer must depend on an evaluation of the arguments below. The basic point concerns whether mandatory testing is designed to prevent the spread of HIV, or to identify and punish certain people for their alternative lifestyles.

Morally Contradictory?

Another argument against mandatory testing involves thinking through what will be done with positive results. Society is largely dependent on the HIV-positive person to refrain from unsafe practices. Can forcing a person to take a test elicit the desired voluntary restraint? The policy of mandatory testing seems internally contradictory. Some states and institutions requiring mandatory testing also require mandatory reporting of results. Thus, society violates a person's privacy twice, once by testing him against his will, and once by reporting his positive results. Then it asks him "to do the moral thing" by voluntarily ceasing his unsafe practices. If society uses moral persuasion, it should be on firm moral ground itself in doing so.

Second, people change their sexual behavior slowly, even with the best of professional counseling. Little money has come forth for drug counseling, much less for counseling those with HIV. When counseling really changes behavior, there must be more than a 1-hour session explaining prevention.

It may be especially difficult with prostitutes, whose income and lifestyle depend on this behavior. Will they easily give up their profession after being tested? Some prostitutes, who make $50,000 a year, tax free, will not easily find other ways to obtain this income. If not, will they quit prostitution?

Changing actual behavior requires months and even years of counseling. Perhaps 90 percent of those who are drug-dependent and HIV-positive and who need extensive counseling may not get it. Only a small portion of money has been allocated for counseling HIV-positive patients. If education is failing to halt the spread of HIV, then society is at a crossroads: either abandon mandatory testing or continue mandatory testing but with counseling.

In one study of over 2000 gay men in Pittsburgh, about 40 percent of the subjects elected not to learn the results of their HIV tests.[32] They tended to be poorly educated, nonwhite, young, and worried that they could not "psychologically" accept a positive result.

Physician Neil Schram also argues against mandatory testing:

> What the political palliatives ignore is human nature. People who want to be tested can be tested now. Those who are most likely to need testing are also most likely to resist the idea, and if coerced, to find a way out. If premarital testing for AIDS is made mandatory, people who are reluctant will simply choose to live together—and to continue high-risk sexual activity....
>
> Politicians have the power to remove the major disadvantages by enacting anti-discrimination legislation, by funding programs to teach health care professionals how to counsel, and by funding mental health and similar support services for those who test positive.

When political leaders, from the President on down, urge widespread testing, they should also guarantee that this will not constitute punishment. It would cost the government nothing to remove such barriers as the Justice Department's opinion that fear—no matter how unjustified—is reason enough to allow an employer to fire an employee who tests positive for the AIDS antibody....

Until there is good post-test counseling, as well as anti-discrimination legislation, wide-scale testing will result in despair and tragedy with very little effect in slowing the spread of the virus. And such testing will have the additional ill effect of lulling Americans into believing that nothing will happen to them because "something" is being done, somewhere, to others.[33]

Privacy

Privacy is a great good. It allows us to control what happens to our bodies, our lives, and to some extent, the opinions others have of us. It is one reason people want to come to America from foreign countries where secret police tap telephones.

Privacy in medicine is perhaps more important than privacy in other areas of life. Medicine often deals with a person's ultimate values. When people see a physician, they are often embarrassed. They may need to expose their genitals to a stranger. They may be forced by pain or disease into revealing details of their life which they would otherwise never reveal to strangers, e.g., that they drink too much or take illegal drugs. Medical privacy protects the core of personal life. Anything which endangers this risks destroying the great value of life.

Mandatory testing runs just such a risk. In some cases, there is no sense in doing mandatory testing if a person is allowed to keep the result confidential, e.g., for prehospital admissions. Mandatory testing may then weaken the right to privacy—not only for those with HIV but for everyone. (If government can mandatorily test for HIV, why not for drug use? Alcoholism? Genetic markers?)

If, and that is a big "if," there is a great definite benefit from violating confidentiality and violating the right to privacy, mandatory HIV testing might be considered. But other arguments would need to prove that such violations would actually stop the spread of HIV. In many cases, that proof is lacking.

Inadequate Tests

Two technical problems present obstacles to mandatory testing: false positives and delayed antibody response. The ELISA and Western Blot tests both have "false positive" results. The ELISA and Western Blot tests were designed for high sensitivity, i.e., to make the "net" of the test as wide as possible so that few HIV carriers escape detection. In general populations, as many as 1 in 3 "positive" results for antibodies to the AIDS virus can be mistaken.[34] This is actually a double false positive, because it is the result of at least one ELISA test and one Western Blot.

A 1987 medical study estimated that of 3.8 million people screened, 1325 would be HIV-positive on the ELISA test.[35] Of those who test positive, 1219 would be repeatedly positive on a Western Blot test. Of these, 382 would really not have the HIV virus. Such tests would cost $23 million. Because some of these couples will have had coitus, about 70 partners would already be infected. So 1150 people with real HIV would be identified by mandatory premarital testing, costing $20,000 each.

Opponents of testing argue that the number of cases of HIV prevented by such testing would be small and that it would be better to spend the $23 million and thousands of hours of labor targeting specific groups. This is especially true because, without real counseling, merely identifying those with HIV does little to stop the spread of HIV.

The problem of false positives is less severe in high-risk populations, where false positives drop to 2 to 5 percent. *The test's accuracy is a function of the true incidence of the virus in a population.* In a high-risk population where 1 in 20 people is infected, a positive ELISA is much more likely to be accurate than in a low-risk population where 1 in 10,000 is infected. In general, the number of false positives varies inversely with the incidence of the virus in the general population, i.e., there are many more false positives in a population with 0.1 percent incidence (the 1987 estimate for the United States population) than with 5 percent incidence. In general populations, i.e., those with less than 1 percent expected incidence, the number of false positive has been high.

The high number of false positives explains why some AIDS counselors stress that being ELISA positive is only being positive for the antibody to HIV and that ELISA does not test for the virus itself. As can be seen from the above account, this advice is both true and false. If a person has no risk factors, chances increase of a false positive. On the other hand, if a person has engaged in risky behavior, chances of false positives decrease.

How is a false positive result detected? There are two ways. First, more sophisticated tests can be done to detect the virus itself (see below). Results of these tests can be compared to the cheaper tests used in screening. Second, researchers can wait to see who does and who does not develop symptoms among those who test HIV-positive. Unfortunately, this takes many years.

From a humane point of view, telling a person she is HIV-positive, when she is not, is cruel. Of 100,000 patients screened from a general population, say for hospital admission, 15 would be expected to test positive twice on the ELISA test and again on the Western Blot. Of these, only ten would truly have the virus, and five would not. From an equally humane point of view, stressing that the test might be a false positive allows people some hope, and such hope may be necessary to reflect on how to live with the results.

Regardless of the number of false positives in general populations, the problem is virtually nonexistent in high-risk populations. Thus, there may be good reasons for mandatory screening in high-risk populations, reasons which do not hold for general populations. It may be that every person using a methadone or sexual-disease clinic should get an HIV test. It may be that a "high risk" profile can be identified, similar to the one used at airports on suspected terrorists. Regardless of the objections to this on other grounds, there would be few false positives if the profile in fact correlated to high-risk factors.

What Are the Goals of Mandatory Testing?

One way to make motives clear is for leaders to emphasize whether such testing will be used to the detriment of those tested. Will premeds be denied admission to medical school? Will tested patients be excluded from high-risk operations? Will expenses be paid for counseling for those who have no medical insurance, or will they simply be told in one counseling session?

In some cases, the goals are sadly clear. Reports abound of hospitals testing patients, scheduling them for surgery, and then transferring patients elsewhere when they come back HIV-positive. Preadmission medical testing may seek to (1) reduce (perceived) risk to staff, (2) reduce losses (the insurance company may refuse to pay when learning of HIV-positive status because patients recently obtained such insurance, or because the policy excludes such costs, leaving the hospital with a very sick, very costly, indigent patient), or (3) decide upon the best long-term medical care. Any, or all, of the above may be used to justify preadmissions testing.

The most prejudicial goal is to reduce the "dirt" in the hospital (we don't want "them" here). Representative William Dannemeyer of California says that, "AIDS victims and all those who have been exposed must be forced to acknowledge the severity of their condition and take responsibility for the consequences of their actions and inactions."[36] For new cases of HIV, Dannemeyer's attitude seems to be, "You knew there was risk and now you are infected. You are going to die, and the least you can do is not complain when we identify you as a person who could kill others."

Mandatory Testing to Prevent Occupational Risk

In one study of residents treating gay AIDS patients at San Francisco General Hospital, 84 percent of male house staff felt anxiety about risks to their health around gay AIDS patients but very few female house staff did.[37] Either male residents knew something that female residents didn't, or irrational anxieties were present.

Nationally known physicians reacted similarly. Dudley Johnson, a leader in coronary bypass surgery, refused to do complex operations on HIV-positive patients. He specialized in patients at high risk and "re-operations." Johnson claims he is sometimes bathed in blood for 8 hours and that his underwear is soaked with blood. "Today I cleaned a dozen specks of blood off my glasses. How many specks of blood can you get in your eye before you're infected?" he said.[38]

Others say that logic requires consistency. In January 1987, Chicago's Cook County Hospital removed a staff physician who tested positive for HIV. Ian Carr, president of the hospital's medical staff, disagreed, saying the physician should continue seeing patients and that patients did not need to be informed. Cook County commissioners defended the public, saying that physicians had never claimed there was no risk, only "minimal risk."[39]

Between 1981 and 1987, roughly 6 percent of AIDS patients were health care workers (roughly 2000 of 32,000 patients). If this holds true, and since there are many more asymptomatic HIV-positive people than ARC or AIDS patients, there are many HIV-positive physicians, nurses, and lab workers. If hospitals have a right to know the HIV status of patients, don't patients have a right to know the HIV status of their attendants? If all patients should be tested to overcome unsafe practices due to ignorance, shouldn't all staff be tested to overcome the same?

Along this line, three authors emphasize that "safer" sex with condoms reduces risk of exposure to HIV in heterosexuals with unknown infected partners to the same magnitude of risk of surgeons of getting HIV from unknown infected patients. The authors then ask:

> If the risks of sexual and surgical contact are of the same order of magnitude, why should we eschew screening in low-risk heterosexual populations but recommend it for low-risk patients awaiting surgery? Arguing that we should screen low-risk patients before surgery implies that preventing HIV infection in a physician, a nurse, or a technician is more important than preventing the infection in others. Is that argument either rational or ethical? Hepatitis B virus is at least an order of magnitude more prevalent and more infectious than HIV, yet we do not routinely screen patients for hepatitis B virus. How many false-positive results are tolerable to protect one health-care worker? What is the joint false-positive rate for HIV testing of hospitalized patients? How many patients should be denied adequate medical care to prevent one hospital-acquired infection?[40]

Someone may reply that the fears are irrational because there is so little risk either from physicians to patients or vice versa. Moreover, an ancient dictum of medical ethics is, *Primum, non nocere*—meaning, first do not harm patients. But mandatory testing may harm some patients (e.g., through false positives). Thus, to prevent a minuscule risk to physicians, some patients are harmed by physicians.

Medical personnel reply that any risk of death from AIDS is not worth taking. At least, they say, they should have a choice about it.

These issues of occupational risk and prejudice are complex. Many medical residents say they would rather not treat AIDS patients, and that it was not unethical to refuse to care for AIDS patients. Residents in New York City hospitals, in 1988, cared for an average of 39 AIDS patients each, and 66 of them had stuck themselves collectively 96 times with HIV-positive blood. Between 1982 and 1987, medical residents in New York, San Francisco, Miami, and Los Angeles cared for perhaps 50 percent of 33,000 AIDS patients.[41] Such cases overwhelmed many residents, as with the following one:

> But in my three years at Bellevue, AIDS grew to engulf the hospital; it dominated my medical training, and now it dominates my memories.

> I remember the weekend when no patient in the intensive care unit was over the age of forty. I remember the intern who tearfully refused to come to the emergency room to see the fourth AIDS patient I had admitted to her in as many hours. She never did meet him; he died before she calmed down. I remember the meal trays, stacked precisely three and four deep, undistributed, outside the closed doors of the private rooms on one of the medical wards. And I remember Nilda, a drug addict who, like many others at the time, had a fever we couldn't explain; one morning, in my usual state of exhaustion, I jammed the needle I had just used to draw her blood, deep into my thumb.[42]

Society may have a right to require some physicians to treat HIV-positive patients, but does it have the right to require residents (such as Abigail Zuger above) to be saints? Doesn't society owe those at the bedside the advantage of knowing who is infected?

All staff are supposed to act "as if" all patients are infected, according to CDC recommendations, but this isn't realistic for harried personnel, e.g., in New York City with a critical shortage of nurses and where one nurse already does the work which three formerly did. Nevertheless, the uncertainties of mass testing and the low risk of accidental transmission imply a low presumed benefit to staff, whereas consequences of false positives and discrimination (loss of medical insurance) imply a much greater evil to infected patients.

Will Mandatory Testing Prevent AIDS?

Mandatory testing is usually justified, not to prevent occupational risk, not to "cleanse" the system, not to reduce costs, and not even to plan for maximal patient care, but to prevent the spread of HIV to more people. This major justification of mandatory testing needs to be evaluated.

In all proposals, it is important to think through what, if anything, is going to happen with infected people to prevent more cases of infection. With couples about to be married today, chances are high that they have already had sex. If so, if one was infected, both may now be infected. If premarital testing is to prevent spread of HIV, such couples either will need to not marry, or marry without having sex.

If a couple does not get married after one is HIV-positive, this does not necessarily mean that the HIV-positive person ceases at-risk behavior. Yet the assumption of premarital testing seems to be that the HIV-positive person would become celibate and drug free. Is this realistic?

Even then things are not simple. Only 40 to 50 percent of HIV-positive babies really have the virus, and for this reason, and because some HIV-positive mothers don't want to be alone in dying, few HIV-positive mothers abort.

Although selfish, the only question relevant to mandatory testing concerns whether such testing would in fact prevent spread of HIV. Would it better to be morally correct about blame and have an extra million people infected, or be morally neutral and have no new infections?

Past experience fighting syphilis teaches a lesson. In the first half of the 20th century, the American antisyphilis movement sharply divided between crusaders opposing sinful sex and crusaders opposing syphilis.[43] Those who believed in virginal marriage preached abstinence and opposed distributing condoms. Generals during World War I worried that more doughboys might die of venereal disease than war and overruled politicians, giving their soldiers newly manufactured latex condoms. The same pattern repeated in World War II, during which penicillin was discovered. Famous physicians such as Thomas Parhan then opposed giving out penicillin because it would remove the "wages of sin" from promiscuity. Sexual behavior during these decades changed little. Instead, generals by fiat gave out penicillin. When the war was over, everyone had become accustomed to the new miraculous drug.

This supports a certain cynicism about the power of education to prevent the spread of AIDS. During the first half of this century, the country could not agree on a way to prevent the spread of syphilis, because it could not agree whether the primary enemy was syphilis or unapproved sex. The population did not change its behavior, probably because the consequences were so remote. A deliberate campaign in posters and movies to produce "syphilophobia" failed to produce the desired chastity.

In 1987, Secretary of Education William Bennett opposed Surgeon General Everett Koop's plan to distribute condoms to prevent AIDS. Bennett urged abstinence; Koop's plan implied that such urging wasn't enough. Koop broke his fundamentalist stereotype and enraged his former supporters by urging discussion of safe sex among junior high school classes. Such safe-sex education accepts the probability of teenage sexual activity, as well as the existence of homosexual sex, anal sex, and oral-anal sex. Russell Baker, a spokesman for the National Conference of Catholic Bishops, opposed such education as encouraging promiscuity. Norman Podhoretz agreed, arguing that when he was a teenager in the 1940s, it was much harder to get condoms, yet there was less teenage pregnancy; whereas today, it is very easy to get condoms, yet there is massive teenage pregnancy. The cause? "Can there be any doubt that it is linked to the moral stigma attached to female promiscuity?"[44] Critics reply: Even if that were the case, isn't it easier to prevent AIDS than to turn "promiscuous" females into virgins?

Crusaders in recent years predictably divided over whether or not to provide clean needles and syringes to drug addicts. Such division raises the spectre of identifying those with HIV in testing programs and being unable to agree about subsequent action. Even though needle-swap programs were successful in Europe, even though it is almost impossible to get IV drug users to reform, and even though 82 percent of AIDS from IV drug use is in the New York metropolis (which has 50 percent of American IV drug users), New York for years resisted swap programs. Mayor Ed Koch said, "How can I support something that the police and law enforcement leaders are totally against"? (Critics said this was a bit disingenuous, since homosexuality was illegal, too.) Politicians resorted to "Just say, 'No'!" New York's Catholic clergy publicly urged sexual abstinence and avoiding drugs, while all around them people used illegal drugs and unmarried teenagers became pregnant. When Ronald Reagan told the nation at the end of his two terms that the corner on the drug war had been turned, his otherwise-loyal HHS secretary and physician Otis Bowen broke ranks and publicly disagreed. He said crack had become a national tragedy, and that only 20 percent of addicts who wanted to quit could get into a rehabilitation program. Indeed, the war against drugs looked so hopelessly lost in 1988 that the mayors of Washington, D.C., and Baltimore stunned their peers by suggesting the legalization of crime-related drugs. In 1988, New York City and Mayor Ed Koch gave in and began a pilot program allowing addicts to swap dirty needles for clean ones.

In sum, the question of prevention at bottom concerns the old division between those against the newer forms of sin and those against the newer forms of deadly microbes. During the years when AIDS has begun to frighten people, mandatory premarital testing for syphilis has been required in all states. Nevertheless, rates of syphilis are rising faster than ever. Because society cannot agree on how to prevent AIDS once someone has been identified as having HIV, why test people?

Mandatory Testing and Insurance

Screening to protect unknowing individuals from lethal risk is one thing; screening for maximal profit is quite another. A 1988 study by the Office of Technology Assessment found that most insurers screen applicants for HIV.[45] Insurers reject anyone admitting to HIV-positive status. Knowingly falsifying HIV status, if it can be proven when claims are later submitted for medical care, results in cancellation of policies and denial of payments. Insurers which presently screen or plan to screen include 77 percent of Blue Cross/Blue Shield (BCBS) plans, 86 percent of commercial insurers, and most health maintenance organizations (HMOs) which allow individual enrollment. Moreover, small employer-based groups are often required by insurers to screen employees for pre-existing conditions and companies which self-insure may legally screen out those with HIV.

Perhaps half of HIV-positive people will not have adequate coverage for AIDS treatment. Only the best policies cover such catastrophes. Young people between school and career, people between jobs, and people who work part-time with no medical benefits are hard hit.

Many individuals not at risk for HIV experience similar problems. One professor saw a psychotherapist after her divorce while insured by her university, which had liberal benefits for mental health. When she left the university to form her own business, she attempted to buy an individual policy from the same BCBS plan, but was first told it would cost $8000 a year and then was denied altogether when she refused to be tested for HIV. Anyone who has ever had substantial medical claims in a group plan and then left to try to buy an individual plan has experienced similar problems. As mentioned in the last chapter, some companies track at-risk people and help insurance companies to deny them coverage. Group plans spread out risk across generations and among people of varying health risks, and no company wants to insure a young person already making substantial claims.

Insurers claim they cannot bear the financial costs of AIDS. In general, the companies which make the most money insure the best risks, offer the lowest premiums, and therefore have the most customers. Some bad risks were able to be added because of subsidies by means of hospital or physician discounts and tax-free status.[46] These arguments may have the greatest weight in states such as New York, New Jersey, California, and Texas with the greatest concentrations of insured people with AIDS and, hence, the greatest threats to equity of insurers.

In 1988, some insurance companies denied coverage to single men employed as hairdressers, florists, interior designers, ballet dancers, and actors. Such denial was an obvious attempt to exclude gay men from medical insurance. In 1988, *60 Minutes* reported on a gay man in San Francisco who had owned his own company and been self-insured. When he developed AIDS, he was allowed to continue his medical insurance, but the company raised the rates each month. When the show aired, his *monthly* premiums had increased from $100 to $200, to $1000, to $2000.

Denial of medical insurance undermines voluntary testing. If a person has been exposed, why should he get tested if there is not only no cure, but if he will immediately lose his insurance? And if he is HIV-positive and doesn't inform his insurance company, it may be considered fraud. So why get tested?

Philosopher Richard Mohr argues that the government should prevent insurers from screening for HIV, just as Wisconsin, the District of Columbia, and California did.[47] Insurers claim it's unfair to raise premiums for others to pay for care for gays. Mohr replies that it's no more unfair than if the majority subsidizes women with multiple sex partners—women who consequently run much higher risks of ovarian cancer: "Does an individual policyholder have a legitimate complaint against this insurance company if this insurance company has not pursued a policy of trying to screen out every imaginable risk group of every imaginable disease that might raise insurance rates? The answer is obviously not." Similarly, government forces higher dairy and food prices on consumers by subsidizing farmers.

Mohr claims insurance companies have traditionally discriminated against gays and thus have "dirty hands." As such, he argues, they "should shoulder some of the burden" as "a matter of compensatory justice." Such an attitude worries insurers, a spokesperson for which accused many people with AIDS of "perpetrating fraud" on the life insurance industry after they knew they were seriously ill, and said that 44 percent purchased life insurance within 2 years of their death when they were "well aware" that they were symptomatic.[48]

Such questions lead one to ponder opposing answers to the question: what is insurance *for?* For companies, it is profit under the name of social service. For individuals, it is protection by sharing risks. On some views of justice (e.g., Rawls), it is a way of reducing the inequalities of life. Such questions also make one ponder the fragmented medical insurance system of this country. In Massachusetts, Governor Michael Dukakis vetoed an attempt to ban HIV testing among insurers, but later signed a bill requiring all employers to purchase medical insurance for employees.

UPDATE

Randy Shilts in an interview in 1989 expressed disappointment that nothing had happened since he wrote *And the Band Played On.* "The bitter irony is, my role as an AIDS celebrity just gives me a more elevated promontory from which to watch the world make the same mistakes in the handling of the AIDS epidemic that I had hoped my work would help to change."[49]

By 1989, a dozen lawsuits were proceeding against blood banks by people who had been infected by blood transfusions between 1983 and 1985.[50] At the same time, and as the relentless toll of AIDS adds up, its face began to change. Gradually, the disease became less of a disease of white gay males and more a disease of minorities and poor people. Intravenous drug usage and prostitution became vectors of HIV's spread and, as such, AIDS disproportionately affected poor communities.

In 1989, scientists discovered, using a new test (polymerase chain reaction) which tested directed for the DNA of HIV itself, that the false negative rate of ELISA and Western Blot tests could be far higher than the (exceedingly small) rate which had been previously claimed.[51] In some gay men, the HIV virus was claimed not to cause antibodies to appear for 35 months after infection. Whether this was a fact, and if so, what significance it would have, was difficult—as always—to figure out. As in the history of AIDS from the beginning, facts about the detection, transmission, and course of this HIV infection were highly politicized and subject to differing interpretations.[52]

Both prejudice and emotion run high about AIDS, and arguments about mandatory testing reflect them. Perhaps the point to keep in mind is that actually the most important thing to do is to *stop the spread of what is really just a virus.* Mandatory testing may or may not do this. The details must be thoroughly and dispassionately analyzed.[53]

FURTHER READING

J. Humber and R. Almeder, *AIDS and Ethics: Biomedical Reviews 1988*, Humana Press, New York, 1989.

Richard Mohr, *Gays/Justice: A Study of Ethics, Society, and Law*, Columbia University Press, New York, 1988.

Susan Sontag, *AIDS and Its Metaphors*, Farrar, Straus and Giroux, New York, 1988.

Randy Shilts, *And the Band Played On*, St. Martin's, New York, 1987.

Notes

The following abbreviations occur in the notes below:

NYT   = *New York Times*
JAMA = *Journal of the American Medical Association*
NEJM = *New England Journal of Medicine*
AMN   = *American Medical News*
HCR   = *Hastings Center Report*
WP   = *Washington Post*
WSJ   = *Wall Street Journal*
AP   = Associated Press
UPI   = United Press International

CHAPTER 1: KAREN QUINLAN

1 The first *NYT* story is September 16, 1975 in the "New Jersey" section, 32 (not duplicated in many photocopying services for libraries, hence no page; page numbers are frequently misleading for newspapers on microfilm since different versions of the day's paper often appear in different parts of the country and world).

2 Joseph Quinlan and Julia Quinlan, with Phyllis Battelle, *Karen Ann: The Quinlans Tell Their Story*, Doubleday Anchor, New York, 1977.

3 Robert Morse, in *In the Matter of Karen Quinlan: The Complete Legal Briefs, Court Proceedings, and Decisions in the Superior Court of New Jersey, Vols. 1 and 2*, University Publications of America, Frederick, Md., 1982, p. 236 (hereafter cited as *Proceedings*).

4 George Daggett, *NYT*, September 20, 1975 (New Jersey section).

5 Julius Korein, in *Proceedings*, 1, pp. 34–35.

6 Joseph and Julia Quinlan, in *Karen Ann*, p. 22.

7 Mary Lou Quinlan, in Quinlan, *Karen Ann*, p. 27.

8 Julia Quinlan, in Quinlan, *Karen Ann*, p. 29.

9 Daniel Coburn, in *Proceedings*, 1, p. 17.

10 Thomas C. Oden, "Beyond an Ethic of Immediate Sympathy," *HCR*, February 1976, p. 12.

11 Daniel Coburn, in *Proceedings*, 1, pp. 196–198.

12 Ralph Porzio, in *Proceedings*, 1, pp. 202–206.

13 Julius Korein, in *Proceedings*, p. 329.

14 Fred Plum, in Quinlan, *Karen Ann*, pp. 188–189.

15 *In the Matter of Karen Quinlan: An Alleged Incompetent*, 137 N.J. Superior (1975).

16 *In re Quinlan*, 70 N.J. 10, 355 A2d 647, 429 U.S. 922 (1976).

17 Julia and Joseph Quinlan, in Quinlan, *Karen Ann*, p. 198.

18 Ibid., pp. 272–273.

19 Gino Corretti, in Quinlan, *Karen Ann*, p. 211.

20 Joseph Fennelly, in Quinlan, *Karen Ann*, p. 284.

21 John Stuart Mill, *On Liberty*, 1859.

22 Peggy Stinson and Robert Stinson , *The Long Dying of Baby Andrew*, Little Brown, Boston, 1983.

23 President's Commission for the Study of Ethical Problems in Medicine and Bio-medical and Behavioral Research, *Defining Death,* Superintendent of Documents, Washington D.C., 1981, p. 14.

24 Christiaan Barnard and Curtiss Bill Pepper, *One Life,* Macmillan, Toronto, Ontario, 1969.

25 Ad Hoc Committee of the Harvard Medical School to Examine the Definition of Brain Death, "A Definition of Irreversible Coma," *JAMA* **205**: 337 (1968).

26 The Reverend and Mrs. Coles, as well as the young man, appeared on the *Donahue Show* in November of 1986 (author's videotape).

27 National Conference of Commission on Uniform Laws, *Uniform Laws Annual,* Vol. 15, Suppl., 1981.

28 Quinlan, *Karen Ann,* p. 87.

29 American Academy of Neurology, Amicus Curiae Brief, *Brophy vs. New England Sinai Hospital, Inc.,* 1986. Quoted in Ronald Cranford, "The Persistent Vegetative State: The Medical Reality (Getting the Facts Straight)," *HCR,* **18** (1): 31 (1988).

30 Robert Veatch, "Whole Brain, Neocortical, and Higher Brain Related Concepts of Death," in Richard Zaner (ed.), *Whole Brain and Neocortical Definitions of Death: A Critical Appraisal,* D. Reidel, Norwell, Mass., 1986.

31 President's Commission for the Study of Ethical Problems in Medicine and Bio-medical and Behavioral Research, *Defining Death,* Superintendent of Documents, Washington D.C., 1981, p. 2.

32 A previous version of this chapter was given at the Alabama Philosophical Asso-ciation meetings at the University of Alabama in Birmingham, in 1984, where sev-eral philosophers, especially George Graham, made useful comments. UAB med-ical professors C. Kirk Avent (Infectious Diseases) and William Goetter (Pulmonary Medicine) made useful comments on this chapter. Alfred N. Garwood also made early, useful suggestions.

CHAPTER 2: ELIZABETH BOUVIA AND VOLUNTARY DEATH

1 The views of both the historical and fictional Socrates are given by his student, Plato, in E. Hamilton, and H. Cairns (eds.), *Plato: Collected Dialogues,* Princeton Uni-versity Press, Princeton, N.J. 1961. Quotations are from the end of the *Phaedo.*

2 Epictetus, *Dissertations,* 1. 9, 16. Quoted from James Rachels, "Euthanasia," in T. Regan (ed.), *Matters of Life and Death,* 2d ed., Random House, New York, 1986, p. 41.

3 Seneca, *De Ira.* Quoted in Rachels, "Euthanasia."

4 Jean Paul Sartre, *Existentialism Is a Humanism,* Philosophical Library, New York, 1947.

5 Alasdair MacIntyre, *A Short History of Ethics,* Macmillan, New York, 1966, pp. 116–117.

6 Frederick Russell, *The Just War in the Middle Ages,* Cambridge University Press, Cambridge, Engl., 1975.

7 Margaret Pabst Battin, *Ethical Issues in Suicide,* Prentice Hall, Englewood Cliffs, N.J., 1982, p. 34.

8 Paul Johnson, *A History of Christianity,* Atheneum, New York, 1983, p. 113.

9 Paul Badham, "Christian Belief and the Ethics of In-Vitro Fertilization and Abor-tion," *Bioethics News* **6** (2): 8 (January 1987).

10 Montaigne. Quoted in James Gutman, "Death and Dying in Western Culture," *Encyclopedia of Bioethics,* Vol. 1, Free Press, New York, 1978, p. 240.

11 Spinoza, *Ethics,* James Gutman (ed.), William White and Amelia Stirling (trans.), Hafner, New York, 1949.

12 John Donne. Quoted in Derek Humphrey and Ann Wickett, *The Right to Die: Understanding Euthanasia,* Harper & Row, New York, 1986, pp. 8–9.

13 David Hume, "On Suicide" (1755), in *Collected Essays of David Hume,* edited by Eugene F. Miller, Liberty Classics, Indianapolis, Ind., 1986.

14 John Stuart Mill, *On Liberty,* 1859.

15 Charlotte Perkins Gillman. Quoted in Humphrey and Wickett, *The Right to Die,* p. 16.

16 Robert Steinbock and Bernard Lo, "The Case of Elizabeth Bouvia: Starvation, Suicide, or Problem Patient?" *Archives of Internal Medicine* **146:** 161 (January 1986).

17 Elizabeth Bouvia, AP story, October 16, 1983.

18 Donald Fischer. Quoted in George Annas, "When Suicide Prevention Becomes Brutality: The Case of Elizabeth Bouvia," *HCR* **14** (2): 20 (April 1984).

19 Steinbock and Lo, "Elizabeth Bouvia," p. 161.

20 Richard Scott, in "Patient's Suicide Wish Troubles Hospital, MDs," *AMN,* January 20, 1984, p. 15.

21 Judge Hews, *Bouvia vs. County of Riverside,* California Superior Court, December 16, 1983.

22 Arthur Hoppe, *San Francisco Examiner,* December 20, 1983.

23 Annas, "When Suicide Prevention...," p. 46.

24 Habeeb Bacchus, in "Patient's Suicide Wish Troubles Hospital, MDs," *AMN,* January 20, 1984, p. 16.

25 Annas "When Suicide Prevention...," p. 20.

26 Steinbock and Lo, "Elizabeth Bouvia," p. 162.

27 George Annas, "Elizabeth Bouvia: Whose Space Is This Anyway?" *HCR* **16** (2): 24–25 (April 1986).

28 Humphrey and Wickett, *The Right to Die,* p. 150.

29 Paul Longmore, "Elizabeth Bouvia, Assisted Suicide, and Social Prejudice," in *Issues in Law and Medicine* **2** (2): 158 (Fall 1987).

30 The hospital's rationale in its brief to Judge Deering is quoted in Annas, "Elizabeth Bouvia."

31 Judge Deering, *Bouvia vs. Glenchur,* Los Angeles Superior Court, *California Reporter* vol. 225, 296–308, 1986.

32 *Bouvia vs. Superior Court* (Glenchur), *California Reporter* Vol. 297 (California Appellate 2 District, 1986).

33 H. Hendin, "Suicide in America," *Miami News,* August 30, 1982, Bl.

34 Art Kleiner, "Life After Suicide," *Co-Evolution Quarterly: The Continuation of the Whole Earth Catalogue,* 30.

35 Derek Humphrey, *Jean's Way,* Harper & Row, New York, 1978.

36 Derek Humphrey, *Let Me Die Before I Wake: Hemlock's Book of Self-Deliverance for the Dying,* Hemlock Society, Los Angeles, Cal., 1984.

37 Nancy Mullen, in Humphrey and Wickett, *The Right to Die,* p. 152.

38 Carol Gill, in ibid., pp. 154–155.

39 Longmore, "Assisted Suicide," p. 156.

40 John Stuart Mill, *On Liberty,* 1859.

41 Longmore, "Assisted Suicide," p. 168.

42 Immanuel Kant, "On Suicide," *Lectures on Ethics*, L. Enfield (trans.), Harper & Row, New York, 1963, pp. 148–154.

43 David Hume, "On Suicide."

44 Battin, *Ethical Issues*, p. 22.

45 James Rachels, *The End of Life*, Oxford University Press, Oxford, Engl., New York 1986, p. 182.

46 Tom Beauchamp, "Suicide," *Matters of Life and Death*, T. Regan (ed.), 2d ed., Random House, New York 1986.

47 I am indebted to philosopher James Rachels of the University of Alabama at Birmingham for comments on this chapter.

CHAPTER 3: MERCY KILLING IN HOLLAND

1 Anonymous resident, "It's Over, Debbie," *JAMA* **259:** 272 (1988).

2 Willard Gaylin, Leon Kass, Edmund Pellegrino, and Mark Seigler, "Doctors Must Not Kill," *JAMA* **259** (14): 2139–2140 (April 8, 1988).

3 S. Wanzer et al., "The Physician's Responsibility toward Hopelessly Ill Patients: A Second Look," *NEJM* **320** (13): 844–849 (March 30, 1989).

4 Ludwig Edelstein, *Ancient Medicine: Collected Essays of Ludwig Edelstein*, O. and L. Temkin (eds.), John Hopkins University Press, Baltimore, Md., 1967.

5 Leo Alexander, "Medical Science Under Dictatorship," *NEJM* **42** (July 14, 1949).

6 Robert Jay Lifton, *The Nazi Doctors*, Basic Books, New York, 1986.

7 David Wheeler, "Euthanasia an Increasingly Pressing Issue for Ethicists and Physicians," *Chronicle of Higher Education*, November 9, 1988, A1, A6.

8 Lucy Davidowicz. Quoted in "Biomedical Ethics in the Shadow of Nazism: Use of the Nazi Analogy in the Euthanasia Debate: Report of a Conference," *HCR* **6** (4) supplement, 1–20 (August 1978).

9 Joseph Fletcher, *Morals and Medicine*, Beacon, Boston, Mass. 1961, pp. 85–86.

10 Elizabeth Kübler-Ross, *On Death and Dying*, Macmillan, New York, 1969.

11 R. Rosenbaum, "Turn On, Tune In, Drop Dead," *Harper's Magazine*, July 1982, pp. 32–42.

12 Stewart Alsop, "The Right to Die with Dignity," *Good Housekeeping*, 1974.

13 Phillip M. Boffey, "Cancer Progress: Are the Statistics Telling the Truth?" *The New York Times*, September 18, 1984.

14 Geertruida Postma. Quoted in Derek Humphrey and Ann Wickett, *The Right to Die: Understanding Euthanasia*, Harper & Row, New York, 1988, p. 172.

15 *Nightline*, April 1987 (author's videotape).

16 Christiaan Barnard, *One Life*, Macmillan, New York, 1965.

17 Karel Gunning, on *Nightline*, April 1987 (author's videotape).

18 Peter Admiraal. Quoted by Alan Parachini, "A Dutch Doctor Carries Out a Death Wish," *Los Angeles Times*, July 5, 1987, section 6, p. 9.

19 Cited by Marcia Angell, "Euthanasia," *NEJM* **319** (20): 1349 (November 17, 1988).

20 Ibid., pp. 1348–1350.

21 Stanley Milgram, *Obedience*, Harper & Row, New York, 1974.

22 American Medical Association, *Opinions of the Judicial Council*, Chicago, Ill., 1973.

23 James Rachels, "Active and Passive Euthanasia," *NEJM* **292:** 78–80 (January 9, 1975).

24 Baruch Brody, "Ethical Questions Raised by the Persistent Vegetative Patient," *Hastings Center Report* **18** (1): 35.

25 Daniel Dinello, "On Killing and Letting Die," *Analysis* **31** (3): 83-86 (January 1971).

26 Holly Goldman, *Analysis* **40** (4): 224 (October 1980).

27 Richard O'Neil, *Analysis* **38** (2): 124–125 (March 1978).

28 Nat Hentoff, "The Deadly Slippery Slope," *Village Voice*, September 1, 1987.

29 Allan Parachini, "The Netherlands Debates the Legal Limits of Euthanasia," *Los Angeles Times*, July 5, 1987, section 6, p. 8.

30 Parachini, "The Netherlands Debates...," p. 1.

31 James Rachels, *The End of Life: Euthanasia and Morality*, Oxford University Press, Oxford, Engl., 1986.

32 Daniel Callahan, "On Feeding the Dying," *HCR* **13** (5): 22 (October 1983).

33 Gilbert Meillander, "On Removing Food and Water: Against the Stream," *HCR* **14** (6): 11–13 (December 1984).

34 James Childress and Joanne Lynn, "Must Patients Always Be Given Food and Water?" *HCR* **13** (5): 17–21 (October 1983).

35 President's Commission for the Study of Ethical Problems in Medicine and Biomedical and Behavioral Research, *Deciding to Forego Life-Sustaining Treatment*, Superintendent of Documents, Washington, D.C., 1983.

36 M. Pabst Battin, "The Least Worst Death," *HCR* **13** (2): 13–16 (April 1983).

37 Council on Judicial Affairs, American Medical Association, *Opinions*, American Medical Association, Chicago, Ill, 1986.

38 "Man Convicted of Killing Wife Who Begged to Die," *NYT*, May 10, 1985.

39 "Doctor Is Cleared in Wife's Death," *Miami Herald*, December 2, 1988, pp. 1, 17; T. Woody, "Was His Act of Mercy Also Murder?" *NYT*, November 7, 1988.

40 "Easeful Death," *British Medical Journal* **293**: 1187 (November 8, 1986).

41 I am indebted to philosophers Margaret Battin of the University of Utah and James Rachels of the University of Alabama at Birmingham for comments on this chapter. A condensed version of this chapter, "Do Not Go Slowly Into That Dark Night: Mercy-Killing in Holland," appeared in the *American Journal of Medicine* **84**: 139–141 (January 1988).

CHAPTER 4: BABY LOUISE BROWN'S IN VITRO FERTILIZATION

1 A. Wilcox et al., "Incidence of Early Loss of Pregnancy," *NEJM* **319** (4): 189–194 (July 28, 1988).

2 John Brown and Lesley Brown, *Our Miracle Called Louise*, Paddington Press, London, 1979, p. 83, 88.

3 Deborah Yaeger, "Doctors Make Progress Treating Infertility, But Costs Are High," *WSJ*, October 12, 1984, p. 1.

4 "Adoption Demand Exceeding Supply," *NYT*, April 5, 1987, p. A1.

5 Eileen Helper. Quoted in Yaegar, "Doctors Make Progress ...," p. 1.

6 Brown and Brown, *Our Miracle*, p. 98.

7 *Newsweek*, August 7, 1978, p. 68.

8 Patrick Steptoe and Robert Edwards, *A Matter of Life: The Story of a Medical Breakthrough*, William Morrow, London, 1980, p. 64.

9 Edwards and Steptoe, *A Matter of Life*, pp. 32–33.

10 Brown and Brown, *Our Miracle*, p. 163.

11 *Time*, August 7, 1978, p. 68.

12 Brown and Brown, *Our Miracle*, p. 75.

13 Jeremy Rifkin and Ted Howard, *Who Shall Play God?*, Dell, New York, 1977.

14 *Newsweek*, August 7, 1978, p. 66.

15 Audrey Smith. Quoted by Robert Edwards, *A Matter of Life*, p. 48.

16 *Newsweek*, August 7, 1978, p. 68.

17 Edwards and Steptoe, *A Matter of Life*, p. 90.

18 James Watson. Quoted in *Newsweek*, August 7, 1978, p. 69.

19 Richard Blandau. Quoted in *Time*, November 13, 1978, p. 89.

20 *Time*, November 13, 1978, p. 89.

21 "Text of Vatican's Statement on Human Reproduction," *NYT*, March 11, 1987, pp. 10ff.

22 Bishop Kelly. Quoted in G. Vecsey, "Religious Leaders Differ on Implant," *NYT*, July 27, 1978, p. A16.

23 Joseph Fletcher, *Ethics of Genetic Control: Ending Reproductive Roulette*, Doubleday Anchor, New York,; reprinted by Prometheus, Buffalo, N.Y., 1984, p. 36.

24 Joseph Fletcher, "Ethical Aspects of Genetic Controls," *NEJM* **285** (14): 776–781 (1971).

25 Ramsey is quoted in *A Matter of Life*, p. 113.

26 Paul Ramsey, *The Ethics of Fetal Experimentation*, Yale University Press, New Haven, Conn., 1975.

27 Michael Bayles, *Reproductive Ethics*, Prentice Hall, Englewood Cliffs, N.J., 1986, p. 13.

28 John Marlow. Quoted in *U.S. News & World Report*, August 7, 1978, p. 24.

29 John Marshall. Quoted in *Time*, July 31, 1978, p. 59.

30 Leon Kass, "The New Biology: What Price Relieving Man's Estate?" *JAMA* **174**: 779–788 (November 19, 1971).

31 James Watson, "Moving Towards Clonal Man," *Atlantic*, May 1971, p. 53.

32 Max Purutz. Quoted in Edwards and Steptoe, *A Matter of Life*, p. 117.

33 Rifkin and Howard, *Who Shall Play God?*, p. 115.

34 Daniel Callahan, *NYT*, July 27, 1978, p. A16.

35 This point is due to G. Lynn Stephens.

36 Hans Tiefel, "In Vitro Fertilization: A Conservative View," *JAMA* **247** (23): 3235–3242 (June 18, 1982).

37 This point is due to E. Haavi Morreim and Derek Parfit.

38 *U.S. News & World Report*, August 7, 1978, p. 70.

39 Leon Kass. Quoted in *Newsweek*, August 7, 1978, p. 71.

40 Paul Ramsey, *Fabricated Man*, Yale University Press, New Haven, Conn., 1970.

41 Mary Anne Warren, "IVF and Women's Interests: An Analysis of Feminist Concerns," *Bioethics* **2** (1): 37–57 (January 1988), p. 44.

42 Kay Honea, lecture, UAB medical ethics course, November 1979.

43 John Rawls, *A Theory of Justice*, Harvard University Press, Cambridge, Mass., 1971.

44 Peter Singer and Deane Wells, "In Vitro Fertilisation: The Major Issues," *Journal of Medical Ethics* **9** (4): 192–199 (1983); plus P. Singer, "Response" to "Comment," by G. D. Mitchell (same issue).

45 *NYT*, July 28, 1978, p. A22; July 27, 1978, p. A16.

46 David Ozar, "The Case for Not Unthawing Frozen Embryos," *HCR* **15** (4): 7–12 (August 1985). A similar article was brought to my attention by George Graham.

47 Singer, "In Vitro...," p. 193.

48 M. Viola, quoted from Howard Brody, *Ethical Decisions in Medicine*, Little Brown, Boston, Mass., 1976, p. 147.

49 Derek Parfit, *Reasons and Persons*, Oxford University Press, New York, 1984.

50 M. Gold, "The Baby Makers," *Science '85*, (April 1985, p. 32).

51 Edwards and Steptoe, Letter, *British Medical Journal* **286**: 1351–1352 (1983).
52 Jean Seligman et al., "The Grueling Baby Chase," *Newsweek*, November 30, 1987, pp. 78–82. *60 Minutes* documented such problems in December 1988.
53 Louise Brown. Quoted in AP story, *Birmingham News*, July 25, 1988, p. B1.

CHAPTER 5: THE BABY M CASE

1 Phillip Parker, "Surrogate Mothers' Motivations: Initial Findings," *American Journal of Psychiatry* **40**:1 (1983).
2 Linda Arking, "Surrogate Motherhood: Searching for a Very Special Woman," *McCall's*, June 1987.
3 "Who Keeps 'Baby M'?," *Newsweek*, January 19, 1987, p. 49.
4 AP story, January 9, 1987.
5 *NYT*, February 5, 1987, p. 15.
6 *In the Matter of Baby M*, New Jersey Superior Court, 313 (1987). See also "Surrogate Deals for Mothers Held Illegal in Jersey," *NYT*, February 3, 1987.
7 "Whose Child Is This?" *Time*, January 19, 1987, pp. 56–58; "Who Keeps 'Baby M'?," *Newsweek*, January 19, 1987, pp. 44–49.
8 William Handel. Quoted in "Jersey Surrogate Ruling Downplayed by Brokers," *NYT*, February 5, 1987, p. A10.
9 Nanette Dembitz. Quoted by Vivian Cadden, "Hard Questions about the Baby M Case," *McCall's*, June 1985, p. 58.
10 Eleanor Smeal, lecture, University Lecture Series, Birmingham, Ala., January 1987.
11 "Testimony Conflicts in Surrogate Trial," AP story, January 10, 1987.
12 "Doctor Backs Baby M Mother," *NYT*, January 15, 1987.
13 Richard McCormick, "Surrogate Motherhood: A Stillborn Idea," *Second Opinion 5*: 130 (1987).
14 Sidney Callahan, "Lovemaking and Babymaking," *Commonweal*, April 24, 1987, p. 238.
15 Hillary Baber, "For the Legitimacy of Surrogate Contracts," *On the Problem of Surrogate Parenthood: Analyzing the Baby M Case*, Edwin Mellen Press, Lewiston, N.Y., 1987 p. 39.
16 M. Schester. Quoted in *In the Matter of Baby M*, p. 52.
17 Lee Salkl *In the Matter of Baby M*, p. 56ff.
18 Judith Grief. Quoted in *In the Matter of Baby M*, p. 64ff.
19 Bonnie Steinbock, "Surrogate Motherhood as Prenatal Adoption," *Law, Medicine & Health Care* **16** (1–2): 45 (Spring 1988).
20 Asa Ruskin, letter to the Editor, *AMN*, May 15, 1987, p. 6.
21 Phyllis Chesler, *Sacred Bond: The Legacy of Baby M*, Vintage, New York, 1989, p. 23.
22 George Annas, "Baby M: Babies (and Justice) for Sale," *HCR* **17** (3): 13–15 (June 1987).
23 Herbert Krimmel, "The Case Against Surrogate Parenting," *HCR* **13** (5): 35–39 (October 1983).
24 Barbara Katz Rothman, "Surrogacy: A Question of Values," *Conscience* **8**: 3 (1987).
25 "Whitehead vs. sperm," *Off Our Backs*, May 1987, pp. 1, 12.
26 Patricia Werhane, "Against the Legitimacy of Surrogate Contracts," *On the Problem . . .*, pp. 21–30.

27 Rosemary Tong, "Feminist Philosophy: Standpoints and Differences," *Newsletter on Feminism and Philosophy*, American Philosophical Association, no. 9 (1988).

28 Carol Gilligan, *In a Different Voice: Psychological Theory and Women's Development*, Harvard University Press, Cambridge, Mass., 1982.

29 Allison Jaggar, *Feminist Politics and Human Nature*, Rowman and Allanheld, Totawa, N. J., 1983. Jaggar's critics were Luce Iriguray, Helene Cixous, and Julia Kristeva. Quoted in Tong, "Feminist Philosophy," p. 10.

30 The reference to "body-mediated" knowledge is to a claim made by Beverly Harrison, *Making the Connections: Essays in Feminist Social Ethics*, Carol Robb (ed.), Beacon Press, Boston, Mass., 1985.

31 George Will, "Surrogate Mother Should Get Child," *Birmingham Post-Herald*, January 22, 1987, p. A4.

32 Edwin Newman, Lecture, University Lecture Series, Birmingham, Ala., March 1987.

33 *In the Matter of Baby M*, p. 70.

34 Ellen Goodman, "Reproduction Slowly Being Separated from Sex," *Birmingham Post-Herald*, April 25, 1986.

35 ABC World News, January 26, 1987.

36 ABC World News, January 26, 1987.

37 Michael Kinsley, "The Moral Logic of Capitalism," *WSJ*, April 16, 1987, p. 31.

38 Kenneth Titmus, *The Gift Relationship: From Altruism to Commerce*, Pantheon, New York, 1971.

39 Baruch Brody, "Surrogate Motherhood," lecture, Berry College, April 1987. Videotape available from Philosophy Department, Berry College, Rome, Ga. 30149.

40 Bonnie Steinbock, "The Logical Case for Wrongful Life," *HCR* **16** (2): 15 (1986).

41 "Text of Vatican's Statement on Human Reproduction," *NYT*, March 11, 1987, p. 10ff.

42 Department of Health and Social Security (Great Britain), *Report of the Committee of Inquiry into Human Fertilisation and Embryology*, Her Majesty's Stationery Office, 1984.

43 Harold Cassidy. Quoted in Mark Rust, "Whose Baby Is It?" *ABA Journal: The Magazine for Lawyers*, June 1, 1987, p. 52.

44 Lee Salk. Quoted in Linda Arking, "Surrogate Motherhood: Searching for a Very Special Woman," *McCall's*, June 1987.

45 *In the Matter of Baby M, New Jersey Supreme Court*, 140 (1987). See also "Excerpts from Decision by New Jersey Supreme Court in the Baby M Case," *NYT*, February 4, 1987.

46 Anthony D'Amato, letter to the editor, *NYT*, February 18, 1988.

47 "Baby M's Mother Wins Broad Visiting Rights," *NYT*, April 7, 1988, p. Al.

48 New York State Task Force on Life and the Law, *Surrogate Parenting: Analysis and Recommendations for Public Policy* (1988).

49 Joan Beck, "Surrogate Motherhood Opponents Have Chosen Wrong Crusade," *Birmingham News*, February 9, 1989.

CHAPTER 6: ABORTION AND THE TRIAL OF KENNETH EDELIN

1 Paul Badham, "Christian Belief and the Ethics of In Vitro Fertilization," *Bioethics News* **6** (2): 10 (January 1987).

2 Paul Johnson, "Faith, Reason, and Unreason, 1648–1870," *A History of Christianity*, Atheneum, New York, 1983.

3 Barbara Ehrenreich and Deirdre English, *For Her Own Good: 150 Years of the Experts' Advice to Women*, Doubleday, New York, 1987, pp. 319–320.

4 *Roe vs. Wade, Supreme Court Reporter* 93, 410 US 151, 709–762.

5 The Boston Women's Health Book Collective, *The New Our Bodies/Our Selves*, Simon & Schuster, New York, 1984, pp. 309–310.

6 U.S. Bureau of the Census, *Statistical Abstract of the United States*, 106th ed., Superintendent of Documents, 1986, pp. 66, 49–52.

7 A. Philipson et al., "Transplacental Passage of Erythromycin and Clindamycin," *NEJM*, **288** (23): 1219–1221 (June 7, 1973).

8 William Nolen, *The Baby in the Bottle*, Coward, McCann, & Geoghegan, New York, 1978.

9 Ibid., p. 203.

10 "The Edelin Trial," transcript of trial for WBGH re-creation for Bill Moyers' documentary. A Project of Legal-Medical Studies, Inc., Box 8219, John F. Kennedy Station, Government Center, Boston, Mass. 12134.

11 Nolen, *The Baby in the Bottle*, p. 150.

12 "The Edelin Trial," transcript, p. 55.

13 William F. Buckley, Jr. *The National Review*, March 14, 1975. Quoted in Nolen, *The Baby in the Bottle*, p. 221.

14 *Commonwealth vs. Kenneth Edelin*, 000 Mass.000, 359 N.E. 2nd 4 (1976).

15 Kenneth Edelin, *Ob. Gyn. News*, January 1, 1977, p. 1.

16 Walter Cronkite. Quoted in Paul Ramsey, *Ethics at the Edges of Life*, Yale University Press, New Haven, Conn., 1978, p. 94.

17 Nolen, *The Baby in the Bottle*, p. 175.

18 Judith Jarvis Thomson, "A Defense of Abortion," *Philosophy & Public Affairs* **1** (1): 47–66 (Fall 1971).

19 Daniel Wikler, "Ought We to Try to Save Aborted Fetuses?" *Ethics* 90: 58–65 (October 1979).

20 Ellen Willis, "Harper's Forum On Abortion," *Harper's Magazine*, July 1986, p. 38.

21 AP story, *Birmingham News*, June 2, 1986, p. 5A.

22 Maggie Scarf, "The Fetus as Guinea Pig," *NYT Magazine*, October 19, 1975, p. 194–200.

23 Sissela Bok. Quoted in Scarf, "The Fetus as Guinea Pig," p. 196.

24 Scarf, "The Fetus as Guinea Pig," pp. 194–195.

25 Paul Ramsey, *The Ethics of Fetal Research*, Yale University Press, New Haven, Conn., 1975.

26 Jeff Lyon, "The Doctor's Dilemma: When Abortion Gives Birth to Life, Physicians Become Troubled Saviors," *Chicago Tribune*, August 15, 1982, section 12, pp. 1, 3.

27 Sandra Day O'Connor. Quoted in *Newsweek*, January 14, 1985, p. 28.

28 "Explosions Over Abortion," *Time*, January 14, 1985, p. 17.

29 A. Bonavoglia, "The Ordeal of Pamela Fae Stewart," *MS* (August 1987); on Donna Piazzi, see T. Thompson, "Augusta Fetus Case Creates Life vs. Death Dilemma," *Atlanta Constitution*, August 6, 1986, p. Al.

30 George Annas, "Forced Caesareans: The Unkindest Cut of All," *HCR* **12** (3): 16–17; (1982); see Annas, "Pregnant Women as Fetal Containers," *HCR* **16** (6): 13–14; (December 1986); Annas, "She's Going to Die: The Case of Angela C," *HCR* **18** (1): 23–25; (February/March 1988).

31 Laurie Abraham, "Debate Follows Ruling for Fetus over Mother," *AMN*, March 1, 1988, p. 1; R. Sandroff, "Invasion of the Body Snatchers," *Vogue*, October 1988, p. 302ff.

32 Eric Schmitt, "Abortion Appeal Is Refused; Woman in Coma Is Readied," *NYT*, February 11, 1989, p. 10.
33 I am indebted to philosopher Baruch Brody of Baylor Medical School, Texas, for comments on this chapter.

CHAPTER 7: THE BABY JANE DOE CASE

Note: A videotape from NBC News, "The Case of Baby Jane Doe," discusses the central case of this chapter and is available from the Society for Health and Human Values, McLean, Virginia.

1 Robert Weir, *Selected Nontreatment of Handicapped Newborns,* Oxford University Press, New York, 1984; John Boswell, *The Kindness of Strangers: The Abandonment of Children in Western Europe from Late Antiquity to the Renaissance,* Pantheon, New York, 1989.
2 William Lecky, *History of European Morals from Augustus to Charlemagne,* 1869; Reprinted by George Braziller, New York, 1955, Vol. II, pp. 25–56.
3 W. L. Langer, "Europe's Initial Population Explosion," *American Historical Review,* **(69):** 1–17 (1963). Quoted in G. Hardin's *Exploring New Ethics for Survival: The Voyage of the Spaceship Beagle,* Viking Press, New York, 1972, pp. 180–183.
4 The film *Who Should Survive?* was produced by the Joseph P. Kennedy, Jr., Foundation. Available from Film Service, 999 Asylum Avenue, Hartford, Conn. 06105.
5 Renée Fox. Quoted in *Who Should Survive?*
6 James Gustafson, "Mongolism, Parental Desires, and the Right to Life," *Perspectives in Biology and Medicine* **16**: 529 (Summer 1973).
7 Ibid., 529.
8 Ibid., 529.
9 John Lorber, "Results of Treatment of Myelomeningocele: An Analysis of 524 Unselected Cases, with Special Reference to Possible Selection for Treatment," *Developmental Medicine & Child Neurology* **13** (3): 279–303 (1971).
10 R. Duff and A. Campbell, "Moral and Ethical Dilemmas in the Special-Care Nursery," *NEJM* **289** (17): 890–894 (October 25, 1973).
11 Shari Staver, "Siamese Twins' Case 'Devastates' MD's," *AMN* October 9, 1981, pp. 15–16.
12 John Robertson, "Dilemma in Danville," *HCR* **11** (5): 7 (October 1981).
13 Adrian Peracchio, "Government in the Nursery: New Era for Baby Doe Cases," *Newsday,* November 13, 1983. This story and Kerr's story below are available from *Newsday* as part of a reprint of the Pulitzer-prize winning stories.
14 Marcia Angell, "Handicapped Children: Baby Doe and Uncle Sam," *NEJM* **309** (11): 659–61 (1983).
15 William Bortz, III, letter to the editor, *NEJM* **309** (24): 1517 December 15, 1983.
16 President's Commission for the Study of Ethical Problems in Medicine and Biomedical and Behavioral Research, *Deciding to Forego Life-Sustaining Treatment,* Superintendent of Documents, Washington, D.C., 1983.
17 Kathleen Kerr, "An Issue of Law and Ethics," *Newsday,* October 26, 1983. Reprinted in "The Baby Jane Doe Story: Winner of the 1984 Pulitzer Prize for Local Reporting." Available from *Newsday.*
18 Kathleen Kerr, "Legal, Medical Legacy of Case," *Newsday,* December 7, 1987.
19 Ibid.

20 Bonnie Steinbock, "Baby Jane Doe in the Courts," *HCR* **14** (1): 15 (February 1984).

21 Kathleen Kerr, "Legal, Medical Legacy...." See also Kathleen Kerr, "Reporting the Case of Baby Jane Doe," *HCR* **14** (4): 14 (August 1984).

22 John Paris, "Right to Life Doesn't Demand Heroic Sacrifice," *WSJ*, November 28, 1983, p. 30.

23 John Fletcher, in *Who Should Survive?*.

24 Robert Weir, *Selective Nontreatment of Handicapped Newborns*, (Quoted above in #1).

25 Fletcher, *Who Should Survive?*; Paul Ramsey, *Ethics at the Edges of Life*, Yale University Press, New Haven, Conn., 1978, p. 146.

26 Peter Singer, *Practical Morality*, Cambridge University Press, Cambridge, Engl., 1979, p. 137; Tristam Engelhardt, "Ethical Issues in Aiding the Death of Young Children," *Beneficent Euthanasia*, Marvin Kohl (ed.), Prometheus, Buffalo, N.Y., 1975; Michael Tooley, "Abortion and Infanticide," *Philosophy & Public Affairs* **2** (1): 37–65 (Fall 1972).

27 J. Rachels, "Active and Passive Euthanasia," *NEJM* **292** (2): 78–80 (January 9, 1976).

28 Hastings Center Project on Imperiled Newborns, ed. Arthur Caplan, "Imperiled Newborns," Section 7, "Conclusion," *HCR* **17** (6): 31 (December 1987).

29 Kathleen Kerr, "Legal, Medical Legacy...."

30 Ellen Goodman, "A Clumsy Intrusion on Parental Pain," *Boston Globe*, November 1, 1983.

31 K. Kerr, "An Issue of Law and Ethics."

32 R. B. Zachary, "Life with Spina Bifida," *British Medical Journal* **2**: 1461 (1977).

33 C. Everett Koop, presented *in idem* in "The Seriously Ill or Dying Child: Supporting the Patient and the Family," D. Horan and D. Mall (eds.) *Death, Dying and Euthanasia*, University Publications of America, Frederick, Md., 1977, pp. 537–539.

34 C. Everett Koop, "The Slide to Auschwitz," *Whatever Happened to the Human Race*, Fleming H. Revell Co., Old Tappan, N.J. 1979.

35 R. McCormick, "To Save or Let Die: The Dilemma of Modern Medicine," *JAMA*, **229** (8): 172–176 (July 1974).

36 David Gibson, "Dimensions of Intelligence," *Down Syndrome: The Psychology of Mongolism*, Cambridge University Press, New York, 1978, 35–77; Janet Carr, "The Development of Intelligence," in David Lane and Brian Stratford (eds.), *Current Approaches to Down Syndrome*, Praeger Publishers, New York, 1985, pp. 167–186.

37 See J. Freeman, "To Treat or Not to Treat: Ethical Dilemmas of Treating the Infant with Myelomeningocele," *Clinical Neurosurgery* **20**: 137 (1973).

38 J. Livermore, C. Malmquist, and P. Meehl, "On the Justification for Civil Commitment," *University of Pennsylvania Law Review* **117**: 75–96 (November 1968).

39 Steinbock, "Baby Jane Doe."

40 George Will, "Baby Jane Doe: Major Expansion of Civil Rights Protection," *Birmingham Post-Herald*, November 1, 1983 .

41 Peter Singer, "Sanctity of Life or Quality of Life?" *Pediatrics* **72** (1): 128–129 (July 1983). Letters in reaction were in *Pediatrics* **73** (2) (February 1984).

42 Peter Geach, *The Virtues*, Cambridge University Press, Cambridge, Engl., 1977.

43 Fred Bruning, "The Politics of Life," *MacLean's* December 12, 1983, p. 17.

44 "Baby Jane Doe," *WSJ*, November 21, 1983.

45 Gregg Levoy, "Birth Controllers," *Omni*, August, 1987, p. 31.

46 *Gleitman vs. Cosgrove*. Quoted in M. Coppenger (ed.), *Bioethics: A Casebook*, Prentice-Hall, Englewood Cliffs, N.J., 1985, pp. 8–12.

47 *Curlender*, 106 California Appellate Court, 3rd District, *California Reporter*, 165, 479–480.

48 Bonnie Steinbock, "Whatever Happened to the Danville Siamese Twins?" *HCR* **17** (4): 3–4 (August/September 1987).

49 "Baby Jane Doe Has Surgery to Remove Water from Brain," *NYT* April 7, 1983, p. 28.

50 Nat Hentoff, "Which Babies Shall Live?" *Washington Post,* October 16, 1981, p. A21.

51 Ronald E. Cranford, "The Persistent Vegetative State: The Medical Reality (Getting the Facts Straight)," *HCR* **18** (1): 29 (February/March 1988).

52 Kathleen Kerr, "Legal, Medical Legacy..."

53 Diane Gianelli, "MDs, not parents, end up making "Baby Doe" decisions—Report," *AMN,* December 2, 1988, p. 33.

54 B. D. Colen, "A Life of Love—and Endless Pain," *Newsday,* October 26, 1983. Reprinted in "The Baby Jane Doe Story," *Newsday.*

55 Steven Baer, "The Half-Told Story of Baby Jane Doe," *Columbia Journalism Review,* November/December 1984, pp. 35–38.

56 B. Steinbock, "Baby Jane Doe...," p. 15.

57 A. Gallo, "Spina Bifida: The State of the Art of Medical Management," *HCR* **14** (1): 10–13 (February 1984).

58 Ibid., p. 11.

59 Spina Bifida Association, Brief Amicus Curiae of the Spina Bifida Association of America, *Weber vs. Stony Brook Hospital,* New York State Supreme Court, Appellate Division, 2nd Department, *New York Law Journal,* October 28, 1983. Quoted in Bonnie Steinbock, "Baby Jane Doe...," p. 19.

60 I am indebted for comments on this chapter to philosophers Loretta Kopelman, East Carolina Medical School, and Bonnie Steinbock of SUNY-Albany, as well as pediatrics professors Paul Palmisano (University of Alabama at Birmingham) and Norman Fost (University of Wisconsin, Madison).

CHAPTER 8: THE PHILADELPHIA HEAD-INJURY STUDIES ON PRIMATES

Note: The controversial, edited videotape of the Gennarelli research is available from PETA (People for the Ethical Treatment of Animals), Washington, D.C.

1 Peter Singer, "Animal Liberation," *New York Review of Books,* 1975, quoting L. Rosenfield, *From Beast-Machine to Man-Machine: The Theme of Animal Soul in French Letters from Descartes to La Mettrie* Oxford University Press, 1940, who in turn is quoting Nichola Fontaine, *Mémoires pour servir a l'histoire de Port-Royal,* vol.2, Cologne, 1738, pp. 52–53.

2 C. S. Lewis, *The Problem of Pain: How Human Suffering Raises Almost Intolerable Intellectual Problems,* Macmillan, New York, 1940, pp. 131–133.

3 David Hume, *A Treatise of Human Nature,* 1789.

4 Office of Technology Assessment, *Animal Usage in the United States,* Superintendent of Documents, Washington, D.C., 1986, 12, "Alternatives to Laboratory Animals," 1984, p. 71; Andrew Rowan, *Of Mice, Models, and Men: A Critical Evaluation of Animal Research,* State University of New York Press, Albany, N.Y., 1984, pp. 67–70; *Newsweek,* December 26, 1988, p. 51.

5 Bernard Rollins, *Animal Rights and Human Morality,* Prometheus, Buffalo, N.Y., 1981, pp. 97–99.

6 W. Robbins, "Animal Rights: A Growing Movement in U.S.," *NYT*, June 15, 1984, p. A16

7 Ibid., p. Al.

8 "The Use of Animals in Research," *NEJM* **313** (6): 395–400.

9 James Kilpatrick, "Animal-Rights Supporters Claim Well-Won Victory," *Birmingham News*, July 23, 1985.

10 *Evaluation of Experimental Procedures Conducted at the University of Pennsylvania Experimental Head Injury Laboratory 1981–1984 in Light of the Public Health Service Animal Welfare Policy*, Office for Protection of Research Risks, National Institutes of Health, 1985, p. 37.

11 Carolyn Compton. Quoted in "Animals in the Middle," in the *Innovation* series on television, sponsored by Johnson & Johnson, on the Arts and Entertainment Network, September 5, 1987.

12 Robert Marshak, dean of University of Pennsylvania School of Veterinary Medicine. Quoted in *NYT*, July 29, 1984, p. A12.

13 Donald Abt, associate dean, University of Pennsylvania School of Veterinary Medicine. Quoted in *NYT*, August 12, 1984, p. B1.

14 *NYT*, December 10, 1984, p. A10.

15 Ibid.

16 Singer, "Animal Liberation."

17 Susan Wolf, "Moral Saints," *Journal of Philosophy* **79**: 8 (August 1982).

18 S. Isen, "Laying the Foundation for Animal Rights: Interview with Tom Regan," *Animals Agenda*, July/August, 1984, pp. 4–5.

19 Tom Regan, *The Case for Animal Rights*, University of California Press, Berkeley, Cal. 1983, p. 246ff.

20 Carl Cohen, "The Case for the Use of Animals in Biomedical Research," *NEJM* **315** (14): 865–870 (October 4, 1986).

21 R. G. Frey, *Rights, Killing, and Suffering*, Basil Blackwell, Oxford, Engl. 1983, p. 65.

22 Charles McArdel and Carol Compton. Quoted in "Animals in the Middle" (videotape).

23 Ingrid Newkirk. Quoted in Katie McCabe, "Who Will Live, Who Will Die?" *Washingtonian Magazine*, April 1986, p. 115.

24 J. Dusheck, "Protestors Prompt Halt in Animal Research," *Science News*, July 27, 1985, p. 53.

25 John Rawls, *A Theory of Justice*, Harvard University Press, Cambridge, Mass., 1971.

26 O. Cusak, "Direct Action for Animals: Interview with England's Marley Jones," *Animals Agenda*, May/June, 1983, pp. 4–5.

27 "Of Pain and Progress," *Newsweek*, December 26, 1988, p. 53.

28 Bernard Levin, "The Animal Lovers Lusting for Blood," *The Times*, July 3, 1985, p. 15.

29 Donald Barnes, "Debating the Values of Animal Research," *Animals Agenda* **7** (3): 32–34 (April 1987).

30 L. Jewell and D. Frazier, "Annual Questionnaire Results," *The Physiologist* **29** (2): 23 (1986).

31 D. Moss and P. Greanville, "The Emerging Face of the Movement," *Animals Agenda*, March/April, 1985, p. 11.

32 F. Ferretti, "Forsaken Vacation Animals," *NYT*, September 5, 1984, p. Cl.

CHAPTER 9: THE TUSKEGEE SYPHILUS STUDY

1 David J. Rothman, "Ethics and Human Experimentation," *NEJM* **317** (19): 1198 (November 5, 1987).

2 Eugene Kogon, *The Theory and Practice of Hell*, Farrar, Straus, and Cudahy, New York, 1950; Berkeley reprint, 1980, p. 166.

3 Ibid., p. 164ff.

4 Gerald Posner and Jerome Ware, *Mengele: The Complete Story*, McGraw-Hill, New York, 1986, p. 11.

5 Vera Alexander, "The Search for Mengele," Home Box Office production, October 1985; interviewed by Central Television (London) and quoted in Posner and Hare, p. 37.

6 Dr. Nyiszli. Quoted in R. J. Lifton "What Made This Man Mengele," *NYT Magazine*, July 21, 1985, 22; Posner and Hare, *Mengele*, p. 39.

7 William Curran, "The Forensic Investigation of the Death of Joseph Mengele," *NEJM* **315**: (17): 1071–1073 (October 23, 1986).

8 Rothman, "Ethics," p. 1198.

9 Gomer, Powell, and Rolino, "Japan's Biological Weapons," and Powell, "A Hidden Chapter in History," *Bulletin of Atomic Scientists*, October 1981, pp. 43, 44.

10 Rothman, "Ethics," p. 1199.

11 Henry Beecher, "Ethics and Clinical Research," *NEJM* **274**: 1354–1360 (1966).

12 M. H. Pappworth, *Human Guinea Pigs*, Beacon, Boston, 1968.

13 Molly Selvin, "Changing Medical and Societal Attitudes toward Sexually Transmitted Diseases: A Historical Overview," in King, Holmes et al. (eds.), *Sexually Transmitted Diseases*, McGraw-Hill, New York, 1984, pp. 3–19.

14 Alan Brandt, *No Magic Bullet: A Social History of Venereal Disease in the United States Since 1880*, Oxford University Press, New York, and Oxford, Engl., 1985.

15 Todd Savitt, *Medicine and Slavery: The Disease and Health of Blacks in Antebellum Virginia*, University of Illinois Press, Champaign, Ill., 1978.

16 James Jones, *Bad Blood*, Free Press, New York, 1981.

17 H. H. Hazen, "Syphilis in the American Negro," *JAMA* **63**: 463 (August 8, 1914).

18 Jones, *"Bad Blood,"* p. 74.

19 Alan Brandt, "Racism and Research: The Case of the Tuskegee Syphilis Study," *HCR* **8** (6): 21–29 (December 1978).

20 Paul De Kruif, *The Microbe Hunters*, Harcourt Brace, New York, 1926, p. 323.

21 R. H. Kampmeier, "The Tuskegee Study of Untreated Syphilis," *Southern Medical Journal* **65** (10): 1247 (October 1972).

22 E. Bruusgaaerd, "Uber das Schicksal der nicht spezifisch behandelten Luektiker" [Fate of Syphilitics Who Are Not Given Specific Treatment], *Archives of Dermatology of Syphilis* **157**: 309–332 (April 1929).

23 William Osler. Quoted by Edmund Tramont, "Syphilis in the AIDS Era," *NEJM* **316** (25): 600–601 (June 18, 1987).

24 R. A. Vonderlehr, T. Clark, and J. R. Heller, "Untreated Syphilis in the Male Negro," *JAMA* **107** (11): 856–860 (September 12, 1936).

25 Letter, Archives of the National Library of Medicine. Quoted in Jones, *Bad Blood*, p. 127.

26 Ibid., pp. 190–193.

27 Ira Myers. Quoted in Jones, *Bad Blood*, p. 196.

28 W. J. Brown et al., *Syphilis and Other Venereal Diseases,* Harvard University Press, Cambridge, Mass., 1970, p. 34.

29 Jean Heller, "Syphilis Victims in U.S. Study Went Untreated for 40 Years," *NYT,* July 26, 1972, pp. 1, 8.

30 Heller, "Syphilis Victims," p. 8.

31 Jones, *Bad Blood,* insert following p. 48.

32 Tuskegee Syphilis Study Ad Hoc Panel to the Department of Health, Education and Welfare, *Final Report,* Superintendent of Documents, Washington, D.C., 1973.

33 Seward Hiltner, "The Tuskegee Syphilis Study Under Review: Seward Hiltren on Human Experimentation," *Christian Century* **90** (2): 1175–1176 (November 28, 1973).

34 Heller, "Syphilis Victims," p. 8.

35 Thomas Benedek, "The 'Tuskegee Study' of Syphilis: Analysis of Moral Aspects Versus Methodological Aspects," *Journal of Chronic Diseases* **31:** 35–50 (1978).

36 Heller, "Syphilis Victims," p. 1.

37 R. H. Kampmeier, "Final Report on the 'Tuskegee Syphilis Study,'" *Southern Medical Journal* **67** (11): 1349–1353 (1974).

38 "Malpractice Suit Settled for 2.7 Million," *Burlington Free Press,* December 21, 1988.

39 "The Tuskegee Study of Untreated Syphilis: The 30th Year of Observation," *Archives of Internal Medicine* **114:** 792–798 (1961).

40 Benjamin Friedman, M.D., letter to author, April 25, 1985.

41 R. H. Kampmeier, "The Tuskegee Study of Untreated Syphilis," editorial, *Southern Medical Journal* **65** (10): 1247–1251 (October 1972).

42 Benedek, "The Tuskegee Study," p. 44.

43 S. Edberg and S. Berger, *Antibiotics and Infection,* Churchill Livingstone, New York, 1983, pp. 141–142. See also K. Holmes et al., *Sexually Transmitted Diseases,* McGraw-Hill, New York, 1984, p. 1352.

44 Dr. Sarah Polt, letter to author, Pathology Department, UAB Medical School. See also John Hotson, "Modern Neurosyphilis: A Partially Treated Chronic Meningitis," *Western Journal of Medicine* **135:** 191–200 (September 1981).

45 UPI, *Birmingham News,* September 11, 1988.

46 W. Seidelman, "Mengele Medicus: Medicine's Nazi Heritage," *Milbank Quarterly* **66** (2): 221–232 (1988).

47 I am indebted to the following physicians for detailed readings of this chapter: from the University of Alabama at Birmingham, Sarah Polt in Pathology and, in Internal Medicine, Benjamin Friedman (Medicine, Emeritus), William Goetter, C. Kirk Avent, Max Michael, and Harriet Dustan. Medical historian Todd Savitt of the East Carolina Medical School also made useful comments on this chapter. A previous version was read at the Alabama Philosophical Association meetings at Spring Hill College, where Max Hocutt made useful comments, and the Southern Philosophy and Psychology Meetings in New Orleans in 1981.

CHAPTER 10: CHRISTIAAN BARNARD'S FIRST HEART TRANSPLANT

1 Richard Howard and John Najarian, "Organ Transplantation: Medical Perspective," *Encyclopedia of Bioethics,* Vol. 3, Free Press, New York, 1978, p. 1160.

2 Ibid., pp. 1160–1165.

3 Phillip Blaiberg, *Looking at My Heart,* Stein & Day, New York, 1968, p. 66.

4 Christiaan Barnard and Curtiss Bill Pepper, *One Life,* , Macmillian, New York, 1969, p. 290.

5 Ibid., p. 210.

6 Ibid., pp. 238–239.

7 Ibid., p. 310.

8 Ibid., p. 332.

9 Ibid., p. 343.

10 Ibid., p. 372.

11 "The Ultimate Operation," *Time,* December 15, 1967, p. 65.

12 "Heart Transplant Keeps Man Alive in South Africa," *NYT* , December 4, 1967, p. A1.

13 Barnard and Pepper, *One Life,* p. 378.

14 Ibid., p. 406.

15 "The Ultimate Operation," p. 66.

16 Barnard and Pepper, *One Life,* p. 444.

17 Werner Forssmann. Quoted in Barnard and Pepper, *One Life,* p. 339.

18 Ibid., p. 360.

19 Robert Veatch, "Whole Brain, Neocortical, and Higher Brain Related Concepts of Death," in R. Zaner (ed.), *Whole Brain and Neocortical Definitions of Death: A Critical Appraisal,* D. Reidel, Norwell, Mass., 1986.

20 "The Ultimate Operation," pp. 65–66.

21 Shimon Glick, letter to author, September 18, 1988.

22 Peter Hawthorne, *The Transplanted Heart,* Keartland Publishers, Johannesburg, South Africa 1968, 188.

23 *NYT,* December 6, 1967, p. A8.

24 Norman Shumway. Quoted in "Pioneers of Surgery," Part IV, NOVA Program, WGBH, Boston, Mass. (Shown during September 1988 and June 1989.)

25 Plato, *Laches,* in E. Hamilton and H. Cairns (eds.), *Collected Dialogues of Plato,* Princeton University Press, Princeton, N.J., 1961.

26 Hawthorne, *The Transplanted Heart,* Princeton, N.J., pp. 84–85.

27 "Heart Surgery: Were Transplants Premature?" *Time,* March 15, 1968.

28 Renée Fox and Judith Swazey, *The Courage to Fail: A Social View of Organ Transplants and Dialysis,* 2d ed., rev., University of Chicago Press, 1978, p. 44.

29 *Time,* March 15, 1988, p. 66.

30 "Organ Transplantation," Department of Health and Human Services, Superintendent of Documents, Washington, D.C., 1988.

31 Oscar Salvatierra, "The Role of Organ Transplantation in Medicine," *Heart Transplantation* **4** (3): 288 (May 1985).

32 I am indebted to surgeon Roy Gandy of Birmingham, and Harriet Dustan, M.D., of the University of Alabama at Birmingham, for comments on this chapter.

CHAPTER 11: BARNEY CLARK'S ARTIFICIAL HEART

1 Shana Alexander, "They Decide Who Lives, Who Dies: Medical Miracle Puts a Burden on a Small Committee," *Life* **53:** 102 (November 9, 1962).

2 Shep Glazer. Quoted in Michael Kroman, "Dialyzing for Dollars," *Reason,* August 1984, pp. 21–30.

3 Michael Strauss, "The Political History of the Artificial Heart," *NEJM* **310** (5): 333 (February 2, 1984).

4 Lewis Thomas, "The Technology of Medicine," *Lives of a Cell*, Viking, New York, 1974, p. 37.

5 Both the Haskell Karp case and the charges against Cooley are described in a *NOVA* videotape, "The Trial of Denton Cooley," produced by WGBH of Boston, as well as in Chapter 6 of Renée Fox and Judith Swazey, *The Courage to Fail: A Social View of Organ Transplants and Dialysis*, 2nd ed., rev., University of Chicago Press, 1978.

6 *Life*, column by managing editor Richard Stolley, February, 1983.

7 Una Clark. Quoted in *WP*, May 1, 1983, p. A2.

8 "The Brave Man with the Plastic Heart," *Life*, February 7, 1983, p. 25.

9 Thomas Preston, "Who Benefits from the Artificial Heart," *HCR* **15** (1): 5 (February 1985); also *NYT*, December 5, 1988, p. 48.

10 Denise Grady, "Summary of Discussion on Ethical Perspectives," from *After Barney Clark*, M. Shaw (ed.), University of Texas Press, Austin, Tex., 1984, p. 52.

11 *NYT*, December 5, 1982, p. 48.

12 *Time*, December 9, 1982, p. 43.

13 *NYT*, December 5, 1982, p. 48.

14 *NYT*, December 3, 1982, p. A1.

15 *NYT*, March 25, 1983, p. A1.

16 *NYT*, December 3, 1982, p. A25.

17 *Time*, March 14, 1983, p. 74.

18 Thomas Preston, "Who Benefits...," p. 6.

19 *WP*, May 1, 1983, p. A2.

20 *NYT*, April, 17, 1983, p. 44.

21 Eric Cassell, "How Is the Death of Barney Clark to Be Understood?," in *After Barney Clark*, pp. 25–41.

22 *NYT*, March 25, 1983, p. A29.

23 *WP*, December 21, 1982.

24 Denise Grady, "Summary of Discussion on Ethical Perspectives," from *After Barney Clark*, p. 48.

25 *WP*, March 25, 1983, p. A14.

26 *NYT*, April 17, 1983, p. 44.

27 *NYT*, editorial, December 16, p. 1982, A26.

28 William Check, "Lessons from Barney Clark's Heart," *Health*, April 1984, p. 25.

29 *NYT*, December 5, 1982, p. 48.

30 Ibid.

31 Preston, "Who Benefits...," p. 5.

32 Ibid., p. 6.

33 Ibid.

34 George Annas, "Consent to the Artificial Heart: The Lion and the Crocodiles," *HCR* (**13**) 2:20–22.

35 Pierre Galetti, "Replacement of the Heart with an Artificial Device: The Case of Dr. Barney Clark," *NEJM* **310** (5): 312–314 (February 2, 1984).

36 *NYT*, April 17, 1983, p. A1.

37 Denise Grady, "Summary of Discussion on Ethical Perspectives," from *After Barney Clark*, p. 46.

38 *NYT*, April 17, 1983.

39 *Time*, April 4, 1983, p. 63.

40 D. P. Lubeck and J. P. Bunker, Office of Technology Assessment, *Case Study #9, The Artificial Heart: Costs, Risks, and Benefits*, U.S. Government Printing Office, Washington, D.C., 1982.

41 Preston, "Who Benefits...," p. 7, quoting an unamed *WP* report.

42 Preston, "Who Benefits...," p. 7.

43 *Progressive*, February 1983, pp. 12–13.

44 Jonathan Glover, *Causing Death and Saving Lives*, Penguin Books, New York, 1977; Leon Trachtman, "Why Tolerate the Statistical Victim?" *HCR* **15** (1): 14 (February 1985).

45 William DeVries, "The Physician, the Media, and the 'Spectacular Case'," *JAMA* **259** (6): 891 (February 12, 1988).

46 *Time*, September 12, 1983, p. 43.

47 *NYT*, December 3, 1982, p. A25.

48 *NYT*, April 17, 1983, p. A44.

49 Arnold Relman, "Artificial Hearts: Permanent and Temporary, *NEJM* **314**: 645 (1986).

50 William Pierce, "Permanent Heart Substitution: Better Solutions Ahead," editorial, *JAMA* **259** (6) 891 (February 12, 1988).

51 Alexander Capron, "The Role of the Lawyer and Legal Advice in the Utah Artificial Heart," in *After Barney Clark*, pp. 91–102.

52 George Annas "Consent...," p. 20.

53 Jay Katz, "Patient Autonomy and the Process of Consent,"in *After Barney Clark*, pp. 11–24.

54 Lawrence Altman, "After Barney Clark: Reflections of a Reporter on Unresolved Issues," in *After Barney Clark*, pp. 113–128.

55 Chase Peterson, "A Spontaneous Reply to Dr. Lawrence Altman," in *After Barney Clark*, pp. 129–138.

56 Renée Fox, "'It's the Same, but Different': A Sociological Perspective on the Case of the Utah Artificial Heart," in *After Barney Clark*, pp. 6–90.

57 William DeVries, p. 889.

58 Stanley Reiser, "The Machine as End and Means: The Clinical Introduction of the Artificial Heart," in *After Barney Clark*, pp. 168–175.

59 Preston, "Who Benefits...," p. 5.

60 Malcomn N. Carter, "The Business Behind Barney Clark's Heart," *Money*, April 1983, pp. 130–144.

61 Clifford Kwan-Gett, personal communication to author, August 1987.

62 Ronni Scheier, "Robert K. Jarvik, M.D.: Inventor, Lecturer, Hero," *AMN*, December 11, 1987, pp. 9–10.

63 Michael Vitez, "Marriage of Two Minds: 'World's Smartest Couple' Nears First Anniversary," Knight-Ridder newspapers, July 3, 1988.

64 Check, "Lessons...," p. 26.

65 Ibid., p. 22.

66 Malcolm Browne, "U.S. Halts Artificial Heart Funds," *NYT*, May 13, 1988, pp. Al, A7.

67 Phillip Boffey, "Federal Agency, in Shift, to Back Artificial Heart," *NYT*, July 3, 1988, p. Al.

68 Gideon Gil, "The Artificial Heart Juggernaut," *HCR* 19:(2): 24–31 (March/April 1989).

69 I am indebted to physicians Roy Gandy (surgery) and Harriet Dustan (medicine) for comments on this chapter.

CHAPTER 12: BABY FAE

1 Renée Fox and Judith Swazey, *The Courage to Fail: A Social View of Organ Transplants and Dialysis*, 2nd ed, rev., University of Chicago Press, 1978; Harmon Smith, "Heart

Transplantation," *Encyclopedia of Bioethics*, Vol. 2, Free Press, New York, 1978, pp. 654–660; Richard Howard and J. Najarian, "Organ Transplantation—Medical Perspective," *Encyclopedia of Bioethics*, Vol.3, Free Press New York, 1978, pp. 1160–1165.

2 Denise Breo, "Interview with 'Baby Fae's' Surgeon," *AMN*, November 16, 1984, 13.

3 "Baby Fae Stuns the World," *Time*, November 12, 1984, p. 70.

4 Breo, "Interview . . . ," p. 18.

5 Tom Regan, "The Other Victim," *HCR* **15** (1): 9–10 (February 1985).

6 "Pro and Con: Use Animal Organs for Human Transplants?—Interview with Tom Regan," *U.S. News & World Report*, November 12, 1984, p. 58.

7 Thomasine Kushner and Raymond Belotti, "Baby Fae: A Beastly Business," *Journal of Medical Ethics* **11:** 178–183 (1985).

8 Dan Chu and Eleanor Hoover, "Helped by a Baboon Heart, An Imperiled Infant, 'Baby Fae, ' Beat the Medical Odds," *People Weekly* **22** (21): 73 (November 19, 1984).

9 "Interview with Dr. Jack Provonsha," *U.S. News & World Report*, November 12, 1984, p. 59.

10 Alexander Capron, "When Well-Meaning Science Goes Too Far," *HCR* **15** (1): 8–9 (February 1985).

11 Breo, "Interview . . . ," p. 18.

12 Jacques Losman, *Journal of Heart Transplantation* **4** (1): 10–11 (November 1984).

13 George Annas, "Baby Fae: The 'Anything Goes' School of Human Experimentation," *HCR* **15** (1): 15–17 (February 1985).

14 Charles Krauthammer, "The Using of Baby Fae," *Time*, December 3, 1984, pp. 87–88.

15 Breo, "Interview . . . ," p. 13.

16 Ibid., p. 14.

17 Ibid.

18 Breo, "Interview . . . ," p. 18.

19 Chu and Hoover, "Helped by a Baboon Heart," p. 74.

20 Breo, "Interview . . . ," 18; see also Leonard Bailey et al., "Cardiac Allotransplantation in Newborns as Therapy for Hypoplastic Helft Heart Syndrome," *NEJM* **315** (15): 951, (October 9, 1986).

21 Chu and Hoover, "Helped by a Baboon Heart," p. 74.

22 Paul Ramsey, "The Enforcement of Morals: Nontherapeutic Research on Children," *HCR* **6** (4): 21–30 (August 1976).

23 Krauthammer, "The Using of Baby Fae," p. 88.

24 Richard McCormick, "Proxy Consent in the Experimentation Situation," *Perspectives in Biology and Medicine* **18** (1): 2–20 (Autumn 1974).

25 *Newsweek*, December 28, 1987, p. 62; *AMN*, January 1, 1988, p. 12. Baby Fae: Ethical Issues Surrounding Cross-Species Organ Transplantation," Scope Note #5, Bioethics Library, Kennedy Institute of Ethics, p. 3; quoted from *Federal Register:* 48, 9816.

26 *Nature:* 88: 312, p. 5990 (November 8, 1984).

27 "Judicial Council Offers New Guidelines," *American Medical News* 27, p. 46, December 14, 1984.

28 Quoted on the "Hard Choices" series on American Public Television, show on "Organ Transplantation." Available from School of Journalism, Columbia University, New York, N.Y.

29 *Newsweek*, December 28, 1987, p. 62; *AMN*, January 1, 1988, p. 12.

30 D. Alan Shewmon, "Anencephaly: Selected Medical Aspects," *HCR* **18** (5): 11–19 (October/November 1988).

31 Alexander Capron, "Anencephalic Donors: Separate the Dead from the Dying," *HCR* **17** (1): 5–8 (February 1987); John Arras, "Anencephalic Newborns as Organ Donors: A Critique," *JAMA* **259** (15): 2284–2285 (April 15, 1988).

32 Shewmon, D. A. et al., "The Use of Anencephalic Infants as Organ Sources," *JAMA* **261** (12): 1773–1781 (March 24/31, 1989).

33 Laurie Abraham, "Anencephalic Organ Donation Stymied by Controversy," *AMN,* September 23/30, 1988), p. 10.

34 *Newsweek,* December 28, 1987, p. 63.

35 Surgeon Roy Gandy made useful comments on this chapter.

CHAPTER 13: MAYOR KOCH, JOYCE BROWN, AND INVOLUNTARY PSYCHIATRIC COMMITMENT

1 Luis R. Marcos, personal communication, citing study by New York City's Human Resources Administration on use of the city's emergency shelters in 1988.

2 Julian Jaynes, *The Origin of Consciousness and the Breakdown of the Bicameral Mind,* Houghton, Mifflin, Boston, 1976.

3 Plato, *The Republic,* in E. Hamilton and H. Cairns (eds.), *Collected Works of Plato,* Princeton University Press, Princeton, N.J., 1961.

4 Thomas Szasz, "Involuntary Mental Hospitalization: A Crime Against Humanity," excerpted from *Ideology and Insanity,* Doubleday, New York, 1970.

5 D. Rosenhan, "On Being Sane in Insane Places," *Science* **179:** 250–258 (1973).

6 *O'Connor vs. Donaldson* 422 U.S. 563. 95 S. Ct. 2486 (June 26, 1975).

7 John Petrila, "Mental Health Therapies," *Biolaw,* University Publications of America, Frederick, Md., 1986, pp. 177–215.

8 John F. Kennedy. Quoted by Charles Krauthammer, "How to Save the Homeless Mentally Ill," *New Republic,* February 8, 1988, p. 24.

9 Saul Feldman, "Out of the Hospitals, onto the Streets: The Overselling of Benevolence," *HCR* **13** (3): 5–7 (June 1983).

10 Paul Chodoff, "The Case for Involuntary Hospitalization of the Mentally Ill," *American Journal of Psychiatry* **133** (5): 496–501 (May 1976).

11 *NYT,* November 7, 1987, p. B1.

12 *NYT,* November 6, 1987, p. B1.

13 *NYT,* November 6, 1987, p. B1.

14 *NYT,* November 13, 1987, p. B21.

15 *NYT,* November 14, 1987, p. B1.

16 *NYT,* November 13, 1987, p. A1.

17 Ibid.

18 Charles Krauthammer, "How to Save the Homeless Mentally Ill," *New Republic,* February 8, 1988, pp. 22–25.

19 J. Livermore, C. Malmquist, and P. Meehl, "On the Justification for Civil Commitment," *University of Pennsylvania Law Review* **117:** 75–96 (November 1968).

20 Virginia Abernethy, "Compassion, Control, and Decisions about Competency," *American Journal of Psychiatry* **141** (1): 53–58.

21 *NYT,* November 13, 1987, p. A1.

22 Donahue Transcript #012788, Multimedia Entertainment, Inc., PO Box 2111, Cincinnati, Ohio 45201.

23 Robert Levy and Robert Gould, "Psychiatrists as Puppets of Koch's Round-Up," *NYT*, November 27, 1987.

24 *NYT*, November 14, 1987, p. 30.

25 A. M. Rosenthal, "Question to a Judge," *NYT*, November 27, 1987.

26 Chodhoff, "The Case for Involuntary Hospitalization," p. 498.

27 Harold Evans, "Joyce Brown's Freedom," *U.S. News & World Report*, May 23, 1988, p. 78.

28 Ellen Goodman, "Before They Die 'With Their Rights On,'" *WP*, November 21, 1987.

29 Livermore, Malmquist, and Meehl, "On the Justification . . . ," p. 95.

30 "Court Backs Treatment of Woman Held Under Koch Plan," *NYT*, December 19, 1987, p. A1.

31 *NYT*, January 20, 1988, p. A16.

32 "New York Woman Rising Up from Anonymity," *NYT*, February 15, 1988.

33 "Back on the Street Again," *Time*, March 21, 1988, p. 33.

34 *Birmingham News*, September 6, 1988, p. A2.

35 Charles Krauthammer, "Billie Boggs Revisited," *New York Daily News*, December 27, 1988, p. 21.

36 Josh Barbarel, "Poll Finds New Yorkers Dissatisfied with help for Homeless," June 29, 1989, p. 11. NYT.

37 I am indebted to Harold Kincaid, G. Lynn Stephens, Luis R. Marcos, and William Ruddick for comments on this chapter.

CHAPTER 14: PREVENTING UNDESIRABLE TEENAGE PREGNANCIES

1 Daniel Kevles, *In the Name of Eugenics: Genetics and the Uses of Human Heredity*, Knopf, New York, 1985, pp. 3–19.

2 Kenneth Ludmerer, "History of Eugenics," *Encyclopedia of Bioethics*, vol.1, Free Press, New York, 1978, p. 460.

3 Robert Lacey, *Ford: The Men and the Machine*, Little, New York, 1987.

4 Kevles, *In the Name of Eugenics*, pp. 93–94.

5 Ibid., p. 110.

6 *Buck vs. Bell*, Superintendent, *United States Supreme Court Reporter*, 1927.

7 Kevles, *In the Name of Eugenics*, p. 53.

8 Richard Hernstein, "I.Q.," *Atlantic*, September 1971, pp. 63–64.

9 Hermann Muller, *Out of the Night: A Biologist's View of the Future*, Vanguard, New York, 1935. Quoted by Kevles, *In the Name of Eugenics*, p. 164.

10 Kevles, *In the Name of Eugenics*, p. 117.

11 Ibid., 116.

12 Ronald W. Clark, *The Life and Work of J. B. S. Haldane*, Coward-McCann, New York, 1968, p. 70. Quoted by Kevles, *In the Name of Eugenics*, p. 127.

13 J. B. S. Haldane, "Toward a Perfected Posterity," *The World Today* 45 (December 1924). Quoted by Kevles, *In the Name of Eugenics*, p. 122.

14 Kevles, *In the Name of Eugenics*, p. 97.

15 J. Huxley and A. C. Haddon, *We Europeans: A Survey of "Racial" Problems*, Jonathan Cape, 1935, p. 184. Quoted by Kevles, *In the Name of Eugenics*, p. 133.

16 This case is in *Bertha*, Joseph P. Kennedy, Jr., Foundation, Film Service, 99 Asylum Ave., Hartford, Conn. 06105. Unfootnoted quotation in the following text is from this film.

17 These quotations—"What are you protecting me from?" and "So?" are from producer Annie Michaels; the rest are from the film itself.

18 Robert Neville, "Sterilizing the Mildly Retarted without Their Consent," in R. Macklin and W. Gaylin (eds.), *Mental Retardation and Sterilization,* Plenum Press, New York, 1981.

19 Barry Hoffmaster, "Caring for Retarded Persons—Ethical Ideals and Practical Choices," in Stanley Hauerwas (ed.) *Responsibility for Devalued Persons,* Charles Thomas, Springfield, Ill., pp. 28–41.

20 Rosalind Pollack Pechchesky. "Reproduction, Ethics, & Public Policy: The Federal Sterilization Regulations," *HCR* **9** (5): 29 (October 1979).

21 John Rawls, *A Theory of Justice,* Harvard University Press, 1971.

22 *NYT,* February 27, 1989.

23 Bureau of Census, *1987 Statistical Abstract of the United States* Superintendent of Documents) Washington, D.C., tables 619, 621–622.

24 ABC World News, June 26, 1989.

25 Charles Murray, *Losing Ground: American Social Policy: 1950–1980,* Basic Books, New York, 1986.

26 *NYT,* March 15, 1989.

27 Sue Miller, *The Good Mother,* Harper & Row, New York, 1986. On the Parillo case, see Ellen Goodman, "Parenthood on Trial in Court and Geraldoland," *Birmingham Post-Herald,* March 24, 1989, p. A5.

28 Stephen Mosher, *Broken Earth,,* Free Press, New York, 1983, p. 553.

29 Hugh LaFollette, "Licensing Parents," *Philosophy & Public Affairs* **9** (2): 182–197, (1979).

30 "Teens and Sex," United Nations Population Division, *Birmingham News,* January 7, 1988.

31 Janet Shibley Hyde, *Human Sexuality,* McGraw-Hill, New York, 1979, p. 15, quoting anthropologist Clellan Ford's and psychologist Frank Beach's study of sexual behavior in 190 societies, *Patterns of Sexual Behavior,* Harper & Row, New York 1951.

32 ABC World News, June 26, 1989.

CHAPTER 15: NANCY WEXLER AND GENETIC MARKERS

1 "Interview with Nancy Wexler," *U.S. News & World Report,* 1985, p. 75.

2 V. A. McKusick, *Mendelian Inheritance in Man: Catalogs of Autosomal Dominant, Autosomal Recessive and X-Linked Disorders, 8th Ed.,* Johns Hopkins University Press, Baltimore, Md., 1988.

3 A. Wilcox et al., "Incidence of Early Loss of Pregnancy," *NEJM* **319** (4): 189–194 (July 28, 1988).

4 Tabitha Powledge, "Genetic Screening," *Encyclopedia of Bioethics,* Free Press, New York, 1978, pp. 567–572.

5 James Thompson and Margaret Thompson, *Genetics in Medicine,* 4th ed., Saunders, Philadelphia, 1986, p. 55.

6 Ibid., p. 53.

7 M. R. Hayden, *Huntington's Chorea,* Springer-Verlag, New York, 1981.

8 Denise Grady, "The Ticking of a Time Bomb in the Genes," *Discover,* June, 1987, p. 34.

9 D. Craufurd and R. Harris, "Ethics of Predictive Testing for Huntington's Disease: The Need for More Information," *British Medical Journal* **293**: 249–251 (July 26, 1986).

10 Len Cooper, "After Her Mother's Death, One Woman Confronts the Risk of Huntington's Disease," *Washington Post*, August 27, 1986, p. 14.

11 Maya Pines, "In the Shadow of Huntington's," *Science 84*, May 1984, p. 34.

12 Ibid., p. 39.

13 J. F. Gusella, N. S. Wexler, P. M. Conneally, et al., "A Polymorphic DNA Marker Genetically Linked to Huntington's Disease," *Nature* **306**: 234–238 (1983).

14 V. A. McKusick, *Mendelian Inheritance in Man*.

15 Pines, "In the Shadow...," p. 33.

16 President's Commission for the Study of Ethical Problems in Medicine and Biomedical and Behavioral Research, *Screening and Counseling for Genetic Conditions: The Ethical, Social, and Legal Implications of Genetic Screening, Counseling and Educational Problems*, U.S. Government Printing Office, Washington, D.C., 1983.

17 G. Meissen et al., "Predictive Testing for Huntington's Disease with Use of a Linked DNA Marker," *NEJM* **318** (9): 538 (March 3, 1988).

18 I am indebted to John Fletcher for this critique of the do-not-tell position.

19 I am indebted to Micheal Connealy for this case-study.

20 Denise Grady, "The Ticking of...," p. 30.

21 Ibid., p. 30.

22 M. Waldohz, "Probing the Cell: The Diagnostic Power of Genetics Is Posing Hard Medical Choices," *WSJ*, April 1986, p. A1.

23 Ibid., p. 20.

24 Grady, "The Ticking of...," p. 30.

25 G. Meissen et al, "Predictive Testing...," p. 538.

26 Letter, "Preclinical Testing in Huntington's Disease," *American Journal of Medical Genetics* 27 (1987), pp. 733–734.

27 Kolata, p. 318.

28 C. Norton, "Absolutely Not Confidential" *Hippocrates* (March/April, 1989), pp. 53–59. See also, *Medical Records: Getting Yours* (Public Citizen, 1986).

29 Waldoz, p. 1.

30 Waldoz, p. 1.

31 D. C. Watt's et al. letter, *Nature* **320**: 6 (March 6, 1986), p. 21.

32 James Gusella, letter, *Nature* **320**: 6 (March 1986), pp. 21–22.

33 James Gusella, letter, *Nature* **323** (11) (September 1986), p. 118.

34 Grady, p. 30.

35 *60 Minutes*, May, 1987 (author's videotape). Diane Sawyer interview Nancy, Alice and Milton Wexler, as well as James Gusella.

36 Harold M. Schmeck, "50% of Colon-Rectal Cancers Tied to Genetic Predisposition," *NYT*, September 1, 1988, p. A1.

37 Marc Lappe, "The Limits of Genetic Inquiry," *HCR* **17** (4): 5–10. (August 1987).

38 P. Gorner and R. Kotulak, "Scientists Foresee Simple Tests for Detecting Genetic Disorders," *Chicago Tribune* (August 30, 1988).

39 G. Meissen et al., pp. 535–542.

40 Nova, "Confronting the Killer Gene," March 28, 1989.

41 Nova, "Confronting the Killer Gene," March 28, 1989.

42 I am indebted to medical geneticist Wayne Finley, M.D. of UAB, as well as medical ethicist John Fletcher of the University of Virginia Medical School, for their comments on this chapter.

CHAPTER 16: MANDATORY TESTING FOR AIDS

1 Susan Sontag, *AIDS and Its Metaphors*, Farrar, Straus and Giroux, New York, 1988, p. 34ff.

2 Daniel Defoe, *Journal of the Plague Year* (1723), Penguin, New American Library, New York, 1960, p. 86.

3 Barbara Tuchman, *A Distant Mirror*, Knopf, New York, 1978, p. 119.

4 A. Zuger and S. Miles, "Physicians, AIDS and Occupational Risk," *JAMA* **258** (14): 1924–1928 (October 9, 1987).

5 Charles Shepard, "Leprosy," *Harrison's Principles of Internal Medicine*, Wintrobe et al. (eds.), McGraw-Hill, New York, 1974, pp. 870–873.

6 C. Rosenberg, *The Cholera Years*, University of Chicago Press, 1962, p. 47ff.

7 A. Brandt, *No Magic Bullet: A Social History of Venereal Disease in the United States Since 1880*, Oxford University Press, New York 1985, pp. 43–44.

8 Randy Shilts, *And the Band Played On*, St. Martin's, New York, 1987, p. 186ff.

9 Centers for Disease Control, *Morbidity and Mortality Report*, June 5, 1981.

10 Institute of Medicine, *Confronting AIDS: Directions for Public Health, Health Care, and Research*, National Academy Press, Washington, D.C., 1986.

11 G. Freidland and Robert Klein, "Transmission of the Human Immunodeficiency Virus," *NEJM* **317** (18): 1127 (October 29, 1987).

12 Shilts, *And the Band Played On*, p. 345.

13 Ibid., p. 433 (quoting the *WSJ*).

14 *Confronting AIDS*, p. 85ff.

15 Shilts, *And the Band Played On*, pp. 529–530.

16 William Masters, Virginia Johnson, and Robert Kolodny, *Crisis: Heterosexual Behavior in the Age of AIDS*, Grove Press, New York, 1988.

17 June Osborne, "AIDS: Politics and Science," *NEJM* **318** (7):444–447 (February 18, 1988).

18 William Dannemeyer, "The AIDS Epidemic," *Congressional Record*, January 7, 1987.

19 Masters, Johnson, and Kolodny, *Crisis*, pp. 177–178.

20 Ann G. Fettner, "The Facts about Straight Sex and AIDS: An Interview with Randy Shilts," *Village Voice*, February 23, 1988, pp. 21–23.

21 "James W. Curran, M.D.," *AMN*, January 15, 1988, pp. 19–21.

22 John Tierney, "Snooping for the Breakout," *Rolling Stone*, November 17, 1988, pp. 124–137.

23 Masters, Johnson, and Kolodny, *Crisis*, pp. 171.

24 Greg Dixon, "Stop Homosexuals Before They Infect Us All," *U.S.A. Today*, January 16, 1983.

25 Charles Stanley, Scripps Howard News Service, *Birmingham Post-Herald*, January 21, 1986.

26 *CrossFire*, Cable News Network, November 16, 1987.

27 Patrick Buchanan. Quoted by Shilts, *And the Band Played On*, p. 311.

28 Socrates probably was bisexual, as indicated by the scene in the *Symposium* where Alcibiades attempts to seduce him and Socrates' argument is not that he doesn't want to, but that higher duties should prevail. Also, the Platonic dialogues constantly refer to young boys, not young girls or women, as objects of lust. On this question, see A. H. Chroust, *Socrates: Man and Myth*, Routledge, London 1957;

Kenneth J. Dover, *Greek Homosexuality*, Cambridge, University Press, New York, 1978; and Eva Keuls, "The Boy Beautiful: Replacing a Woman or Replacing a Son?" *The Reign of the Phallus: Sexual Politics in Ancient Athens*, Harper & Row, New York, 1985.

On Frederick II, see P. M. Dale, *Medical Biographies*, University of Oklahoma Press, Norman, Okla, 1987. On Emperor Hadrian and other Roman emperors, see John Boswell, *Christianity, Social Tolerance and Homosexuality*, University of Chicago Press, 1980, pp. 61–91.

29 John Boswell, *Christianity, Social Tolerance, and Homosexuality*, University of Chicago Press, Chicago and London, 1980.

30 Alfred Kinsey, *Sexual Behavior in the Human Male*, J. B. Lippincott Co., Phil., Pa., 1948.

31 Richard Mohr, *Gays/Justice: A Study of Ethics, Society, and Law*, Columbia University Press, 1988, pp. 251, 262.

32 D. Lyter et al., "The HIV Antibody Test: Why Gay and Bisexual Men Want or Do Not Want Their Results," *Public Health Reports* **102**: 468–474.

33 Neil Schram, "Leadership, Not Expediency, Needed in AIDS Crisis," *AMN*, November 13, 1987, p. 33.

34 "Screening for HIV: Can We Afford the False Positive Rate?" *NEJM* **317** (4): 238–241 (July 23, 1987).

35 P. Cleary et al., "Compulsory Premarital Screening for HIV," *JAMA* **258** (13): 1757–1762 (October 2, 1987).

36 Dannemeyer, "The AIDS Epidemic."

37 Sari Staver, "'Very Normal' for Health Care Workers to Fear Caring for AIDS Patients," *AMN*, October 2, 1987, pp. 27–28.

38 *Newsweek*, August 3, 1987, p. 58.

39 Raymond Coffey, "Should Physician with AIDS Continue Work in a Hospital?" *Chicago Tribune*, January 14, 1987.

40 Michael Hagen et al., "Routine Preoperative Screening for HIV," *JAMA* **259**: 1359 (March 4, 1988).

41 Abigail Zuger, "AIDS on the Wards," *HCR* **17**: 3 (June 1987). See also M. Wachter, "Impact of AIDS on Medical Residency Training," *NEJM* **314** (5): 177–178 (June 16, 1986).

42 Zuger, "AIDS on the Wards," p. 16.

43 Brandt, *No Magic Bullet*, p. 163ff.

44 Norman Podhoretz, "Control Sexual Epidemics with Moral Standards, Not Condoms," *Minneapolis Star-Tribune*, November 4, 1986.

45 Health Program, Office of Technology Assessment, staff paper no.2, "AIDS and Health Insurance," U.S. Government Printing Office, Washington, D.C., (February 1988).

46 G. Oppenheimer and R. Padgug, "AIDS: The Risks to Insurers, the Threat to Equity," *HCR* **16** (5): 18–22 (October 1986).

47 Sari Staver, "Insurance Attorney Alleges 'Fraud' with AIDS Coverage," *AMN*, May 8, 1987, p. 2.

48 Mohr, *Guys/Justice*, p. 246.

49 Randy Shilts, "Talking *AIDS* to Death," *Esquire*, March 1989, p. 124.

50 Joshua Hammer, "AIDS, Blood and Money," *Newsweek*, January 23, 1989, p. 43.

51 David Imagawa et al., "Human Immunodeficiency Virus Type I Infection in Homosexual Men Who Remain Seronegative for Prolonged Periods," *New England Journal of Medicine*, **320** (22): 1458–1462.

52 Gregory E. Pence, "Evaluative Assumptions and Facts about AIDS," *Biomedical Reviews 1988: AIDS,* ed. J. Humber and R. Almeder, Humana Press, Clifton, N.J., 1988.

53 I am indebted for comments on this chapter to Richard Mohr of the University of Illinois, and David Ozar of Loyola University of Chicago, as well as my colleagues Scott Arnold and Harold Kincaid.

Name Index

Subject Index